MALARIA

Obstacles and Opportunities

Stanley C. Oaks, Jr., Violaine S. Mitchell,
Greg W. Pearson, and Charles C. J. Carpenter, *Editors*

A Report of the
Committee for the Study on Malaria Prevention and
Control: Status Review and Alternative Strategies
Division of International Health

INSTITUTE OF MEDICINE

NATIONAL ACADEMY PRESS
Washington, D.C.   1991

National Academy Press • 2101 Constitution Avenue, N.W. • Washington, D.C. 20418

NOTICE: The project that is the subject of this report was approved by the Governing Board of the National Research Council, whose members are drawn from the councils of the National Academy of Sciences, the National Academy of Engineering, and the Institute of Medicine. The members of the committee responsible for the report were chosen for their special competences and with regard for appropriate balance.

This report has been reviewed by a group other than the authors according to procedures approved by a Report Review Committee consisting of members of the National Academy of Sciences, the National Academy of Engineering, and the Institute of Medicine.

The Institute of Medicine was established in 1970 by the National Academy of Sciences to secure the services of eminent members of appropriate professions in the examination of policy matters pertaining to the health of the public. The Institute acts under the responsibility given to the National Academy of Sciences by its congressional charter to be an adviser to the federal government and, upon its own initiative, to identify issues of medical care, research, and education. Dr. Samuel O. Thier is president of the Institute of Medicine.

Funding for this study was provided by the Agency for International Development, the U.S. Army Medical Research and Development Command, and the National Institute of Allergy and Infectious Diseases of the National Institutes of Health.

Printed in the United States of America

The serpent has been a symbol of long life, healing, and knowledge among almost all cultures and religions since the beginning of recorded history. Ths image adopted as a logotype by the Institute of Medicine is based on a relief carving from ancient Greece, now held by the Staatlichemuseen in Berlin.

PEDRO L. TAUIL, Assistant Professor, Faculty of Medicine, University of Brasilia, and Health Advisor to the Federal Senate, Brasilia, Brazil

TERRIE E. TAYLOR, Assistant Professor, Department of Community Health Science, Michigan State University, College of Osteopathic Medicine, East Lansing, Michigan

AWASH TEKLEHAIMANOT, Malaria Unit, Control of Tropical Diseases, World Health Organization, Geneva, Switzerland

McWILSON WARREN, Director, Office of Scientific Services, Center for Infectious Diseases, Centers for Disease Control, Atlanta, Georgia

THEODORE F. WOODWARD, Professor of Medicine Emeritus, University of Maryland School of Medicine, Baltimore, Maryland

Institute of Medicine Staff

STANLEY C. OAKS, JR., Study Director

VIOLAINE S. MITCHELL, Program Officer

SHARON SCOTT-BROWN, Senior Secretary

POLLY F. HARRISON, Director, Division of International Health

STEPHANIE R. SAGEBIEL, Senior Program Officer, Division of International Health

KATHERINE B. EDSALL, Administrative Assistant, Division of International Health

Preface

Despite heroic efforts to eradicate malaria in the 1950s and 1960s, this disease not only has prevailed but has made a dramatic resurgence within the past two decades. Morbidity and mortality from malaria are at almost unprecedented levels, particularly in Africa south of the Sahara, where the disease claims more than 1 million lives per year. To address this dilemma, the Institute of Medicine (IOM) was asked by the U.S. Agency for International Development (USAID) to conduct a study and present recommendations that relevant U.S. government funding agencies could use to focus their efforts in malaria research, prevention, and control. Funding for the study came from USAID, from the U.S. Army Medical Research and Development Command, and from the National Institute of Allergy and Infectious Diseases of the National Institutes of Health.

In response to the request, IOM formed the 19-member Committee for the Study on Malaria Prevention and Control. Its membership included international expertise in infectious diseases, epidemiology, economics, parasite biology, vector biology and control, clinical tropical medicine, drug and vaccine development and evaluation, molecular biology, immunology, control program management, anthropology, and ecology. The committee's recommendations evolved from its deliberations and the analysis of information from a wide range of sources, including articles from peer-reviewed journals, material published in book form, commissioned background papers, academic dissertations, unpublished case studies, presentations by and interviews with experts, and relevant conferences and workshops. The full committee met three times during the 18-month study; the final meeting was held in January 1991.

To supplement its efforts, the committee sponsored a symposium on ethical issues in malaria research, prevention, and control at the 1990 annual meeting of the American Society for Tropical Medicine and Hygiene. In addition, several working groups were formed. The epidemiologic paradigms described in Chapter 10 were drafted by a working group composed of several committee members, IOM staff, and representatives of the World Health Organization (WHO). Another working group was convened to address more fully some of the issues related to host immunology and vaccine development. Finally, nine-and six-member subcommittees were constituted and tasked to refine the conclusions and recommendations developed at the third committee meeting and to respond to the comments of the National Research Council's Report Review Committee.

The committee sees its report as a source of information and guidance that can be used in several ways, depending on the reader's perspective and interests. Readers who seek only the committee's conclusions and recommendations are directed to Chapter 1. Chapters 2 and 3 will be of particular interest to readers who are unfamiliar with malaria. Those who wish to delve still deeper into the biomedical aspects of the disease can read Chapters 4 through 12, which provide state-of-the-science information as well as research agendas that offer more precise avenues for advancing knowledge in specific areas.

As an appendix to this report, the reader will find a statement of dissent by committee member Awash Teklehaimanot. Overall, the committee believes that most of the concerns expressed by Dr. Teklehaimanot are, in fact, addressed in the report. The committee's charge was to assess the status of malaria research and control and make recommendations as to how the United States, as the largest single supporter of malaria research and control activities worldwide, could best contribute to global efforts to control the disease. Writing a "how-to" manual on malaria research and control was not a part of that charge. Rather, over the course of 18 months, the committee identified major challenges and obstacles in the science base and in the implementation of the current armamentarium of interventions for prevention and control. It then formulated specific recommendations on how U.S. support could be most effective in stemming the world's growing malaria problem.

The committee calls for sustained U.S. and international support for malaria control activities; a renewed commitment by donor agencies to support national programs; and extensive support for training of individuals from malaria-endemic countries in research, prevention, and control. The committee firmly believes that the United States' most effective contribution will come from support of a balanced agenda for both research and control: to develop the new tools that are desperately needed, to test and apply those tools appropriately and economically, and to utilize more contextually specific and rigorous approaches to U.S.-supported malaria control activities in countries where the disease is endemic.

The committee is hopeful that the conclusions and recommendations it offers will provide the impetus for critical decisions and for needed research, which will allow progress to be made in the global fight against malaria.

Charles C. J. Carpenter, *Chair*
Committee on Malaria Prevention and Control

Acknowledgments

This is perhaps the most difficult portion of the report to write, for fear of failing to acknowledge an individual or organization. Many people outside of the committee contributed to this study in various ways. Some prepared commissioned papers or provided relevant funding information; others participated in the symposium, the joint World Health Organization/Institute of Medicine effort to draft the paradigms, or the Immunology and Vaccine Development Working Group. Still others provided organizational information as members of the Liaison Panel. All of these contributors and others who provided the committee and staff with material for use in the study are listed on the following pages. To all of you, we offer our sincere appreciation.

The committee is particularly grateful to the following individuals, who took time from their busy schedules (and, in some cases, traveled great distances) to express their viewpoints and answer the many questions posed by the committee: Carlos C. Campbell of the Centers for Disease Control; Udom Chitprarop of the Malaria Center in Chiangmai, Thailand; Deberati Guha-Sapir of the University of Louvain, Brussels; Bernhard Liese of the World Bank; and Milton Tam of DiaTech, Program for Appropriate Technology in Health. Thanks are also due to the staff of the American Association for the Advancement of Science's project on malaria in Africa, directed by the Sub-Saharan Africa Program, for their cooperation and coordination with the Institute of Medicine study staff.

LIAISON PANEL

WILLIAM H. BANCROFT, Military Disease Hazards Research Program, U.S. Army Medical Research and Development Command, Fort Detrick, Frederick, Maryland

CARLOS C. CAMPBELL, Malaria Branch, Centers for Disease Control, Atlanta, Georgia

TORE GODAL, United Nations Development Programme/World Bank/World Health Organization Special Programme for Research and Training in Tropical Diseases, World Health Organization, Geneva, Switzerland

SCOTT B. HALSTEAD, Health Sciences Division, The Rockefeller Foundation, New York, New York

STEPHANIE L. JAMES, Parasitic and Tropical Diseases Branch, Division of Microbiology and Infectious Diseases, National Institute of Allergy and Infectious Diseases, National Institutes of Health, Bethesda, Maryland

BERNHARD LIESE, Health Services Department, The World Bank, Washington, D.C.

FRANCISCO LOPEZ-ANTUNANO, Tropical Disease Program, Pan American Health Organization, Washington, D.C.

NANCY PIELEMEIER, Office of Science and Technology/Health, Agency for International Development, Washington, D.C.

JAMES D. SHEPPERD, Bureau for Africa, Agency for International Development, Washington, D.C.

CONTRIBUTORS TO THE STUDY

ANDREW ARATA, Vector Biology and Control Project, Medical Service Corporation International, Arlington, Virginia

JOHN H. AUSTIN, Bureau of Science and Technology, Office of Health, Agency for International Development, Washington, D.C.

MICHELE BARRY, Tropical Medicine and International Traveler's Clinic, Yale University School of Medicine, New Haven, Connecticut

C. A. W. BATE, Department of Immunology, University College and Middlesex School of Medicine, London, United Kingdom

FREDERICK BATZOLD, Clinical Research Management Branch, National Institutes of Health, Bethesda, Maryland

JAY BERZOFSKY, Molecular Immunogenetics and Vaccine Research Section, Metabolism Branch, National Cancer Institute, National Institutes of Health, Bethesda, Maryland

GRAHAM BROWN, The Walter and Eliza Hall Institute of Medical Research, Royal Melbourne Hospital, Melbourne, Victoria, Australia

CARLOS C. CAMPBELL, Malaria Branch, Centers for Disease Control, Atlanta, Georgia

VICENTE I. CANO, Malaria Program, World Health Organization, Geneva, Switzerland

DENNIS CARROLL, Bureau of Science and Technology, Office of Health, Agency for International Development, Washington, D.C.

UDOM CHITPRAROP, Malaria Center, Chiangmai, Thailand

JANE COOLEY, International Health Programs, Centers for Disease Control, Atlanta, Georgia

CARTER DIGGS, Bureau of Science and Technology, Office of Health, Agency for International Development, Washington, D.C.

MARY ETTLING, Department of Population Sciences, Harvard School of Public Health, Boston, Massachusetts

RONALD GERMAINE, Lymphocyte Biology Section, Laboratory of Immunology, National Institute of Allergy and Infectious Diseases, National Institutes of Health, Bethesda, Maryland

DEBERATI GUHA-SAPIR, Department of Epidemiology, School of Public Health, University of Louvain, Brussels, Belgium

ROBERT W. GWADZ, Medical Entomology Unit, Malaria Section, Laboratory of Parasitic Diseases, National Institute of Allergy and Infectious Diseases, National Institutes of Health, Bethesda, Maryland

FABIENNE HARIGA, Department of Epidemiology, School of Public Health, University of Louvain, Brussels, Belgium

BRUCE HARRISON, Office of International Affairs, National Academy of Sciences, Washington, D.C.

J. DAVID HAYNES, Department of Immunology, Division of Communicable Diseases and Immunology, Walter Reed Army Institute of Research, Washington, D.C.

STEPHEN HEMBREE, Headquarters, U.S. Army Biomedical Research and Development Laboratory, Fort Detrick, Frederick, Maryland

PUSHPA HERATH, Malaria Program, World Health Organization, Geneva, Switzerland

DAVID KASLOW, Laboratory of Parasitic Diseases, National Institute of Allergy and Infectious Diseases, National Institutes of Health, Bethesda, Maryland

URIEL D. KITRON, Department of Veterinary Pathobiology, College of Veterinary Medicine, University of Illinois at Urbana-Champaign, Urbana, Illinois

JOHN LAMONTAGNE, Division of Microbiology and Infectious Diseases, National Institute of Allergy and Infectious Diseases, National Institutes of Health, Bethesda, Maryland

ELLI LEONTSINI, Center for International Community-Based Health Research, Department of International Health, Johns Hopkins University School of Hygiene and Public Health, Baltimore, Maryland

CAROL LEVINE, Citizens Commission on AIDS, New York, New York

TAMARA LEWIN, Center for International Health Information, USAID Health Information System, Arlington, Virginia

BERNHARD LIESE, Health Services Department, The World Bank, Washington, D.C.

A. DENNIS LONG, Bureau of Science and Technology, Office of Health, Agency for International Development, Washington, D.C.

WILLIAM H. LYERLY, JR., Bureau for Africa, Agency for International Development, Washington, D.C.

AJOY MATHEW, National Coalition of Hispanic Health and Human Services Organizations, Washington, D.C.

LAURA MEAGHER, Agricultural Molecular Biology Center, Rutgers University, New Brunswick, New Jersey

KIRK D. MILLER, Bureau of Science and Technology, Office of Health, Agency for International Development, Washington, D.C.

LOUIS H. MILLER, Laboratory of Parasitic Diseases, National Institute of Allergy and Infectious Diseases, National Institutes of Health, Bethesda, Maryland

BEVERLY MIXON, Parasitic Diseases Division, Center for Infectious Diseases, Centers for Disease Control, Atlanta, Georgia

LOUIS MOLINEAUX, Malaria Program, World Health Organization, Geneva, Switzerland

MALCOLM E. MOLYNEUX, Department of Tropical Medicine and Infectious Diseases, Liverpool School of Tropical Medicine, Liverpool, United Kingdom

JONATHAN MOSLEY, Center for International Health Information, USAID Health Information System, Arlington, Virginia

J. A. NAJERA, Division of Control of Tropical Diseases, World Health Organization, Geneva, Switzerland

RUTH S. NUSSENZWEIG, Department of Medical and Molecular Parasitology, New York University School of Medicine, New York, New York

VICTOR NUSSENZWEIG, Department of Pathology, Division of Immunology, New York University School of Medicine, New York, New York

RICHARD OBERST, Military Disease Hazards Research Program, U.S. Army Medical Research and Development Command, Fort Detrick, Frederick, Maryland

LORRIN PANG, Malaria Program, World Health Organization, Geneva, Switzerland

JOHN H. L. PLAYFAIR, Department of Immunology, University College and Middlesex School of Medicine, London, United Kingdom

LYMAN ROBERTS, Department of Entomology, Division of Communicable Diseases and Immunology, Walter Reed Army Institute of Research, Washington, D.C.

JERALD SADOFF, Division of Communicable Diseases and Immunology, Walter Reed Army Institute of Research, Washington, D.C.

ALAN SHAPIRA, Malaria Program, World Health Organization, Geneva, Switzerland

EDGAR SMITH, Entomology Consultant, Alexandria, Virginia

ANDREW SPIELMAN, Department of Tropical Public Health, Harvard School of Public Health, Boston, Massachusetts

MILTON TAM, DiaTech, Program for Appropriate Technology in Health, Seattle, Washington

J. TAVERNE, Department of Immunology, University College and Middlesex School of Medicine, London, United Kingdom

KARL WESTERN, Office of Tropical Medicine and International Research, National Institute of Allergy and Infectious Diseases, National Institutes of Health, Bethesda, Maryland

PETER WINCH, Center for International Community-Based Health Research, Department of International Health, Johns Hopkins University School of Hygiene and Public Health, Baltimore, Maryland

ROBERT WRIN, Bureau of Science and Technology, Office of Health, Agency for International Development, Washington, D.C.

Contents

MALARIA

Obstacles and Opportunities

1

Conclusions and Recommendations

DEFINING THE PROBLEM

The outlook for malaria control is grim. The disease, caused by mosquito-borne parasites, is present in 102 countries and is responsible for over 100 million clinical cases and 1 to 2 million deaths each year. Over the past two decades, efforts to control malaria have met with less and less success. In many regions where malaria transmission had been almost eliminated, the disease has made a comeback, sometimes surpassing earlier recorded levels. The dream of completely eliminating malaria from many parts of the world, pursued with vigor during the 1950s and 1960s, has gradually faded. Few believe today that a global eradication of malaria will be possible in the foreseeable future.

Worldwide, the number of cases of malaria caused by *Plasmodium falciparum*, the most dangerous species of the parasite, is on the rise. Drug-resistant strains of *P. falciparum* are spreading rapidly, and there have been recent reports of drug resistance in people infected with *P. vivax*, a less virulent form of the parasite. Furthermore, mosquitoes are becoming increasingly resistant to insecticides, and in many cases, have adapted so as to avoid insecticide-treated surfaces altogether.

In large part because of the spread of drug and insecticide resistance, there are fewer tools available today to control malaria than there were 20 years ago. In many countries, the few remaining methods are often ap-

1

plied inappropriately. The situation in many African nations is particularly dismal, exacerbated by a crumbling health infrastructure that has made the implementation of any disease control program difficult.

Malaria cases among tourists, business travelers, military personnel, and migrant workers in malarious areas have been increasing steadily in the last several years, posing new concerns that the disease will be introduced to currently nonmalarious areas. Recent epidemics have claimed tens of thousands of lives in Africa, and there is an increasing realization that malaria is a major impediment to socioeconomic development in many countries. Unless practical, cost-effective strategies can be developed and successfully implemented, malaria will continue to exact a heavy toll on human life and health around the world.

Although often considered a single disease, malaria is more accurately viewed as many diseases, each shaped by subtle interactions of biologic, ecologic, social, and economic factors. The species of parasite, the behavior of the mosquito host, the individual's immune status, the climate, human activities, and access to health services all play important roles in determining the intensity of disease transmission, who will become infected, who will get sick, and who will die.

Gem miners along the Thailand-Cambodia border, American tourists on a wildlife safari in East Africa, villagers living on the central highlands in Madagascar, residents of San Diego County, California, a young pregnant woman in Malawi, Swiss citizens living near Geneva International Airport, children in Africa south of the Sahara, and a U.S. State Department secretary in Tanzania seem to have little in common, yet they are all at risk of contracting malaria. Because of the disease's variable presentations, each will be affected differently, as illustrated below.

- For the hundreds of thousands of Thai seasonal agricultural workers who travel deep into the forest along the Thailand-Cambodia border to mine for gems, malaria is the cost of doing business. These young men are exposed to aggressive forest mosquitoes, and within two to three weeks after arriving, almost every miner will get malaria. Many gem miners seek medications to prevent and self-treat mild cases of the disease. But because malaria in this part of the world is resistant to most antimalarial drugs, the few effective drugs are reserved for the treatment of confirmed cases of malaria. To complicate matters, there are no health services in the forest to treat patients, and the health clinics in Thailand are overburdened by the high demand for treating those with severe malaria, most of whom are returning gem miners. A similar scenario involving over 400,000 people exists among gold miners in Rondonia, Brazil.

- Each year, over seven million U.S. citizens visit parts of the world where malaria is present. Many, at the recommendation of their travel agent or physician, take antimalarial medications as a preventive measure, but a significant number do not. Tourists and other travelers who have never been exposed to malaria, and therefore have never developed protective immunity, are at great risk for contracting severe disease. Ironically, it is not the infection itself that poses the biggest danger, but the chance that treatment will be delayed because of misdiagnosis upon the individual's return to the United States. Most U.S. doctors have never seen a patient with malaria, are often confused by the wide array of symptoms, and are largely unaware that malaria in a nonimmune person can be a medical emergency, sometimes rapidly fatal.

• Prior to 1950, malaria was the major cause of death in the central highlands of the African island nation of Madagascar. In the late 1950s, an aggressive program of indoor insecticide spraying rid the area of malaria-carrying mosquitoes, and malaria virtually disappeared. By the 1970s, confident of a victory in the battle against malaria, Madagascar began to phase out its spraying program; in some areas spraying was halted altogether. In the early 1980s, the vector mosquitoes reinvaded the central highlands, and in 1986 a series of devastating epidemics began. The older members of the population had long since lost the partial immunity they once had, and the younger island residents had no immunity at all. During the worst of the epidemics, tens of thousands of people died in one three-month period. The tragedy of this story is that it could have been prevented. A cheap antimalarial drug, chloroquine, could have been a powerful weapon in Madagascar, where drug resistance was not a significant concern. Because of problems in international and domestic drug supply and delivery, however, many people did not receive treatment and many died. In the last 18 months, surveillance has improved, spraying against the mosquito has resumed, and more effective drug distribution networks have been established. Malaria-related mortality has declined sharply as a result.

• Malaria, once endemic in the southern United States, occurs relatively infrequently. Indeed, there have been only 23 outbreaks of malaria since 1950, and the majority of these occurred in California. But for each of the past three years, the San Diego County Department of Health Services has had to conduct an epidemiologic investigation into local transmission of malaria. An outbreak in the late summer of 1988 involved 30 persons, the largest such outbreak in the United States since 1952. In the summer of 1989, three residents of San Diego County—a migrant worker and two permanent residents—were diagnosed with malaria; in 1990, a teenager living in a suburb of San Diego County fell ill with malaria. All of the cases were treated successfully, but these incidents raise questions about the possibility of new and larger outbreaks in the future. Malaria transmission in San Diego County (and in much of California) is attributed to the presence of individuals from malaria-endemic regions who lack access to medical care, the poor shelter and sanitation facilities of migrant workers, and the ubiquitous presence of *Anopheles* mosquitoes in California.

• A 24-year-old pregnant Yao woman from the Mangochi District in Malawi visited the village health clinic monthly to receive prenatal care. While waiting to be seen by the health provider, she and other women present listened to health education talks which were often about the dangers of malaria during pregnancy, and the need to install screens around the house to keep the mosquitoes away, to sleep under a bednet, and to take a chloroquine tablet once a week. Toward the end of her second trimester of pregnancy, the woman returned home from her prenatal visit with her eight tablets of chloroquine wrapped in a small packet of brown paper. She promptly gave the medicine to her husband to save for the next time he or one of their children fell ill. The next week she developed a very high malarial fever and went into labor prematurely. The six-month-old fetus was born dead.

• Over a two-week period in the summer of 1989, five Swiss citizens living within a mile of Geneva International Airport presented at several hospitals with acute fever and chills. All had malaria. Four of the five had no history of travel to a malarious region; none had a history of intravenous drug use or blood transfusion. Apart from their symptoms, the only thing linking the five was their proximity to the airport. A subsequent epidemiologic investigation suggested that the malaria miniepidemic was caused by the bite of stowaway mosquitoes en route from a malaria-endemic country. The warm weather, lack of systematic spraying of aircraft, and the close proximity of residential areas to the airport facilitated the transmission of the disease.

• Malaria is a part of everyday life in Africa south of the Sahara. Its impact on children is particularly severe. Mothers who bring unconscious children to the hospital often report that the children were playing that morning, convulsed suddenly, and have been unconscious ever since. These children are suffering from the most frequently fatal complication of the disease, cerebral malaria. Other children succumb more slowly to malaria, becoming progressively more anemic with each subsequent infection. By the time they reach the hospital, they are too weak to sit and are literally gasping for breath. Many children are brought to hospitals as a last resort, after treatment given for "fever" at the local health center has proved ineffective. Overall, children with malaria account for a third of all hospital admissions. A third of all children hospitalized for malaria die. In most parts of Africa, there are no effective or affordable options to prevent the disease, so children are at high risk until they have been infected enough times to develop a partial immunity.

• A 52-year-old American woman, the secretary to the U.S. ambassador in Tanzania, had been taking a weekly dose of chloroquine to prevent malaria since her arrival in the country the year before. She arrived at work one morning complaining of exhaustion, a throbbing headache, and fever. A blood sample was taken and microscopically examined for malaria parasites. She was found to be infected with *P. falciparum*, and was treated immediately with high doses of chloroquine. That night, she developed severe diarrhea, and by morning she was found to be disoriented and irrational. She was diagnosed as having cerebral malaria, and intravenous quinine treatment was started. Her condition gradually deteriorated—she became semicomatose and anemic, and approximately 20 percent of her red blood cells were found to be infected with malaria parasites. After continued treatment for several days, no parasites were detected in her blood. Despite receiving optimal care, other malaria-related complications developed and she died just nine days after the illness began. The cause of death: chloroquine-resistant *P. falciparum*.

These brief scenarios give a sense of the diverse ways that malaria can affect people. So fundamental is this diversity with respect to impact, manifestation, and epidemiology that malaria experts themselves are not unanimous on how best to approach the disease. Malariologists recognize that malaria is essentially a local phenomenon that varies greatly from region to region and even from village to village in the same district. Consequently, a single global technology for malaria control is of little use for specific conditions, yet the task of tailoring strategies to each situation is daunting. More important, many malarious countries do not have the resources, either human or financial, to carry out even the most meager efforts to control malaria.

These scenarios also illustrate the dual nature of malaria as it affects U.S. policy. In one sense, it is a foreign aid issue; a devastating disease is currently raging out of control in vast, heavily populated areas of the world. In another sense, malaria is of domestic public health concern. The decay of global malaria control and the invasion of the parasite into previously disease-free areas, coupled with the increasing frequency of visits to such areas by American citizens, intensify the dangers of malaria for the U.S. population. Tourists, business travelers, Peace Corps volunteers, State Department employees, and military personnel are increasingly at risk, and our ability to protect and cure them is in jeopardy. What is desperately needed is a better application of existing malaria control tools and new methods of containing the disease.

In most malarious regions of the world, there is inadequate access to malaria treatment. Appropriate health facilities may not exist; those that do exist may be inaccessible to affected populations, may not be supplied with effective drugs, or may be staffed inappropriately. In many countries, the expansion of primary health care services has not proceeded according to expectations, particularly in the poorest (and most malarious) nations of the tropical world.

In some countries, antimalarial interventions are applied in broad swaths, without regard to underlying differences in the epidemiology of the disease. In other countries, there are no organized interventions at all. The malaria problem in many regions is compounded by migration, civil unrest, poorly planned exploitation of natural resources, and their frequent correlate, poverty.

During the past 15 years, much research has focused on developing vaccines for malaria. Malaria vaccines are thought to be possible in part because people who are naturally exposed to the malaria parasite acquire a partial immunity to the disease over time. In addition, immunization of animals and humans by the bites of irradiated mosquitoes infected with the malaria parasite can protect against malaria infection. Much progress has been made, but current data suggest that effective vaccines are not likely to be available for some time.

Compounding the difficulty of developing more effective malaria prevention, treatment, and control strategies is a worldwide decline in the pool of scientists and health professionals capable of conducting field research and organizing and managing malaria control programs at the country level. With the change in approach from malaria eradication to malaria control, many malaria programs "lost face," admitting failure and losing the priority interest of their respective ministries of health. As external funding agencies lost interest in programs, they reduced their technical and financial support. As a consequence, there were fewer training opportunities, decreased contacts with international experts, and diminished prospects for improving the situation. Today, many young scientists and public health specialists, in both the developed and developing countries, prefer to seek higher-profile activities with better defined opportunities for career advancement.

THE REPORT

Background

It is against this backdrop of a worsening worldwide malaria situation that the Institute of Medicine was asked to convene a multidisciplinary committee to assess the current status of malaria research and control and to make recommendations to the U.S. government on promising and feasible strategies to address the problem. During the 18-month study, the committee reviewed the state of the science in the major areas of malariology, identified gaps in knowledge within each of the major disciplines, and developed recommendations for future action in malaria research and control.

Organization

Chapter 2 summarizes key aspects of the individual state-of-the-science chapters, and is intended to serve as a basic introduction to the medical and scientific aspects of malaria, including its clinical signs, diagnosis, treatment, and control. Chapter 3 provides a historical overview of malaria, from roughly 3000 B.C. to the present, with special emphasis on efforts in this century to eradicate and control the disease. The state-of-the-science reviews, which start in Chapter 4, begin with a scenario titled "Where We Want To Be in the Year 2010." Each scenario describes where the discipline would like to be in 20 years and how, given an ideal world, the discipline would have contributed to malaria control efforts. The middle section of each chapter contains a critical review of the current status of knowledge in the particular field. The final section lays out specific directions for future research based on a clear identification of the major gaps in scientific understanding for that discipline. The committee urges those agencies that fund malaria research to consult the end of each state-of-the-science chapter for suggestions on specific research opportunities in malaria.

Sponsorship

This study was sponsored by the U.S. Agency for International Development, the U.S. Army Medical Research and Development Command, and the National Institute of Allergy and Infectious Diseases of the National Institutes of Health.

CONCLUSIONS AND RECOMMENDATIONS

A major finding of the committee is the need to increase donor and public awareness of the growing risk presented by the resurgence of malaria. Overall, funding levels are not adequate to meet the problem. The committee believes that funding in the past focused too sharply on specific technologies and particular control strategies (e.g., indiscriminate use of insecticide spraying). Future support must be balanced among the needs outlined in this report. The issue for prioritization is not whether to select specific technologies or control strategies, but to raise the priority for solving the problem of malaria. This is best done by encouraging balanced research and control strategies and developing a mechanism for periodically adjusting support for promising approaches.

This report highlights those areas which the committee believes deserve the highest priority for research or which should be considered when U.S. support is provided to malaria control programs. These observations and suggestions for future action, presented below in four sections discussing policy, research, control, and training, represent the views of a multidisciplinary group of professionals from diverse backgrounds and with a variety of perspectives on the problem.

Policy

The U.S. government is the largest single source of funds for malaria research and control activities in the world. This investment is justified by the magnitude of the malaria problem, from both a foreign aid and a public health perspective. The increasing severity of the threat of malaria to residents of endemic regions, travelers, and military personnel, and our diminishing ability to counter it, should be addressed by a more comprehensive and better integrated approach to malaria research and control. However, overall U.S. support for malaria research and control has declined over the past five years. The committee believes that the amount of funding currently directed to malaria research and control activities is inadequate to address the problem.

Over the past 10 years, the majority of U.S. funds available for malaria research have been devoted to studies on immunity and vaccine development. Although the promise of vaccines remains to be realized, the committee believes that the potential benefits are enormous. At the same time, the relative paucity of funds available for research has prevented or slowed progress in other areas. Our incomplete knowledge about the basic biology of malaria parasites, how they interact with their mosquito and human hosts, and how human biology and behavior affect malaria transmission and control remains a serious impediment to the development and implementation of malaria control strategies. The committee believes that this situation must be addressed without reducing commitment to current research initiatives. The committee further believes that such research will pay long-term dividends in the better application of existing tools and the development of new drugs, vaccines, and methods for vector control.

The committee recommends that increased funds be made available so that U.S. research on malaria can be broadened according to the priorities addressed in this report, including laboratory and field research on the biology of malaria parasites, their mosquito vectors, and their interaction with humans.

The committee believes that the maximum return on investment of funds devoted to malaria research and control can be achieved only by rigorous review of project proposals. The committee further believes that the highest-quality review is essential to ensure that funding agencies spend their money wisely. The committee believes that all U.S.-supported malaria field activities, both research and control, should be of the highest scientific quality and relevance to the goals of malaria control.

The committee recommends decisions on funding of malaria research be based on scientific merit as determined by rigorous peer review, consistent with the guidelines of the National Institutes of Health or the United Nations Development Program/World Bank/ World Health Organization Special Programme for Research and Training in Tropical Diseases, and that all U.S.-supported malaria field projects be subject to similar rigorous review to ensure that projects are epidemiologically and scientifically sound.

Commitment and Sustainability

For malaria control, short-term interventions can be expected to produce only short-term results. The committee believes that short-term interventions are justified only for emergency situations. Longer-term interventions should be undertaken only when there is a national commitment to support sustained malaria surveillance and control.

The committee recommends that malaria control programs receive sustained international and local support, oriented toward the development of human resources, the improvement of management skills, the provision of supplies, and the integration of an operational research capability in support of an epidemiologically sound approach to malaria control.

Surveillance

During the major effort to eradicate malaria from many parts of the world that began in the late 1950s and ended in 1969, it was important to establish mechanisms to detect all malaria infections. As a result, systems were established in many countries to collect blood samples for later microscopic examination for the presence of parasites. Each year, the results from more than 140 million slides are reported to the World Health Organization, of which roughly 3 to 5 percent are positive for malaria. This approach seeks to answer the question posed 30 years ago: How many people are infected with the malaria parasite? It does not answer today's questions: Who is sick? Where? Why? The committee concludes that the mass collection of blood slides requires considerable resources, poses serious biosafety hazards, deflects attention from the treatment of ill individuals, and has little practical relevance for malaria control efforts today. Instead of the mass collection of slides, the committee believes that the most effective surveillance networks are those that concurrently measure disease in human populations, antimalarial drug use, patterns of drug resistance, and the intensity of malaria transmission by vector populations. The committee believes that malaria surveillance practices have not received adequate recognition as an epidemiologic tool for designing, implementing, and evaluating malaria control programs.

The committee recommends that countries be given support to orient malaria surveillance away from the mass collection and screening of blood slides toward the collection and analysis of epidemiologically relevant information that can be used to monitor the current situation on an ongoing basis, to identify high-risk groups, and to detect potential epidemics early in their course.

Inter-Sectoral Cooperation

The committee believes that insufficient attention has been paid to the impact that activities in non-health-related sectors, such as construction, industry, irrigation, and agriculture, have on malaria transmission. Conversely, there are few assessments of the impact of malaria control projects on other public health initiatives, the environment, and the socioeconomic status of affected populations. Malaria transmission frequently occurs in areas where private and multinational businesses and corporations (e.g., hotel chains, mining operations, and industrial plants) have strong economic interests. Unfortunately and irresponsibly, some local and multinational businesses contribute few if any resources to malaria control in areas in which they operate.

The committee recommends greater cooperation and consultation between health and nonhealth sectors in the planning and implementation of major development projects and malaria activities. It also recommends that all proposed malaria control programs be analyzed for their potential impact on other public health programs, the environment, and social and economic welfare, and that local and multinational businesses be recruited by malaria control organizations to contribute substantially to local malaria control efforts.

New Tools for Malaria Control

The committee believes that, as a policy directive, it is important to support research activities to develop new tools for malaria control. The greatest momentum for the development of new tools exists in vaccine and drug development, and the committee believes it essential that this momentum be maintained. The committee recognizes that commendable progress has been made in defining the characteristics of antigens and delivery systems needed for effective vaccines, but that the candidates so far tested fall short of the goal. Much has been learned which supports the hope that useful vaccines can be developed. To diminish activity in vaccine development at this stage would deal a severe blow to one of our best chances for a technological breakthrough in malaria control.

The committee recommends that vaccine development continue to be a priority of U.S.-funded malaria research.

Only a handful of drugs are available to prevent or treat malaria, and the spread of drug-resistant strains of the malaria parasite threatens to reduce further the limited pool of effective drugs. The committee recognizes that there is little economic incentive for U.S. pharmaceutical companies to undertake antimalarial drug discovery activities. The committee is concerned that U.S. government support of these activities, based almost entirely at the Walter Reed Army Institute of Research (WRAIR), has decreased and is threatened with further funding cuts. The committee concludes that the WRAIR program in antimalarial drug discovery, which is the largest and most successful in the world, is crucial to international efforts to develop new drugs for malaria. The benefits of this program in terms of worldwide prevention and treatment of malaria have been incalculable.

The committee strongly recommends that drug discovery and development activities at WRAIR receive increased and sustained support.

The next recommendation on policy directions reflects the committee's concern about the lack of involvement in malaria research by the private sector. The committee believes that the production of candidate malaria vaccines and antimalarial drugs for clinical trials has been hampered by a lack of industry involvement. Greater cooperation and a clarification of the contractual relationships between the public and private sectors would greatly enhance the development of drugs and vaccines.

The committee recommends that mechanisms be established to promote the involvement of pharmaceutical and biotechnology firms in the development of malaria vaccines, antimalarial drugs, and new tools for vector control.

Coordination and Integration

The committee is concerned that there is inadequate joint planning and coordination among U.S.-based agencies that support malaria research and control activities. Four government agencies and many nongovernmental organizations in the United States are actively involved in malaria-related activities. There are also numerous overseas organizations, governmental and nongovernmental, that actively support such activities worldwide.

The complexity and variability of malaria, the actual and potential scientific advances in several areas of malariology, and most important the worsening worldwide situation argue strongly for an ongoing mechanism to assess and influence current and future U.S. efforts in malaria research and control.

The committee strongly recommends the establishment of a national advisory body on malaria.

In addition to fulfilling a much needed coordinating function among U.S.-based agencies and between the U.S. and international efforts, the national advisory body could monitor the status of U.S. involvement in malaria research and control, assess the relevant application of knowledge, identify areas requiring further research, make recommendations to the major funding agencies, and provide a resource for legislators and others interested in scientific policy related to malaria. The national advisory body could convene specific task-oriented scientific working groups to review research and control activities and to make recommendations, when appropriate, for changes in priorities and new initiatives.

The committee believes that the national advisory body should be part of, and appointed by, a neutral and nationally respected scientific body and that it should actively encourage the participation of governmental and nongovernmental organizations, industry, and university scientists in advising on the direction of U.S. involvement in malaria research and control.

The increasing magnitude of the malaria problem during the past decade and the unpredictability of changes in human, parasite, and vector determinants of transmission and disease point strongly to the need for such a national advisory body, which can be responsive to rapidly changing problems, and advances in scientific research, relating to global efforts to control malaria.

Malaria Research Priorities

Malaria control is in crisis in many areas of the world. People are contracting and dying of severe malaria in unprecedented numbers. To address these problems, the committee strongly encourages a balanced research agenda. Two basic areas of research require high priority. Research that will lead to improved delivery of existing interventions for malaria, and the development of new tools for the control of malaria.

Research in Support of Available Control Measures

Risk Factors for Severe Malaria People who develop severe and complicated malaria lack adequate immunity, and many die from the disease. Groups at greatest risk include young children and pregnant women in malaria endemic regions; nonimmune migrants, laborers, and visitors to endemic regions; and residents of regions where malaria has been recently reintroduced. For reasons that are largely unknown, not all individuals within these groups appear to be at equal risk for severe disease. The committee believes that the determinants of severe disease, including risk factors associated with a population, the individual (biologic, immunologic, socioeconomic, and behavioral), the parasite, or exposure to mosquitoes, are likely to vary considerably in different areas.

The committee recommends that epidemiologic studies on the risk factors for severe and complicated malaria be supported.

Pathogenesis of Severe and Complicated Malaria Even with optimal care, 20 to 30 percent of children and adults with the most severe form of malaria—primarily cerebral malaria—die. The committee believes that a better understanding of the disease process will lead to improvements in preventing and treating severe forms of malaria. The committee further believes that determining the indications for treatment of severe malarial anemia is of special urgency given the risk of transmitting the AIDS virus through blood transfusions, the only currently available treatment for malarial anemia. Physicians need to know when it is appropriate to transfuse malaria patients.

The committee recommends greater support for research on the pathogenesis of severe and complicated malaria, on the mechanisms of malarial anemia, and on the development of specific criteria for blood transfusions in malaria.

Social Science Research The impact of drugs to control disease or programs to reduce human-mosquito contact is mediated by local practices and beliefs about malaria and its treatment. Most people in malaria-endemic countries seek initial treatment for malaria outside of the formal health sector. Programs that attempt to influence this behavior must understand that current practices satisfy, at some level, local concerns regarding such matters as access to and effectiveness of therapy, and cost. These concerns may lead to practices at odds with current medical practice. Further, many malaria control programs have not considered the social, cultural, and behavioral dimensions of malaria, thereby limiting the effectiveness of measures undertaken. The committee recognizes that control programs often fail to incorporate household or community concerns and resources into program design.   In most countries, little is known about how the demand for and utilization of health services is influenced by such things as user fees, location of health clinics, and the existence and quality of referral services.   The committee concludes that modern social science techniques have not been effectively applied to the design, implementation, and evaluation of malaria control programs.

> **The committee recommends that research be conducted on local perceptions of malaria as an illness, health-seeking behaviors (including the demand for health care services), and behaviors that affect malaria transmission, and that the results of this research be included in community-based malaria control interventions that promote the involvement of communities and their organizations in control efforts.**

Innovative Approaches to Malaria Control   Malaria control programs will require new ideas and approaches, and new malaria control strategies need to be developed and tested.   There is also a need for consistent support of innovative combinations of control technologies and for the transfer of new technologies from the laboratory to the clinic and field for expeditious evaluation.   Successful technology transfer requires the exchange of scientific research, but more importantly, must be prefaced by an improved understanding of the optimal means to deliver the technology to the people in need (see Chapter 11).

> **The committee recommends that donor agencies provide support for research on new or improved control strategies and into how new tools and technologies can be better implemented and integrated into on-going control efforts.**

Development of New Tools

Antimalarial Immunity and Vaccine Development   Many people are able to mount an effective immune response that can significantly mitigate symptoms of malaria and prevent death.   The committee believes that the development of effective malaria vaccines is feasible, and that the potential benefits of such vaccines are enormous.   Several different types of malaria vaccines need to be developed: vaccines to prevent infection (of particular use for tourists and other nonimmune visitors to endemic countries), prevent the progression of infection to disease (for partially immune residents living in endemic areas and for nonimmune visitors), and interrupt transmission of parasites by vector populations (to reduce the risk of new infections in humans).   The committee believes that each of these directions should be pursued.

> **The committee recommends sustained support for research to identify mechanisms and targets of protective immunity and to exploit the**

use of novel scientific technologies to construct vaccines that induce immunity against all relevant stages of the parasite life cycle.

Drug Discovery and Development Few drugs are available to prevent or treat malaria, and the spread of drug-resistant strains of malaria parasites is steadily reducing the limited pool of effective chemotherapeutic agents. The committee believes that an inadequate understanding of parasite biochemistry and biology impedes the process of drug discovery and slows studies on the mechanisms of drug resistance.

> The committee recommends increased emphasis on screening compounds to identify new classes of potential antimalarial drugs, identifying and characterizing vulnerable targets within the parasite, understanding the mechanisms of drug resistance, and identifying and developing agents that can restore the therapeutic efficacy of currently available drugs.

Vector Control Malaria is transmitted to humans by the bites of infective mosquitoes. The objective of vector control is to reduce the contact between humans and infected mosquitoes. The committee believes that developments are needed in the areas of personal protection, environmental management, pesticide use and application, and biologic control, as well as in the largely unexplored areas of immunologic and genetic approaches for decreasing parasite transmission by vectors.

> The committee recommends increased support for research on vector control that focuses on the development and field testing of methods for interrupting parasite transmission by vectors.

Malaria Control

Malaria is a complex disease that, even under the most optimistic scenario, will continue to be a major health threat for decades. The extent to which malaria affects human health depends on a large number of epidemiologic and ecologic factors. Depending on the particular combination of these and other variables, malaria may have different effects on neighboring villages and people living in a single village. All malaria control programs need to be designed with a view toward effectiveness and sustainability, taking into account the local perceptions, the availability of human and financial resources, and the multiple needs of the communities at risk. If community support for health sector initiatives is to be guaranteed, the public needs to know much more about malaria, its risks for epidemics and severe disease, and difficulties in control.

Unfortunately, there is no "magic bullet" solution to the deteriorating worldwide malaria situation, and no single malaria control strategy will be applicable in all regions or epidemiologic situations. Given the limited available financial and human resources and a dwindling pool of effective antimalarial tools, the committee suggests that donor agencies support four priority areas for malaria control in endemic countries.

The committee believes that the first and most basic priority in malaria control is to prevent infected individuals from becoming severely ill and dying. Reducing the incidence of severe morbidity and malaria-related mortality requires a two-pronged approach. First, diagnostic, treatment, and referral capabilities, including the provision of microscopes, training of technicians and other health providers, and drug supply, must be enhanced. Second, the committee believes that many malaria-related deaths could be averted if individuals and caretakers of young children knew when and how to seek appropriate treatment and if drug vendors, pharmacists, physicians, nurses, and other health care providers were provided with up-to-date and locally appropriate treatment and referral guidelines. The development and implementation of an efficient information system that provides rapid feedback to the originating clinic and area is key to monitoring the situation and preventing epidemics.

The committee believes that the second priority should be to promote personal protection measures (e.g., bednets, screens, and mosquito coils) to reduce or eliminate human-mosquito contact and thus to reduce the risk of infection for individuals living in endemic areas. At the present time, insecticide-treated bednets appear to be the most promising personal protection method.

In many environments, in addition to the treatment of individuals and use of personal protection measures, community-wide vector control is feasible. In such situations, the committee believes that the third priority should be low-cost vector control measures designed to reduce the prevalence of infective mosquitoes in the environment, thus reducing the transmission of malaria to populations. These measures include source reduction (e.g., draining or filling in small bodies of water where mosquito larvae develop) or the application of low-cost larval control measures. In certain environments, the use of insecticide-impregnated bednets by all or most members of a community may also reduce malaria transmission, but this approach to community-based malaria control remains experimental.

The committee believes that the fourth priority for malaria control should be higher cost vector control measures such as large-scale source reduction or widespread spraying of residual insecticides. In certain epidemiologic situations, the use of insecticides for adult mosquito control is appropriate and represents the method of choice for decreasing malaria transmission and preventing epidemics (see Chapter 7 and Chapter 10).

The committee recommends that support of malaria control programs include resources to improve local capacities to conduct prompt diagnosis, including both training and equipment, and to ensure the availability of antimalarial drugs.

The committee recommends that resources be allocated to develop and disseminate malaria treatment guidelines for physicians, drug vendors, pharmacists, village health workers, and other health care personnel in endemic and non-endemic countries. The guidelines should be based, where appropriate, on the results of local operational research and should include information on the management of severe and complicated disease. The guidelines should be consistent and compatible among international agencies involved in the control of malaria.

The committee recommends that support for malaria control initiatives include funds to develop and implement locally relevant communication programs that provide information about how to prevent and treat malaria appropriately (including when and how to seek treatment) and that foster a dialogue about prevention and control.

Organization of Malaria Control

One of the major criticisms of malaria control programs during the past 10 to 15 years has been that funds have been spent inappropriately without an integrated plan and without formal evaluation of the efficacy of control measures instituted. In many instances, this has led to diminished efforts to control malaria.

The committee strongly encourages renewed commitment by donor agencies to support national control programs in malaria-endemic countries.

The committee recommends that U.S. donor agencies develop, with the advice of the national advisory body, a core of expertise (either in-house or through an external advisory group) to plan assistance to malaria control activities in endemic countries.

The committee believes that the development, implementation, and evaluation of such programs must follow a rigorous set of guidelines. These guidelines should include the following steps:

I. Identification of the problem
    A. Determine the extent and variety of malaria. The paradigm approach described in Chapter 10 should facilitate this step.
    B. Analyze current efforts to solve malaria problems.
    C. Identify and characterize available in-country resources and capabilities.
II. Development of a plan
    A. Design and prioritize interventions based on the epidemiologic situation and the available resources.

B. Design a training program for decision makers, managers, and technical staff to support and sustain the interventions.

C. Define specific indicators of the success or failure of the interventions at specific time points.

D. Develop a specific plan for reporting on the outcomes of interventions.

E. Develop a process for adjusting the program in response to successes and/or failures of interventions.

III. Review of the comprehensive plan by a donor agency review board

IV. Modification of the plan based on comments of the review board

V. Implementation of the program

VI. Yearly report and analysis of outcome variables

To guide the implementation of the activities outlined above, the committee has provided specific advice on several components, including an approach to evaluating malaria problems and designing control strategies (the paradigm approach), program management, monitoring and evaluation, and operational research.

Paradigm Approach

Given the complex and variable nature of malaria, the committee believes that the epidemiologic paradigms (see Chapter 10), developed in conjunction with this study, may form the basis of a logical and reasoned approach for defining the malaria problems and improving the design and management of malaria control programs.

The committee recommends that the paradigm approach be field tested to determine its use in helping policymakers and malaria program managers design and implement epidemiologically appropriate and cost-effective control initiatives.

The committee recognizes that various factors, including the local ecology, the dynamics of mosquito transmission of malaria parasites, genetically determined resistance to malaria infection, and patterns of drug use, affect patterns of malaria endemicity in human populations and need to be considered when malaria control strategies are developed. In most endemic countries, efforts to understand malaria transmission through field studies of vector populations are either nonexistent or so limited in scope that they have minimal impact on subsequent malaria control efforts. The committee recognizes that current approaches to malaria control are clearly inadequate. The committee believes, however, that malaria control strategies are sometimes applied inappropriately, with little regard to the underlying differences in the epidemiology of the disease.

> The committee recommends that support for malaria control programs include funds to permit a reassessment and optimization of antimalarial tools based on relevant analyses of local epidemiologic, parasitologic, entomologic, socioeconomic, and behavioral determinants of malaria and the costs of malaria control.

Management

Poor management has contributed to the failure of many malaria control programs. Among the reasons are a chronic shortage of trained managers who can think innovatively about health care delivery and who can plan, implement, supervise, and evaluate malaria control programs. Lack of incentives, the absence of career advancement options, and designation of responsibility without authority often hinder the effectiveness of the small cadre of professional managers that does exist. The committee recognizes that management technology is a valuable resource that has yet to be effectively introduced into the planning, implementation, and evaluation of most malaria control programs.

> The committee recommends that funding agencies utilize management experts to develop a comprehensive series of recommendations and guidelines as to how basic management skills and technology can be introduced into the planning, implementation, and evaluation of malaria control programs.

> The committee recommends that U.S. funding of each malaria control program include support for a senior manager who has responsibility for planning and coordinating malaria control activities. Where such an individual does not exist, a priority of the control effort should be to identify and support a qualified candidate. The manager should be supported actively by a multidisciplinary core group with expertise in epidemiology, entomology, the social sciences, clinical medicine, environmental issues, and vector control operations.

Monitoring and Evaluation

Monitoring and evaluation are essential components of any control program. For malaria control, it is not acceptable to continue pursuing a specific control strategy without clear evidence that it is effective and reaching established objectives.

> The committee recommends that support for malaria control programs include funds to evaluate the impact of control efforts on the magnitude of the problem and that each program be modified as necessary on the basis of periodic assessments of its costs and effectiveness.

Problem Solving (Operational Research) and Evaluation

At the outset of any malaria prevention or control initiative and during the course of implementation, gaps in knowledge will be identified and problems will arise. These matters should be addressed through clearly defined, short-term, focused studies. Perhaps the most difficult aspects of operational research are to identify the relevant problem, formulate the appropriate question, and design a study to answer that question.

The committee recommends that a problem-solving (operational research) component be built into all existing and future U.S.-funded malaria control initiatives and that support be given to enhance the capacity to perform such research. This effort will include consistent support in the design of focused projects that can provide applicable results, analysis of data, and dissemination of conclusions.

Training

The committee concludes that there is a need for additional scientists actively involved in malaria-related research in the United States and abroad. To meet this need, both short- and long-term training at the doctoral and postdoctoral levels must be provided. This training will be of little value unless there is adequate long-term research funding to support the career development of professionals in the field of malaria.

The committee recommends support for research training in malaria.

Whereas the curricula for advanced degree training in basic science research and epidemiology are fairly well defined, two areas require attention, especially in the developing world: social sciences and health management and training.

The committee recommends that support be given for the development of advanced-degree curricula in the social sciences, and in health management and training, for use in universities in developing and developed countries.

The availability of well-trained managers, decision makers, and technical staff is critical to the implementation of any malaria prevention and control program. The development of such key personnel requires a long term combination of formal training, focused short courses, and a gradual progression of expertise.

The committee recommends support for training in management, epidemiology, entomology, social sciences, and vector control. Such training for malaria control may be accomplished through U.S.-funded grant programs for long-term cooperative relationships

between institutions in developed and developing countries; through the encouragement of both formal and informal linkages among malaria-endemic countries; through the use of existing training courses; and through the development of specific training courses.

The committee recommends further that malaria endemic countries be supported in the development of personnel programs that provide long-term career tracks for managers, decision makers, and technical staff, and that offer professional fulfillment, security, and competitive financial compensation.

2

Background

MALARIA AS A DISEASE

Malaria in humans is caused by four species of protozoan parasites of the genus *Plasmodium*: *P. falciparum*, *P. vivax*, *P. ovale*, and *P. malariae*. Although *P. vivax* is responsible for most malaria infections in the world, the most severe form of malaria is caused by *P. falciparum*. The severity of malarial illness depends largely on the immunological status of the person who is infected. Partial immunity develops over time through repeated infection, and without recurrent infection, immunity is relatively short-lived.

The distinction between infection and disease is particularly important in malaria, since infection with the parasite does not necessarily result in disease. Many infected people in areas where malaria is endemic are asymptomatic: they may harbor large numbers of parasites yet exhibit no outward signs and symptoms of the disease. Asymptomatic individuals are major contributors to the transmission of malaria parasites, however.

For reasons not fully understood, the epidemiology of malaria transmission and the severity of the disease vary greatly from region to region, village to village, and even from person to person within a village. Some of these differences are due to the particular species of parasite. The degree of compliance with an antimalarial drug regimen, local patterns of drug resistance, and an individual's age, genetic makeup, and duration of exposure to infective mosquitoes may also influence the severity of the disease.

Clinical Aspects

The clinical manifestations of malaria are varied. The classic description of an individual progressing episodically from shaking chills through intense fevers to drenching sweats is characteristic but not universal. In areas where malaria is common, infected individuals may have symptoms that mimic other diseases, making a correct diagnosis difficult. The problem of diagnosis is especially difficult in children, who may have high blood levels of parasites but relatively mild symptoms. In areas where health workers are unfamiliar with malaria, or with patients in whom the range of symptoms may not point clearly to malaria, misdiagnosis is a serious problem.

Severe and complicated malaria, generally due to infection with *P. falciparum*, is a medical emergency. In the absence of prompt intervention, the patient's condition can deteriorate rapidly, often ending in death (Figure 2-1). About 80 percent of deaths from the disease result from cerebral malaria, a state of altered consciousness, sometimes including coma, in patients infected with *P. falciparum*. Renal failure, hypoglycemia, severe anemia, pulmonary edema, and shock may also play a role in fatal malaria.

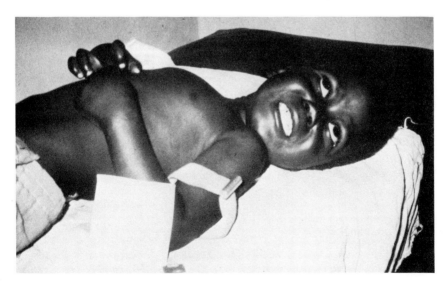

FIGURE 2-1 An African child with severe malaria. (Photo courtesy of Dr. Terrie Taylor, IOM Malaria Committee member)

Malaria during pregnancy can cause miscarriages, fetal death, intrauterine growth retardation, low birth weight, and premature delivery. Women pregnant for the first time and in their third trimester are at particular risk for severe anemia and sometimes even death. The impact of malaria during pregnancy on infant and child development is unknown.

Malarial anemia is an important contributor to *P. falciparum*-associated morbidity and mortality. Because of the risk of transmitting the human immunodeficiency virus (HIV) and other blood-borne pathogens (including hepatitis B virus and the bacterium that causes syphilis) through contaminated blood, the treatment of malarial anemia with blood transfusions raises serious clinical and safety questions. This risk is of particular concern in areas where screening of donated blood for the presence of HIV and other pathogens is not routine and where blood transfusion equipment is reused without being sterilized.

Immunity

Assuming they survive childhood, people in areas of endemic malaria often acquire a moderate level of immunity to malaria by being infected repeatedly. Although they may experience mild symptoms of the disease, including recurrent fevers, they rarely suffer the more severe and potentially fatal consequences. Without repeated exposure, however, this immunity is relatively short-lived, and although it almost always protects against life-threatening malaria, it does not prevent occasional episodes of fever and chills.

Role of Genetics

Some population groups have genetic characteristics that render them resistant to certain forms of malaria. For example, persons of African descent who lack the so-called Duffy blood group surface antigens cannot be infected with *P. vivax*. The heterozygous sickle cell trait, often present in people of African descent, partially protects against infection with *P. falciparum*. Other hereditary abnormalities, such as glucose-6-phosphate dehydrogenase deficiency, are partially protective against malaria.

DIAGNOSIS

Medical personnel should suspect malaria in anyone with a fever who has recently been in a malaria-endemic region. A definitive diagnosis of malaria infection is made by microscopic examination of stained blood smears for the presence of parasites (Figure 2-2). In the early stages of infection and at all stages of infection with *P. falciparum*, when parasites

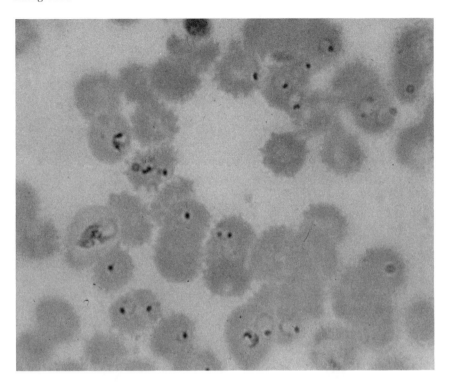

FIGURE 2-2 Photomicrograph of a stained smear of *Plasmodium falciparum*-infected red blood cells, magnification approximately 1,200×. (Photo courtesy of Dr. Terrie Taylor, IOM Malaria Committee member)

disappear from the peripheral blood during schizogony, few or no parasites may be present in a blood smear; examination of blood smears taken at frequent intervals may be necessary to establish a diagnosis. A positive blood smear taken from a feverish patient living in an endemic region does not conclusively implicate malaria as the cause of illness, because many asymptomatic individuals have circulating parasites in their blood and the fever may be due to other infectious agents.

THE PARASITE

Life Cycle

The life cycle of the malaria parasite is complex (Figure 2-3). The process—three phases in the mosquito and two in the human host—has been divided by scientists into nearly a dozen separate steps. The parasite

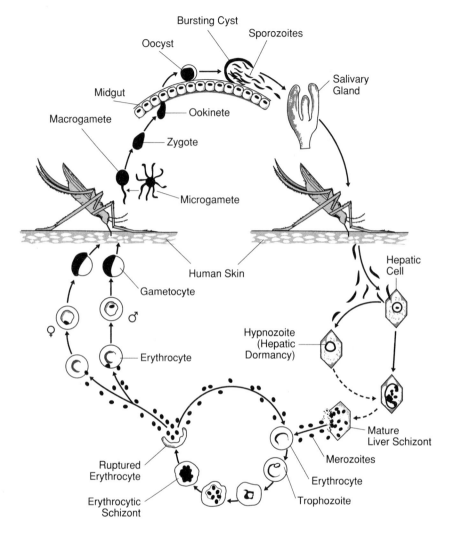

FIGURE 2-3 The life cycle of the malaria parasite. (Adapted from *Hospital Practice*, September 15, 1990, by permission of HP Publishing, New York)

is transmitted to humans by the sporozoite forms in the saliva of infected female mosquitoes of the genus *Anopheles*. Soon after entering the human host, the sporozoites invade liver cells, where during the next 5 to 15 days they develop into schizonts. Each schizont contains 10,000 to 30,000 "daughter" parasites called merozoites, which are released and invade the red blood cells. Once inside the red blood cells, each merozoite matures into a schizont containing 8 to 32 new merozoites. The red blood cell eventually ruptures and releases the merozoites, which are then free to invade additional red blood cells. The rupturing of red blood cells is associated with fever and signals the clinical onset of malaria.

Some merozoites differentiate into sexual forms, gametocytes, which are ingested by a mosquito during its next blood meal. Once in the mosquito, the sexual forms leave the blood cells, and male and female gametes fuse to form a zygote. Over the next 12 to 48 hours, the zygote elongates to form an ookinete. The ookinete penetrates the wall of the insect's stomach and becomes an oocyst. Over the next week or more, depending on the parasite species and ambient temperature, the oocyst enlarges, forming more than 10,000 sporozoites. When the oocyst ruptures, the sporozoites migrate to the mosquito salivary glands, from where they may be injected back into the human host, thus completing the cycle.

Relapse and Recrudescence

Malarial illness may recur months to years after apparently successful treatment. In patients infected with *P. vivax* and *P. ovale*, this phenomenon is known as relapse. Relapse is caused by dormant liver-stage forms of the parasite that resume their developmental cycle and release merozoites into the bloodstream. The recurrence of malaria caused by *P. falciparum* and *P. malariae* is due to recrudescence, which is caused by surviving blood-stage parasites from an earlier infection.

THE MOSQUITO

Of the more than 2,500 known species of mosquitoes worldwide, only a sub-group of 50 to 60 species belonging to the genus *Anopheles* are capable of transmitting malaria. Female anophelines require blood meals to reproduce (Figure 2-4). Some anopheline species are indiscriminant feeders; others prefer to feed on animals (zoophilic) or humans (anthropophilic).

Anopheline mosquitoes breed in relatively clean water, with certain species having very specific preferences as to their aquatic environment (Figure 2-5). Understanding these preferences is crucial for targeting effective malaria control interventions. For example, *An. stephensi* can breed in tin cans and water cisterns, while *Anopheles gambiae*, the most important malaria vector in Africa south of the Sahara, prefers small, sunlit pools.

Life Cycle

The mosquito undergoes four stages of growth: egg, larva, pupa, and adult (imago). Adult females mate once and store the sperm. The female

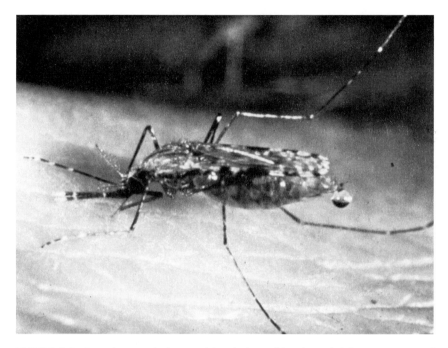

FIGURE 2-4   Female *Anopheles gambiae* during a blood meal. (Photo courtesy of Dr. Robert Gwadz, NIAID, NIH)

may deposit a total of 200 to 1,000 eggs in three or more batches. Actual egg production is dependent on blood consumption. After hatching, anopheline larvae lie along the water-air interface, where it is thought that they feed on organisms along the surface film. Adult mosquitoes develop from the pupal stage within 2 to 4 days. An adult mosquito will emerge from the egg stage in 7 to 20 days, depending on the species of mosquito and environmental conditions.

Female anopheline mosquitoes can survive at least a month under favorable conditions of high humidity and moderate temperatures. That is sufficient time for them to take a blood meal, for the parasite to develop, and for the mosquito to take another blood meal and thus transmit the parasite to a second human host.

Host-Seeking and Feeding Behavior

Mosquitoes are rarely found more than a few miles from their larval development site. They are readily blown short distances by the wind and have been transported internationally as unintended stowaways on airplanes.

Mosquitoes seek their host in response to a combination of chemical and physical stimuli, including carbon dioxide plumes, certain body odors, warmth, and movement.

Anopheline mosquitoes feed most frequently at night and occasionally in the evening, or in heavily shaded or dark areas during the early morning. During feeding, the mosquito injects a minute amount of salivary fluid into the host to increase blood flow to the area. Sporozoites are transmitted to the host in the salivary fluid.

Anopheles mosquitoes are readily distinguished from other genera by their characteristic stance, in which they appear to be standing on their heads. (Most mosquitoes hold their bodies relatively parallel to the surface on which they are resting.) After feeding, some engorged females seek out cool and humid areas of a house, such as walls and the undersides of furniture, while others find dark, secluded spots outdoors near the ground. Some mosquitoes have modified their resting behavior so as to avoid surfaces treated with pesticides.

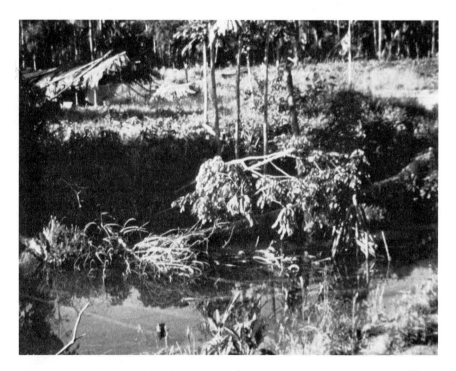

FIGURE 2-5 Ideal larval development site for some anopheline mosquitoes. (Photo courtesy of Dr. Pedro Tauil, IOM Malaria Committee member)

THE ENVIRONMENT

Environmental conditions help determine the intensity of malaria transmission. The optimal climate for sporogony, or parasite development in the mosquito, is a temperature of between 20°C and 30°C with humidity in excess of 60 percent. Sporogony ceases at temperatures below 16°C. Temperature also has a significant effect on mosquito development, and consequently affects vector density. Indeed, development from egg to adult may occur in 7 days at 31°C (88°F) but takes about 20 days at 20°C (68°F).

Mosquitoes benefit from rainfall. Even large amounts that flush away mosquito larvae can produce pools of water that serve as future larval development sites. In areas of unstable malaria transmission, such conditions often bring about an explosion of anopheline mosquitoes and frequently contribute to epidemics.

Human modification to the environment also can create larval development sites and "man-made" malaria. For example, massive logging in West Africa has resulted in a proliferation in certain areas of sunlit pools of water, an ideal habitat for *An. gambiae*. Road building and other types of infrastructure projects, as well as agriculture and irrigation, are among a number of human activities that can spread malaria and other vector-borne diseases. In some regions, human activities can have the opposite effect. For example, deforestation in Thailand has led to the disappearance of malaria in some areas.

EPIDEMIOLOGY

Despite being spread over large regions of the world, malaria is a "focal" disease. That is, because of the complex interactions among the human host, mosquito vector, malaria parasite, and the local environment, malaria affects discrete population groups in different ways. This lack of uniformity is a major reason why it is so difficult to design effective and all-encompassing control strategies.

Geographic Distribution

Malaria is primarily a disease of the tropics, but it is also found in many temperate regions of the world, including parts of the Middle East and Asia. Outbreaks are rare in temperate climates where eradication programs have been successful and in regions where environmental conditions are unfavorable for the anopheline mosquitoes, the malaria parasite, or both (Figure 2-6).

Of the four types of human malaria, that caused by *P. vivax* is the most widely distributed and the most common variety observed in temperate

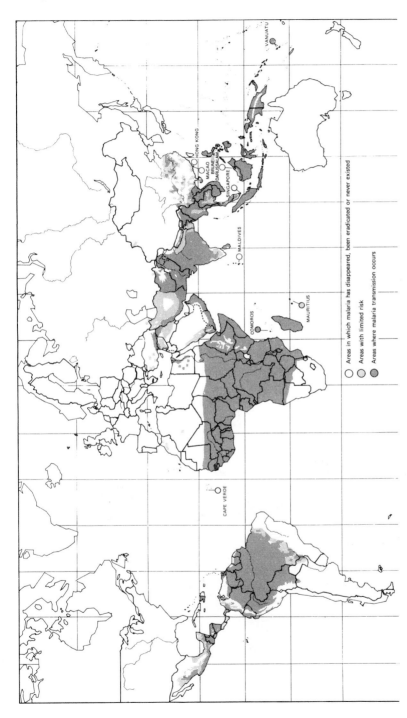

FIGURE 2-6 Epidemiological assessment of the status of malaria, 1989. (Reproduced, by permission of the World Health Organization, from: World malaria situation in 1989, Parts I and II. 1991. Weekly Epidemiological Record 66(22/23):157-163/167-170)

regions of the world. *Plasmodium falciparum*, the most clinically dangerous of the malaria parasites, is most widespread in Africa south of the Sahara and throughout the world's tropics. *Plasmodium ovale* is found almost exclusively in Africa. *Plasmodium malariae* has the same geographic range as *P. falciparum*, although it is much less prevalent and occurs in more restricted zones.

An estimated 2.8 billion people—nearly 60 percent of the world's population—live in areas free from malaria, either because the disease never existed there, because it disappeared as an unintended consequence of human activities, such as road building and urbanization, or because it was eliminated intentionally through eradication efforts. Another 1.7 billion, or slightly more than 30 percent of the population, live in areas where the malaria incidence declined because of eradication efforts but now is making a comeback. Malaria transmission has remained essentially unchanged for 9 percent of the world's inhabitants, about 445 million people. Most in this latter group live in Africa south of the Sahara.

The distribution of malaria within and between geographic regions is greatly influenced by the human population itself. Biological factors such as immune response and genetics, as well as socioeconomic status, living and working conditions, exposure to vectors, and human behavior, all play a critical role in determining a person's risk of infection and illness (Figure 2-7).

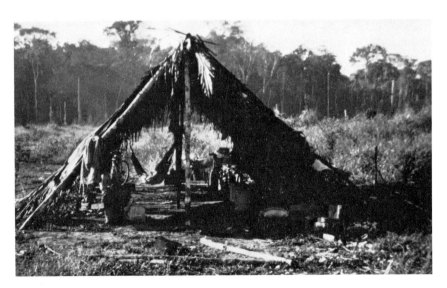

FIGURE 2-7 Lean-to housing provides ideal access for mosquitoes. (Photo courtesy of Dr. Pedro Tauil, IOM Malaria Committee member)

Transmission

Epidemiologists have devised a number of ways of classifying the type of malaria transmission in a particular area. Two of the most common are based on levels of endemicity and stability. In contrast to epidemic malaria, in which there is a sudden rise in the number of cases in a defined population, endemic malaria is characterized by a relatively constant and measurable incidence of cases over a number of years. Since there is great variation in the intensity of transmission between and within malaria-endemic regions, regions are categorized as follows:

- *Holoendemic:* regions of intense year-round malaria transmission, where the population's level of immunity is high, particularly among adults.
- *Hyperendemic:* regions with seasonal transmission, where the population's level of immunity does not confer adequate protection from disease for all age groups.
- *Mesoendemic:* regions that have some malaria transmission, although occasional epidemics constitute a heavy public health burden due to low levels of immunity.
- *Hypoendemic:* regions of limited malaria transmission, where the population has little or no immunity to the parasite.

The level of endemicity in a region can be quantified by determining the percentage of children with enlarged spleens and malaria parasites in their blood (Table 2-1). Although widely used, spleen and parasite indices have various limitations. For one, they are poor indicators of morbidity and mortality, which are increasingly recognized to be important measures of the actual burden of disease. In areas where malaria is just one of a number of parasitic diseases, not all enlarged spleens are due to malaria infection. Finally, in holoendemic regions, blood parasite levels can be affected by both the use of antimalarial drugs and the age of the children being tested.

In a holoendemic area, where malaria transmission is intense, virtually everyone in the population is repeatedly infected. Babies are born with maternal protection to the malaria parasite and retain this passive immunity until about six months of age. As passive immunity wanes and as the infant becomes infected with malaria, the risk of severe disease increases. Indeed, malaria-induced morbidity and mortality in holoendemic regions is greatest in children between the ages of one and four. After repeated bouts of infection, children who survive gradually develop a partial immunity to malaria. Although they may have occasional episodes of illness, adults and children over five years of age rarely suffer severe malarial illness. By comparison, in regions of hyperendemic malaria, both children

TABLE 2-1 Classifications of Malaria Endemicity as Defined by Rates in Children Two to Nine Years Old

Classification	Spleen Rate[a] (%)	Parasite Rate[b] (%)
Holoendemic	>75	>75 (in infants)
Hyperendemic	51-75	51-75
Mesoendemic	11-50	11-50
Hypoendemic	0-10	<10

[a]Originally proposed at the WHO Malaria Conference in Equatorial Africa (1951) and subsequently amended by Molineaux (1988).
[b]Metselaar and van Thiel (1959), as found in Molineaux (1988).

and adults suffer severe disease. In meso- and hypoendemic regions, the frequency of infection is generally low, but epidemics may be devastating.

By definition, stable malaria transmission is intense, robust, and very difficult to interrupt. This type of disease transmission can occur where there are very low densities of mosquitoes, particularly anthropophilic and long-lived vectors such as *An. gambiae* and those with similar characteristics. In stable malaria transmission, the human population generally acquires a partial immunity to malaria, and morbidity and mortality are largely limited to young children and pregnant women. Conversely, unstable malaria occurs in regions of intermittent malaria transmission where there is little or no acquired population immunity and the risk of epidemic malaria is high. As a rule, as endemicity decreases, transmission becomes less stable and the risk of epidemics increases.

MALARIA CONTROL

Malaria control efforts traditionally have relied on the provision of proven antimalarial drugs, on environmental sanitation, and on the application of insecticides.

Drugs

Antimalarial drugs are used to prevent the onset of disease, to treat clinical cases in individuals, and to prevent disease transmission within populations. Some drugs, including doxycycline, proguanil, pyrimethamine, and primaquine, attack the liver stage, preventing the release of parasites into the bloodstream. Others, such as chloroquine, quinine, sulfadoxine-pyrimethamine, and mefloquine, kill the parasite within red blood cells.

The emergence and spread of drug resistant strains of the most dangerous of the four human malaria parasites, *P. falciparum*, has reemphasized concerns about the use and efficacy of other available antimalarial drugs. Chloroquine-resistant *P. falciparum*, first noted in Thailand and Colombia in the 1960s, has since spread to most areas of the world except the Middle East, Central America, and the Caribbean. An additional concern, however, is recent reports of chloroquine-resistant *P. vivax*. There is also widespread and increasing resistance to other antimalarial drugs.

Source Reduction

Eliminating larval development sites by modifying and manipulating the environment is particularly effective in areas where the spread of malaria has been aided by human activities, such as irrigation, public works, and construction projects. One common but expensive technique is to drain and fill in bodies of water.

Larviciding

There are chemical and biological methods for killing mosquitoes in the larval stage. Chemical larvicides include petroleum oils (Paris green) and pesticides such as temephos and fenthion. Biological methods employ larvivorous fish, such as *Gambusia* species (minnows) or *Lebistes* species (guppies), and *Bacillus thuringiensis israeliensis*, a toxin-producing bacterium.

Spraying

Any intervention that shortens the mosquito's life span should also reduce the likelihood of disease transmission. Residual insecticides applied to the interior of houses are very effective against some mosquitoes but have no effect on those that rest primarily outdoors. For these insects, localized outdoor spraying is sometimes warranted in densely populated areas or where the threat of a malaria epidemic is great. The arsenal of pesticides available includes chlorinated hydrocarbons (DDT, dieldrin), organophosphate compounds (malathion, fenitrothion), carbamates (propoxur), pyrethrins, and pyrethroids. Unfortunately, mosquitoes in many parts of the world have become resistant to some pesticides, and some have adapted so as to avoid insecticide-treated surfaces altogether.

Contact Reduction

Protective clothing, insect repellents, mosquito coils, and bednets can help reduce human-mosquito contact. Pyrethrin-impregnated bednets have been shown recently to reduce cases of clinical malaria in some areas by 50 percent or more, and further evaluations are ongoing.

Vaccines

Much recent research has focused on developing effective malaria vaccines (see Chapter 9). The effort has proved more difficult than anticipated, and it appears unlikely that effective vaccines for widespread use will be available during the next decade.

BIBLIOGRAPHY

The following reference materials are provided as suggested reading for those interested in a more comprehensive examination of the topics discussed in this chapter.

Bruce-Chwatt, L. J. 1985. Essential Malariology, 2nd ed. London: Heinemann.

Metselaar, D., and P. M. van Thiel. 1959. Classification of malaria. Tropical and Geographical Medicine 11:157-161.

Molineaux, L. 1988. The epidemiology of human malaria as an explanation of its distribution, including some implications for its control. Pp. 913-998 in Malaria: Principles and Practice of Malariology, Wernsdorfer, W. H., and I. McGregor, eds. Edinburgh: Churchill Livingstone.

Wernsdorfer, W. H., and I. McGregor, eds. 1988. Malaria: Principles and Practice of Malariology, 1st ed. New York: Churchill Livingstone.

World Health Organization, Division of Control of Tropical Diseases. 1990. World malaria situation, 1988. Rapport Trimestriel de Sanitares Mondiales 43:68-79.

3

Overview

Through its direct impact on health and its indirect effects on such factors as economic development, migration, and military conflict, malaria has played and continues to play an important role in human history. The literature of ancient and modern civilizations contains repeated references to "intermittent" and "malignant" fevers and "agues" consistent with a diagnosis of malaria. As far back as 2700 B.C., the Chinese Canon of Medicine, the Nei Ching, discussed malaria-like symptoms and the relationship between fevers and enlarged spleens. Similarly, cuneiform tablets excavated from Assurbanapli's royal library in Nineveh (what is now Iraq) in the 6th century B.C. mention deadly malaria-like fevers that afflicted the populace of ancient Mesopotamia. The writings of Homer, Aristotle, Plato, Socrates, Horace, Tacitus, Carus, Varro, Chaucer, Pepys, and Shakespeare all mention fevers that were undoubtedly malaria related (Bruce-Chwatt, 1988).

The Greek physician Hippocrates was the first to make a connection between the proximity of stagnant bodies of water and the occurrence of fevers in the local population. The Romans also associated marshes with fever and pioneered early efforts at swamp drainage. Appropriately, the role of standing bodies of water and marshes in causing fevers was described by the Italians as "aria cattiva" (spoiled air) or "mal'aria" (bad air) beginning in the mid-sixteenth century, and the latter term entered the English language as "malaria" some 200 years later. Likewise, the French coined the word "paludisme," whose root means swamp, to refer to malaria.

Saint Augustine, the first archbishop of Canterbury, died from what was almost certainly malaria in 597 A.D. Dante Alighieri, the Italian poet, died of malignant fever in 1321 A.D. Peter the Great was so upset by the fever-related illness and death that plagued his Russian army in Persia in the early 1720s that he ordered them to stop eating melons, which he believed caused the sickness.

Kings, popes, and paupers alike have been stricken by this parasite-caused disease. Holy Roman Emperor Charles V died of malaria in a monastery in Yuste, Spain, in 1558. Pope Sixtus V died of "marsh fever" in 1590, as did his successor, Urban VII. During the Conclave of 1623, 8 cardinals and 30 scribes and secretaries died of malaria-induced fever, while other members in attendance fell ill (Celli, 1925). In England, King James I, King Charles II, and Cardinal Wolsey all suffered from intermittent fevers consistent with malaria.

PRE-COLUMBIAN HISTORY

Malaria may or may not have been present in the pre-Columbian New World. Some scholars argue that the disease was introduced to the Americas by people who migrated from malaria-endemic regions in Asia, across the now submerged land bridge, into North America. Early European visitors to South America noted the Indian use of cinchona bark, a natural source of quinine, to treat fevers, further supporting the view that malaria may have predated European expeditions to the New World. Whether or not European exploration and colonization of the Americas introduced malaria, they most certainly facilitated the spread of the disease.

MALARIA IN AMERICA

Malaria was one of the most widespread and debilitating diseases of early North America, significantly impeding the development of the colonies (Duffy, 1953). The English introduced two species of malaria, *Plasmodium vivax* and *P. malariae*, when they settled Jamestown, Virginia, in 1607, but it was the importation of African slaves beginning in 1620 that brought the more virulent *P. falciparum* to the continent (Russell, 1968). Indeed, it is thought that the decision in 1699 to move the capital from Jamestown to Williamsburg was motivated by the desire to escape the effects of malaria.

Boston was particularly hard hit by malaria-related illness and death in the seventeenth century. In 1699, Samuel Maverick of New York wrote, "The flux, agues, and fevers, have much rained both in cittie and country,

& many dead, but not yet soe many as last yeare. The like is all N.Engld. over, especially about Boston, where have dyed verry many" (quoted in Duffy, 1953). In 1723, George Hume, a Scottish settler in Virginia, wrote home to his family that "I am now & then troubled with ye fever & ague wch. is a very violent distemper here. . . . This place is only good for doctors & ministers who have good encouragement here" (quoted in Duffy, 1953).

As the pioneers spread into the interior of the country, so did malaria. In the eighteenth and nineteenth centuries, malaria was endemic in the southern and western portions of the colonies. Most settlers in those regions considered it inevitable that they would contract the disease (Ackernecht, 1945). In New England, malaria was less of a problem, primarily because swamps and marshlands were being drained.

During the Civil War, 8,000 combatants died of malaria and there were more than 1.2 million recorded cases of the disease among Confederate and Union troops (Ognibene and Barrett, 1982; Bruce-Chwatt, 1988). As recently as the early 1900s, 500,000 cases of malaria were reported each year in the United States, the majority occurring in the South.

DISCOVERY OF QUININE

South American Indians used cinchona bark as a traditional remedy for malarial fevers long before any treatment was available in Europe. In 1639, Jesuit missionaries brought some of the bark back with them to Europe, where it eventually became the treatment of choice for fevers. It was not until 1820, however, that Pierre Joseph Pelletier and Joseph Bienaime Caventou, two French chemists, identified the alkaloid quinine as the bark's active ingredient (Russell, 1955). Shortly after this discovery, the demand for and use of quinine spread rapidly throughout Europe, North America, and Asia.

DISCOVERY OF THE MALARIA PARASITE AND ITS LIFE CYCLE

In 1846, the Italian physician Giovanni Rasori proposed that a parasite was responsible for the fever and other symptoms associated with the disease we now call malaria. In 1880, a French Army medical officer, Charles Louis Alphonse Laveran, observed live parasites in blood taken from a feverish soldier in Algeria.

Some of the greatest advances in understanding the complex life cycle of malaria parasites were made by the Italians around the turn of the century. In 1898, Giovanni Battista Grassi, Amico Bignami, and Guiseppe Bastianelli documented the transmission of human malaria parasites in

Anopheles claviger and soon after they described the developmental stages of *P. falciparum* and *P. vivax*, two of the most important malaria parasite species.

A bitter debate surrounded the discovery that malaria parasites are transmitted by anopheline mosquitoes. Both Grassi and his co-workers, as well as Sir Ronald Ross, a British military doctor working in India, were doing research on the problem at the same time and were influenced by another British scientist, Patrick Manson, who stimulated the working hypothesis that mosquitoes were responsible for malaria transmission. Using avian malaria as a model, Ross was the first to demonstrate the cycle of malaria in mosquitoes. But it was the Italians who definitively documented that only *Anopheles* mosquitoes can transmit human malaria, and a classic monograph by Grassi in 1900 details the complete development cycle of the parasite in these mosquitoes. In 1902, Ross was awarded the Nobel Prize in Medicine for his work on malaria.

MALARIA AND THE MILITARY

Malaria remains a disease of tremendous concern to the military. Its debilitating effects can often do more damage than the enemy. In a major outbreak during World War I, for example, more than 100,000 British and French troops on the Macedonian front were sidelined. Responding to a 1916 order to attack, an exasperated French general sent a telegram to Paris complaining, "Mon armee est immobilisee dans les hopitaux." His army had malaria (Wenyon et al., 1921 quoted in Bruce-Chwatt, 1988).

In World War II, both Allied and Axis troops felt the effects of malaria. The U.S. Army alone recorded over 500,000 cases during the war; the Navy and Marine Corps recorded another 90,000 (Ognibene and Barrett, 1982; D. Robinette, Institute of Medicine, personal communication, 1991). "This will be a long war, if for every division I have facing the enemy, I must count on a second division in the hospital with malaria, and a third division convalescing from this debilitating disease," said General Douglas MacArthur from the Pacific theater (Russell et al., 1946).

Malaria had a major impact on the American war effort in Vietnam, especially at the beginning of the conflict. In late 1965, nearly 10 percent of soldiers had the disease. "During that period, rates for certain units operating in the Ia Drang valley were as high as 600 per 1,000 per year, and at least two maneuver battalions were rendered ineffective by malaria," General Spurgeon Neel reported in 1973 (Neel, 1973). Over 80,000 cases of malaria were diagnosed in American troops in Vietnam from 1965 to 1971. The overall mortality rate of 1.7 per 1,000 was low, however, because of rapid diagnosis and treatment of cases as they occurred (Canfield, 1972).

MALARIA CONTROL

Credit for the first efforts at malaria control properly belongs to the Greeks and Romans, who in the sixth century B.C. undertook major engineering projects to drain marshy areas. This practice continued well into the Middle Ages and spread throughout Europe and the Middle East. By and large, however, efforts to control malaria prior to the twentieth century met with minimal success. One of the most successful modern attempts at malaria control occurred under the leadership of General William C. Gorgas, who joined the U.S. Army Medical Corps in 1880, shortly after receiving his medical degree. During construction of the Panama Canal (1904-1914), Gorgas oversaw an integrated program of malaria control that included drainage, application of larvicide, and prophylactic treatment with quinine that resulted in the virtual elimination of malaria from the Canal Zone by 1910.

ERADICATION

Background

Starting in the mid-1940s and continuing through the mid-1950s, public health officials began to consider eradicating malaria from all parts of the world. Successful attempts to eradicate the Mediterranean fruit fly from Florida (1930-1931) and *An. gambiae* from Brazil (1934-1940) and Egypt (1948) made a large campaign against malaria seem feasible. The greatest impetus for malaria eradication came with the development of the powerful insecticide DDT during World War II.

Serious attempts to wipe out malaria in the United States began in 1943. That year, a proposal to eradicate the disease based on a strategy of indoor residual spraying with DDT was presented to the National Malaria Society by the U.S. Public Health Service (PHS) (Mountin, 1944). The result was the National Eradication Program, initiated in 1947 with $7 million in federal funds. Five years later, malaria morbidity and mortality in the United States had dropped to near zero and the program was abandoned (Bradley, 1966).

The years following World War II were unparalleled for the level of international cooperation devoted to combating endemic malaria. The United Nations Rehabilitation and Relief Administration, formed in 1943 as an international emergency organization with the United States as the principal financial backer, was very active in malaria control projects (Russell, 1968). The first Expert Committee on Malaria, established by the Interim Commission of the World Health Organization, met in 1947 (Najera, 1989); the World Health Organization (WHO) was officially formed in 1948.

One of the earliest broad-based proposals for eradication came in 1950 from the Pan American Sanitary Conference (PASC), which later merged with the Pan American Health Organization. In 1954, PASC declared a hemispheric eradication program and solicited support from the United Nations International Children's Emergency Fund (UNICEF), which led to an endorsement of the concept by a joint UNICEF/WHO Health Policy Committee (Soper, 1960). Worldwide malaria eradication seemed truly within reach when George MacDonald, of the Ross Institute in London, developed a mathematical model suggesting that malaria transmission could be interrupted simply by shortening the life span of the mosquito vector, thereby preventing the parasite from developing fully. This approach meant that the total number of mosquitoes could be ignored and justified a strategy of focused, residual insecticide spraying. Accordingly, domestic application of DDT emerged as the single most effective intervention tactic.

Eradication Campaign

In 1955, the Eighth World Health Assembly adopted a plan for worldwide malaria eradication, officially launching the initiative (World Health Organization, 1955). The effort was shadowed from the start by the fear that the vector mosquitoes would develop insecticide resistance before the disease could be wiped out. Historically, resistance developed within 5 to 10 years after an insecticide was in widespread use. Eradication, therefore, was recognized as a time-limited operation. Still, there was optimism. Medical entomologists believed in the efficacy of DDT and expected that their expertise would one day no longer be needed.

The eradication program that finally took shape would last about eight years: a preparatory phase of one year, an attack phase of at least four years, and a consolidation phase of three years. This would be followed by an indefinite maintenance phase (World Health Organization Expert Committee on Malaria, 1957). It was estimated that eradication, using DDT residual spraying, could be accomplished at a cost of 25 cents per person per year and that the cost for the first five years would total $519 million (International Development Advisory Board, 1956).

As the eradication program progressed, serious problems emerged. For one, planning activities often did not adequately address the attitudes of the local populations toward the disease. Often, regional differences in vector behavior, and the earmarking of local and national health resources for the task, were not taken into account (World Health Organization, 1969). In many areas, research could have provided better design strategies, but given the amount already committed to eradication, it was difficult to justify additional expenditures.

Although the eradication effort generated impressive results in North America and Europe, by the mid-1960s there was growing concern that eradication was not technically or economically feasible in many areas (World Health Organization Expert Committee on Malaria, 1967). In fact, Africa south of the Sahara had been excluded from the eradication plan altogether because of the perceived magnitude of the region's malaria problem and the lack of technological capability within those countries (Lepes, 1974). The number of malaria cases decreased dramatically in some regions, but most of these successes were recorded in less threatened temperate zones or on island nations, not in the continental tropical countries, where by the late 1960s malaria was still a serious health threat (Brown et al., 1976).

Research had almost no role in the initial years of the eradication effort. Indeed, there was little interest in involving scientists in a field many thought would soon be obsolete. It was only as the complexity of malaria became apparent that research assumed a more prominent place in eradication programs. Recognizing this, WHO in 1965 began to actively encourage malaria research. In 1969, the World Health Assembly passed a formal resolution to stimulate and intensify multidisciplinary malaria research.

The deemphasis of science combined with a decline in the number of malariologists left countries ill prepared for two major, interrelated changes in international health policy: the shift from malaria eradication to malaria control, and the move toward integration of health services.

Financial Support for Eradication

Many countries invested heavily in the eradication effort. In 1958, two powerful U.S. senators, Hubert H. Humphrey from Minnesota and John F. Kennedy from Massachusetts, attached legislation to the Mutual Securities Act that committed the United States for five years to the goal of worldwide malaria eradication (Spielman and Kitron, 1990). An annual appropriation of $23 million was provided, an enormous investment for the time. The United States spent $85 million in just three years (1957-1960), and the worldwide commitment to the project exceeded $100 million in 1960 alone (International Cooperation Administration Expert Panel on Malaria, 1961). WHO obligations to malaria eradication jumped from $768,000 in 1955 to almost $8 million in 1964 (Gramiccia and Beales, 1988). A number of countries also shifted funds within their own health budgets to accommodate the eradication goal. During the mid-1960s, for instance, India devoted 35 percent of its health dollars to malaria. The tremendous resources devoted to malaria eradication throughout the world meant that less could be spent on other important public health projects (Farid, 1980).

Eradication to Control

In 1969, the World Health Assembly revised its global malaria eradication strategy. The new approach emphasized strategies that could be justified on the basis of health grounds as well as economic considerations, and it encouraged control where eradication was not feasible (World Health Organization, 1969). The shift from malaria eradication to control necessitated a long-term commitment of personnel and financial resources and, unlike eradication, did not offer the potential for time-limited and dramatic results. Politicians were often reluctant to embrace the concept of control, which was not well understood.

The World Health Assembly also urged that malaria control strategies be integrated into the basic health services programs of each country. For some countries, where national malaria services had been run by a centralized organization and a single strategy, this proved to be particularly difficult. The result of this integration was a dramatic decrease in funding for malaria; money was shifted into programs for family planning, smallpox eradication, and multipurpose health services (Farid, 1980). By the early 1970s, changing priorities and responsibilities within the nations that had supported eradication caused a further erosion of support for malaria-related activities. The U.S. Agency for International Development (USAID), with the assistance of the PHS, contributed $375 million to 26 nations over a 20-year period (Howard, 1972). By 1974, the PHS had stopped funding eradication efforts in all but two countries, Nepal and Haiti (Smith, 1974). Similarly, UNICEF's contribution to eradication, which had risen to as much as $8.8 million in one year, began to be phased out by 1973 (Brown et al., 1976).

The combined withdrawal of international funding meant that the financial and technical responsibilities for malaria control would rest almost entirely within individual nations, many of which did not have adequate resources, technical expertise, or the administrative infrastructure to effectively carry out such programs. The situation was particularly serious for countries or regions that had made progress against malaria and for which a drop in technical and financial support would ultimately lead to a resurgence of the disease.

After the 1978 International Congress on Primary Health Care, the responsibility for malaria control in many countries was shifted further to those in the basic health services and to peripheral health workers. This integration was, for the most part, not smooth. Peripheral health workers were overburdened with other tasks and often lacked the technical competence to monitor and direct malaria control operations.

1970 to Present

As the international pool of funding for malaria eradication and control was drying up, a movement in the United States to halt the use of DDT was taking shape. In 1972, under pressure from environmental and conservation groups, the United States banned use of the pesticide for all non-public health uses. By 1982, production of DDT in the United States had ceased altogether. The removal of this cheap and effective antimalaria weapon from the U.S. marketplace had a negative impact on malaria control efforts worldwide. Subsequent pesticides (e.g., malathion) have proved to be more expensive and more toxic.

Beginning in the early 1970s and continuing to the present, resistance to important antimalarial drugs has become increasingly prevalent. Particularly disturbing is the resistance to chloroquine, once the treatment of choice for *P. falciparum* malaria. The progressive spread of *P. falciparum* into areas where other species of the parasite once predominated adds an unfortunate complication to control efforts. Multidrug resistance has become such a problem in some parts of the world, such as Thailand, that malaria control personnel are hard pressed to institute any effective preventive or treatment regimen.

Political and social instability around the world have played a central role in malaria's comeback. From the decades-long civil war in Ethiopia, with its attendant cycles of famine and drought, to the devastation of Brazil's rain forest by urban resettlement, human impact on and interaction with the environment have facilitated the resurgence of the disease. Matters are made worse by the fact that there is a dwindling pool of technically competent malariologists, both nationally and internationally, equipped to manage the complexities of malaria research and control in the coming years.

On the positive side, important research discoveries, such as the development in 1975 of an in vitro culture system for the blood stage of *P. falciparum*, have facilitated scientific understanding of the malaria parasite (Trager and Jensen, 1976). A series of studies in the early and mid-1970s proved that humans could be protected for short periods of time from infection after being inoculated with irradiated sporozoites, lending considerable support to the notion that a vaccine against malaria is possible. Much of the early vaccine-related work in the United States has been supported by the USAID, which by the mid-1970s established a formal malaria vaccine research project. The agency continues to be the major source of U.S. malaria vaccine research funding. During this same period and continuing into the 1980s, a number of new antimalarial drugs, such as mefloquine and halofantrine, were discovered and developed, adding to the available chemotherapeutic options for treating and preventing the disease. The Special Programme for Research and Training in Tropical Diseases (TDR), founded in 1976 as a joint project of the United Nations Development Programme (UNDP), the World Bank, and WHO, has added both scientific direction and consistent financial and organizational support to worldwide activities in the area of malaria research and control.

U.S. AND INTERNATIONAL SUPPORT
FOR MALARIA ACTIVITIES

A number of governmental and nongovernmental organizations around the world actively support malaria research, prevention, and control programs. No two programs are alike, and each operates within a specific policy framework that governs the choice and level of funding for malaria-related activities.

The United States is just one of many countries that support malaria research and control initiatives. Malaria-endemic countries also fund malaria-related projects, which, as one might expect, are geared overwhelmingly to controlling the spread of the disease within national borders.

In general, for industrialized countries, the national agencies in charge of scientific research have tended to focus on issues of domestic concern, while support for tropical diseases research and control has largely been left to government entities involved in foreign aid and international cooperation. For example, the Overseas Development Administration is the largest and most consistent government supporter of tropical disease research and control activities in the United Kingdom, while the Medical Research Council, the government's health research arm, concentrates primarily on issues of domestic concern.

Multilateral organizations, including the World Bank, the European Commission, and WHO support both malaria control and research activities. The WHO, which contributed almost 30 percent of its annual budget to malaria during the eradication years, currently allocates slightly over 4 percent of its total annual budget to malaria activities. This has amounted to almost $12 million per year for the 15 years 1973-1988. Some programs, like the TDR, predominantly support research and training activities. Out of a total 1990-1991 TDR budget of $73 million, approximately 21 percent or $15 million, is allocated to funding laboratory and field research on malaria (World Health Organization, 1991). A number of non-governmental entities, such as the Rockefeller Foundation, also contribute to both malaria control and research activities; others, like the MacArthur Foundation and the Wellcome Trust (United Kingdom), support both research and training.

Two studies on the funding of malaria activities were commissioned for this report, and both confronted similar problems in data collection and analysis (Ettling, 1990; Guha-Sapir and Hariga, 1991). While the absolute and relative funding allocated to a particular program is a prime indicator of an organization's priorities and interests, few governments or independent funding agencies tally their expenditures for malaria in the same way. Many, for instance, do not separate spending for particular diseases from spending for health in general. The problem of assessing relative contributions to malaria research and control is further compounded by the variability in the quality and accuracy of the data that are available. Even if accurate data were widely and easily available, they would likely fail to answer three critical questions: Was the amount spent insufficient, sufficient, or excessive? Was it spent well? Did it have an effect?

For all of the reasons discussed above, the committee decided that the danger of presenting somewhat erratic information outweighed any possible benefit. Because the data were easier to obtain and verify, and because U.S. government funding of malaria activities was of particular interest to the committee, the limited discussion that follows focuses on U.S. government funding of malaria.

United States

Four U.S. government agencies fund malaria activities: USAID, the Centers for Disease Control (CDC), the Department of Defense (DOD), and the National Institute of Allergy and Infectious Diseases (NIAID) of the National Institutes of Health (NIH).

U.S. Agency for International Development

Established in 1961 within the Department of State, USAID is the foreign assistance arm of the U.S. government. Highly decentralized, the various USAID offices and regional bureaus involved in malaria projects around the globe include the Office of Health in the Bureau of Science and Technology, and the Health, Nutrition, and Population Offices in the four regional bureaus for Africa, Asia, Latin America and the Caribbean, and the Near East. In addition to the bureaus, USAID has overseas "missions," each supervised by a mission director, the U.S. country ambassador, and, in Washington, the respective regional bureau. Malaria projects are supported from one or more funding accounts, including the Health Account, Child Survival Fund, the Development Fund for Africa, the Economic Support Fund, Population Account, and the Agriculture, Rural Development, and Nutrition Account. In addition, USAID relies on an estimated 10,000 nongovernmental organizations, consultants, and contractors worldwide to help implement all of its projects.

In fiscal year (FY) 1989, USAID allocated $421 million to health, child survival, and AIDS activities, of which nearly $22 million (5.2 percent) was obligated to malaria research and control. This is fairly consistent with the pattern for each of the last seven fiscal years, during which the agency has allocated between 5 and 7 percent of its health budget to malaria-related activities (Table 3-1).

From 1985 through 1989, a little more than half of USAID malaria funds

TABLE 3-1 USAID Funding for Malaria Research and Control as a Percentage of Overall Obligations for Health[a]

	Funding ($000)						
Category	FY 85	FY 86	FY 87	FY 88	FY 89	FY 90	FY 91
Overall health	354,433	332,733	304,887	309,517	421,278	341,326	363,219
Malaria	25,524	17,595	21,243	20,117	21,793	16,309	27,978
Malaria as a percentage of overall health	7.2	5.3	7.0	6.5	5.2	4.8	7.7

Note: Figures for FY 85 through FY 89 are actual obligations; those for FY 90 and FY 91 are projected obligations. The funding amounts reported here are calculated amounts, based on fiscal year obligations reported in the congressional presentation and on percentage attributions for malaria reported in the annual Health and Child Survival Questionnaires and in the USAID Activity Code/Special Interest System.
[a]All funding accounts
SOURCE: Center for International Health Information/ISTI, USAID Health Information System.

went to support bilateral programs, all of which targeted some aspect of malaria control. Of the bilateral programs funded in FY 1988 and FY 1989, just over a quarter included a small malaria research component as part of their overall control activities. From 1985 through 1989, nearly 48 percent of USAID malaria money was obligated to vaccine and immunity research (Figure 3-1). As a group, countries in Asia and the Near East receive the greatest share of USAID bilateral malaria funding; African nations received the smallest (Figure 3-2). The geographic allocation of funds is consistent with overall USAID funding, whereby the bulk of the resources are targeted to regions of particular U.S. strategic or political interest.

Centers for Disease Control

CDC is charged with protecting and monitoring the health of U.S. citizens. Over 7 million U.S. citizens travel abroad each year to malarious regions, according to CDC. Over each of the past several years, there have been more than 1,000 cases of malaria reported in the United States, most in U.S. nationals and nearly all acquired overseas.

From FY 1985 through FY 1989, CDC spent approximately $5.5 million for malaria surveillance activities and laboratory investigations (Table 3-2). In addition to its own resources, CDC receives funds from USAID for other malaria-related activities, including vaccine and immunity research, child survival projects, and other malaria research and control activities in malaria-endemic countries. CDC has also received funds from WHO on an intermittent basis (Figure 3-3).

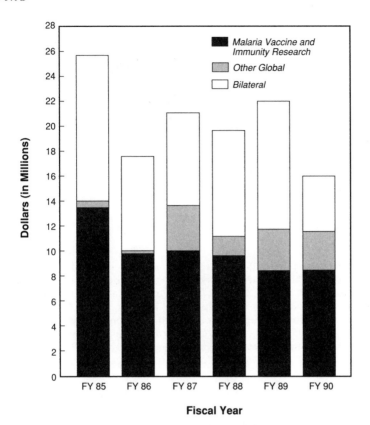

FIGURE 3-1 USAID malaria funding, all accounts (FY 1985 to FY 1990). Note: "Other Global" refers to those projects funded from all accounts, including the Vector Biology and Control Project, Diagnostic Technology for Community Health, Primary Health Care Operations Research, Maternal/Neonatal Health and Nutrition, and Communication for Child Survival, to name but a few. Data source: Center for International Health Information/ISTI, USAID Health Information System.

Department of Defense

DOD's interest in malaria stems from its commitment to protect the health of U.S. military personnel. Malaria exacted a heavy toll on U.S. troops during World War I, World War II, and both the Korean and Vietnam conflicts.

In 1982, Congress directed the United States Army Medical Research and Development Command (USAMRDC) at Fort Detrick, Maryland, to oversee all research on infectious diseases, including malaria, for the military. The Walter Reed Army Institute of Research (WRAIR), part of USAMRDC, and the Naval Medical Research Institute both have active

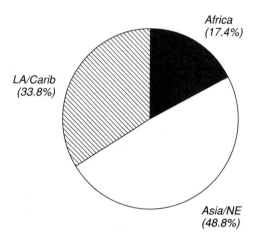

FIGURE 3-2 USAID bilateral malaria program funding (FY 1985 to FY 1989). Note: Over the period 1985-1989, the following countries and areas received funds for malaria activities: Africa (Burkina Faso, Cameroon, Ghana, Kenya, Liberia, Malawi, Mali, Niger, Nigeria, Senegal, Togo, Uganda, Zaire, Zimbabwe); Asia/Near East Region (Afghanistan, Burma, Egypt, India, Morocco, Nepal, Pakistan [received bulk of the funds for this region], South Pacific Region, Sri Lanka, Yemen); and Latin America Region (Belize, Bolivia, Costa Rica, Dominican Republic, Eastern Caribbean Region, Ecuador, Guatemala, Haiti, Honduras, Jamaica, Peru). Source: Center for International Health Information/ISTI, USAID Health Information System.

malaria research programs. In fact, WRAIR is home to the largest antimalarial drug screening program in the world.

The DOD malaria research programs concentrate on vaccine and drug development and, to a lesser extent, vector control. DOD has established field laboratories in Thailand, Kenya, Brazil, Peru, Indonesia, and the Philippines, all of which are involved in the study of malaria and other tropical diseases and are partially supported by malaria vaccine research funds.

Over the four years spanning 1986 through 1989, DOD allocated almost $38 million to malaria activities, including malaria vaccine development, drug development, and vector biology research and control. While funds for vector research and control have held fairly constant over the six years from 1985 to 1990, malaria vaccine funding was reduced by 26 percent between 1988 and 1989, and funds allocated for drug development have been decreasing steadily since 1985 (Table 3-3).

National Institute of Allergy and Infectious Diseases

NIAID is one of 13 institutes at NIH, the medical research branch of the PHS. Like other NIH institutes, NIAID supports both intramural and

TABLE 3-2 CDC Malaria Spending as a Percentage of Total Budget

Category	Spending ($000)					
	FY 85	FY 86	FY 87	FY 88	FY 89	FY 90
Malaria[a]	1,330	1,758	1,938	2,157	1,985	2,508
Total budget	410,000	452,000	587,000	772,000	982,000	1,121,000
Malaria as a percentage of total budget	0.32	0.39	0.33	0.28	0.20	0.22

[a]Includes funds received from USAID and WHO.
SOURCES: Office of Financial Management, Division of Parasitic Diseases, and the International Health Program Office, CDC.

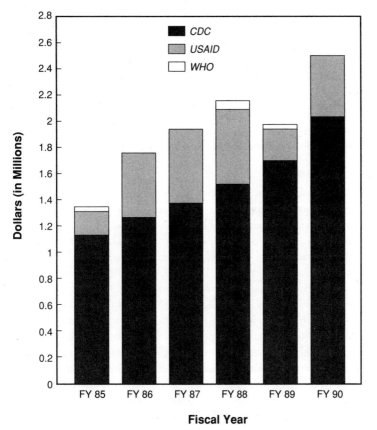

Fiscal Year

FIGURE 3-3 CDC spending on malaria, by account (FY 1985 to FY 1990). Sources: Division of Parasitic Diseases, Center for Infectious Diseases, and International Health Program Office, CDC.

TABLE 3-3 DOD Malaria Program Funding

Category	Funding ($000)				
	FY 86	FY 87	FY 88	FY 89	FY 90
Vaccines					
Technical base					
Army-in-house	1,352	1,252	1,210	914	785
Army-field sites	822	950	738	703	817
Navy-in-house	1,138	706	1,147	996	809
Navy-field sites	220	142	193	245	286
Extramural	452	457	435	402	425
Advanced development					
In-house	587	1,321	1,164	270	330
Extramural	458	834	923	0	0
Total vaccine funding	**5,029**	**5,662**	**5,810**	**3,530**	**3,452**
Drugs	**2,400**	**2,200**	**2,000**	**1,900**	**1,700**
Vectors					
Research					
In-house	210	220	230	240	250
Overseas	320	340	360	380	400
Control	281	189	231	253	212
Total vector funding	**811**	**749**	**821**	**873**	**862**
Total malaria program	**8,240**	**8,611**	**8,631**	**6,303**	**6,014**
Percent vaccines	61.0	65.8	67.3	56.0	57.4
Percent drugs	29.1	25.5	23.2	30.1	28.3
Percent vectors	9.8	8.7	9.5	13.9	14.3

SOURCES: USAMRDC and U.S. Army Biomedical Research and Development Laboratory, Fort Detrick; Division of Experimental Therapeutics and Department of Entomology, WRAIR.

extramural researchers in the basic and clinical sciences and is the only federal entity that actively supports basic research on tropical diseases.

Consistent with overall NIAID and NIH funding patterns, about 20 percent of all tropical disease research monies are spent in-house, with most of the remainder going to U.S. investigators outside NIH through a competitive grants award system. Grants from NIAID to foreign investigators for tropical disease research are relatively rare. Out of a total FY 1989 budget of $831 million, NIAID allocated $8.3 million (1 percent) to malaria (Table 3-4). While funding for tropical diseases as a proportion of the overall NIAID budget has declined over the past four years (largely because of the rapid influx of AIDS research funding), funding for malaria as a proportion of tropical diseases has increased. The bulk of NIAID extramural malaria research support during FY 1987 through FY 1989 went to studies on vaccines and immunity, while research on parasite biology received the next largest share of funds (Figure 3-4).

Overall, the U.S. government has invested nearly $140 million on malaria research and control activities over the past four years (Table 3-5). More than half of that amount was spent by USAID.

TABLE 3-4 NIAID Funding for Tropical Diseases and Malaria, 1986-1990

Category	Funding ($000)			
	FY 87	FY 88	FY 89	FY 90
NIAID	545,433	638,521	740,239	831,181
Tropical diseases[a]	34,118	34,440	32,633	38,765
Malaria	6,122	6,803	7,467	8,337
Tropical diseases as a percentage of NIAID	6.3	5.4	4.4	4.7
Malaria as a percentage of tropical diseases	17.9	19.8	22.9	21.5

[a]This category includes the six tropical diseases (malaria, schistosomiasis, filariasis, trypanosomiasis, leishmaniasis, and leprosy) selected for special emphasis by the UNDP/World Bank/TDR, and training and career development in tropical diseases.
SOURCES: U.S. Department of Health and Human Services, NIH, "NIAID Combined Intramural and Extramural Tropical Medicine Activities," FY 87, FY 88, FY 89, FY 90 (mimeographs).

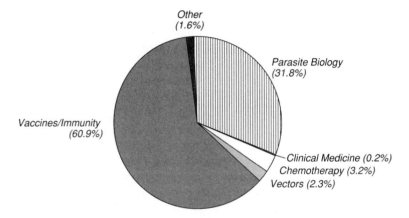

FIGURE 3-4 NIAID extramural malaria funding, by research area (FY 1987 to FY 1989). Source: Office of Tropical Medicine and International Research, NIAID.

TABLE 3-5 Overall U.S. Government Support of Malaria Activities

Agency	Funding ($000)					
	FY 87	FY 88	FY 89	FY 90	Total	%
USAID	21,243	20,117	21,793	16,309	79,462	57.01
NIAID	6,122	6,803	7,467	8,337	28,729	20.61
DOD	7,862	7,810	5,430	5,152	26,254	18.84
CDC	1,105	1,151	1,214	1,471	4,941	3.54
Total	36,332	35,881	35,904	31,269	139,386	100.00

SOURCE: Compiled using information from other tables in this report.

REFERENCES

Ackerknecht, E. H. 1945. Malaria in the Upper Mississippi Valley, 1760-1900. Baltimore: Johns Hopkins Press.

Bradley, G. H. 1966. A review of malaria control and eradication in the United States. Mosquito News 26:462-470.

Brown, A. W. A., J. Haworth, and A. R. Zahar. 1976. Malaria eradication and control from a global standpoint. Journal of Medical Entomology 13:1-25.

Bruce-Chwatt, L. J. 1988. History of malaria from prehistory to eradication. Pp. 1-59 in Malaria: Principles and Practice of Malariology, Wernsdorfer, W. H., and I. McGregor, eds. Edinburgh: Churchill Livingstone.

Canfield, C. J. 1972. Malaria in U.S. military personnel 1965-1971. Proceedings of the Helminthological Society of Washington 39:15-18.

Celli, A. 1925. Storia della malaria nell'agro romano. Academia dei Lincei, Roma.

Duffy, J. 1953. Epidemics in Colonial America. Baton Rouge: Louisiana State University Press.

Ettling, M. B. 1990. Financing of Anti-Malaria Activities in Selected Countries. A paper commissioned by the Committee on Malaria Prevention and Control of the Institute of Medicine, Washington, D.C.

Farid, M. A. 1980. The Malaria Programme—from euphoria to anarchy. World Health Forum 1:8-33.

Gramiccia, G., and P. F. Beales. 1988. The recent history of malaria control and eradication. Pp. 1335-1378 in Malaria: Principles and Practice of Malariology, Wernsdorfer, W. H., and I. MacGregor, eds. Edinburgh: Churchill Livingstone.

Guha-Sapir, D., and F. Hariga. 1991. The Funding of Malaria Research: Where It Goes and Why. A paper commissioned by the Committee on Malaria Prevention and Control of the Institute of Medicine, Washington, D.C.

Howard, L. M. 1972. Basic research priorities from the perspective of national malaria programs in developing countries. Proceedings of the Helminthological Society of Washington 39:10-18.

International Cooperation Administration Expert Panel on Malaria. 1961. Report and recommendations on malaria: a summary. American Journal of Tropical Medicine and Hygiene 10:451-502.

International Development Advisory Board. 1956. Malaria Eradication: Report and Recommendations of the International Development Advisory Board. April 13, 1956.

Lepes, T. 1974. Present status of the Global Malaria Eradication Programme and prospects for the future. Journal of Tropical Medicine and Hygiene 77:47-53.

Mountin, J. W. A. 1944. A program for the eradication of malaria from continental America. Journal of the National Malaria Society 3:69-73.

Najera, J. A. 1989. Malaria and the work of the WHO. Bulletin of the World Health Organization 67(3):229-243.

Neel, S. 1973. Medical Support of the U.S. Army in Vietnam, 1965-70. Vietnam Studies. Washington, D.C.: Office of the Surgeon General and Center for Military History, U.S. Army.

Ognibene, A. J., and O. Barrett, eds. 1982. Internal Medicine in Vietnam. Vol. 2.

Washington, D.C.: Office of the Surgeon General and Center for Military History, U.S. Army.

Russell, P. F. 1955. Man's Mastery of Malaria. London: Oxford University Press.

Russell, P. F. 1968. The United States and malaria: debits and credits. Bulletin of the New York Academy of Medicine 44:623-653.

Russell, P. F., C. S. West, and R. D. Manwell. 1946. Practical Malariology. Philadelphia: W.B. Saunders Company.

Smith, E. A. 1974. AID policy on malaria. From a paper presented at the Forty-second Annual Conference of the California Mosquito Control Association, Inc., and the Thirtieth Annual Meeting of the American Mosquito Control Association, Inc., February 24-27, 1974.

Soper, F. L. 1960. The epidemiology of a disappearing disease: malaria. American Journal of Tropical Medicine and Hygiene 9:357-366.

Spielman, A., and U. Kitron. 1990. Rationale and Conceptual Framework for Malaria Eradication: A Historical Overview with an Emphasis on Time-Limitation and the Role of Research. A paper commissioned by the Committee on Malaria Prevention and Control of the Institute of Medicine, Washington, D.C.

Trager, W., and J. B. Jensen. 1976. Human malaria parasites in continuous culture. Science 193:673-675.

World Health Organization. 1955. WHA8.30 Malaria Eradication, from the Ninth Plenary Meeting, May 26, 1955. WHO Official Records No. 63, pp. 31-32. Geneva: World Health Organization.

World Health Organization. 1969. Re-examination of the Global Strategy of Malaria Eradication. A report by the Director-General to the 22nd World Health Assembly, May 30, 1969. Annex 13, Part I. WHO Official Records No. 176.

World Health Organization. 1991. Tropical Diseases, Progress in Research 1990-91. Tenth Programme Report of the UNDP/World Bank/WHO Special Programme for Research and Training in Tropical Diseases (TDR). Geneva: World Health Organization.

World Health Organization Expert Committee on Malaria. 1957. Sixth Report. World Health Organization Technical Report Series No. 123. Geneva: World Health Organization.

World Health Organization Expert Committee on Malaria. 1967. Thirteenth Report. WHO Technical Report Series, No. 357. Geneva: World Health Organization.

4

Clinical Medicine and the Disease Process

WHERE WE WANT TO BE IN THE YEAR 2010

There will be a worldwide drop in deaths and debilitating illness resulting from many important changes in the way health providers around the world prevent, diagnose, and treat the disease. Unlike the situation at present, health providers will be able to identify and offer preventive therapy for persons at risk for severe and complicated malaria. Further, health providers will be able to quickly identify and treat individuals who do become infected, even if they live in an area far from a fully equipped health post. Anemia and hypoglycemia, important and potentially life-threatening complications of malaria, will be diagnosed and treated promptly. The threat of transmitting AIDS through contaminated blood transfusions, a major problem in the 1980s and 1990s, particularly in Africa, will be significantly lessened with the advent of inexpensive and stable blood substitutes. Efforts to take into account area-specific drug sensitivities when designing local treatment policies will result in a much more effective use of chemotherapeutic agents and containment of the spread of drug resistance. Research on malaria pathogenesis will give physicians new points of attack for treating particularly difficult cases. Health providers in areas of the world where malaria is not a problem will know enough about the disease to recommend effective preventive regimens to those who plan to visit malarious areas and to recognize the disease in returning travelers.

56

WHERE WE ARE TODAY

Despite advances in the understanding of the pathogenic and clinical aspects of malaria, clinicians still do not know why some people tolerate malaria infections with few or no symptoms, whereas others are severely affected. Indeed, it remains a mystery why some people die of malaria but others do not.

Clinical Aspects of Malaria

It is important to distinguish between the *disease* caused by malaria parasites and the frequently asymptomatic *infection* caused by the same parasites. It is important to recognize that one may be infected without having the disease. The disease affects individuals who lack certain anti-illness immunity factors acquired by exposure to malaria or conferred by maternal antibodies transferred across the placenta (World Health Organization, 1990). The specific components of this immunity have yet to be determined, but at-risk groups include those in whom immunity has not yet developed (young children in endemic areas, travelers, and military personnel) and those in whom established immunity has lapsed (pregnant women, inhabitants of an endemic area who leave and then return, and residents of an area in which a successful malaria control program has stopped). Any one of four species of malaria parasite can cause illness, but *Plasmodium falciparum* causes almost all severe and complicated disease. Malarial illness is frequently several different, often overlapping syndromes.

Severe Malaria

Among the best known and serious complications of severe malaria, occurring particularly although not exclusively in children, are cerebral malaria, hypoglycemia, and anemia.

Cerebral Malaria   Cerebral malaria can be defined as altered consciousness in a patient who has *P. falciparum* parasites in the blood and in whom no other cause of altered consciousness can be found (World Health Organization, 1990). Cerebral malaria is frequently the only manifestation of a severe falciparum infection in children (Molyneux et al., 1989a); adults with the syndrome commonly have problems in other organ systems, usually the lungs and the kidneys (Warrell, 1987). Between 10 and 50 percent of people with cerebral malaria die, depending on the level of endemicity, how the syndrome is defined, the level of care available, and the age of the patient (Rey et al., 1966; Bernard and Combes, 1973; Stace et al., 1982; Warrell et al., 1982).

Cerebral malaria may develop very rapidly. In a study of 131 Malawian children with cerebral malaria, for example, symptoms such as fever, malaise, or cough had been present for an average of 47 hours prior to admission, and altered consciousness had been present for a mean of 8 hours. Eighty-two percent of the patients had a history of convulsions, and the level of consciousness had often deteriorated dramatically following the initial convulsion (Molyneux et al., 1989a). The speed with which this syndrome progresses has obvious implications for treatment strategies.

In cerebral malaria, the level of consciousness can vary from mild confusion to profound coma. Some clinical findings suggest a diffuse involvement of the entire brain, while others are consistent with a theory of impairment of specific cerebral functions (Guignard, 1965; Dumas et al., 1986; Molyneux et al., 1989a; Brewster et al., 1990). Cerebral malaria can present with a variety of neurological symptoms such as seizures, increased muscle tone, hyperreflexia (sometimes with clonus), extensor plantar reflexes, and extensor posturing. In some patients, the clinical picture suggests increased intracranial pressure as a possible pathogenetic mechanism (Newton et al., 1991). Among survivors, particularly children, recovery is surprisingly rapid. In the previously mentioned Malawian study, full consciousness was regained over a period ranging from 1 to 152 hours (mean, 31 hours). After 24 hours of treatment with intravenous quinine, half of the children had recovered fully; by 48 hours, 80 percent had recovered completely (Molyneux et al., 1989a). The rapidity of the descent into unconsciousness and, in survivors, of the ascent into full awareness are unique, distinguishing, and intriguing features of cerebral malaria.

The detection of *P. falciparum* parasites in peripheral blood would seem to be a sine qua non for cerebral malaria, but it is not. There are reports of patients in whom repeated attempts to demonstrate *P. falciparum* parasitemia were unsuccessful, yet postmortem examination showed unequivocal evidence of *P. falciparum* infection with parasitized red blood cells sequestered in the tissues (World Health Organization, 1990). The absolute level of parasitemia has some prognostic significance: the higher the parasite count, the more likely the patient is to die or develop neurological sequelae (Field and Niven, 1937; Molyneux et al., 1989a). However, many patients with cerebral malaria have scanty parasitemias, and many children with very high parasite densities have fairly mild symptoms.

Current evidence suggests that mechanical obstruction of the microcirculation by parasitized red blood cells is the most likely cause of cerebral malaria. In patients with malaria, sequestration of parasitized red blood cells is seen in various human tissues, including brain, heart, liver, lung, and kidney. Patients dying of cerebral malaria show the same general pattern of sequestration, but the parasite densities in the brain are higher than in those dying of noncerebral malaria. The resulting reduction in cerebral blood flow may lead to anaerobic cerebral glycolysis and increased cerebral lactateproduction. Lactate levels are elevated both in arterial blood and in cerebrospinal fluid (CSF). Since lactate in the blood does not cross the blood-brain barrier into the CSF (Posner and Plum, 1967), this finding suggests that lactate is being independently generated in both fluid systems. The magnitude of CSF lactate elevation is higher in fatal than in nonfatal cases of cerebral malaria (White et al., 1985). Lactate is also a building block utilized by the liver in the synthesis of glucose. Hepatic gluconeogenesis may be impaired in severe malaria, and this could contribute to elevated plasma levels of lactate (Taylor et al., 1988). Another potential source of high plasma lactate levels is the metabolism of the parasites: *P. falciparum* consumes glucose and generates lactate as a by-product. A mass of sequestered parasites may cause localized hypoglycemia (low blood sugar) and elevated lactate concentrations in the brain.

Another potential contributor to the pathogenesis of cerebral malaria is tumor necrosis factor (TNF), a cytokine. Plasma levels of TNF are elevated in adults with severe malaria (Kern et al., 1989) and in children with acute *P. falciparum* infections (Grau et al., 1989; Kwiatkowski et al., 1990). TNF is produced by monocytes and macrophages in response to a number of stimuli (Carswell et al., 1975; Cuturi et al., 1987) and has been shown to cause a wide variety of physiological effects in humans (Tracey et al., 1986). Some of these, such as fever and hypoglycemia, are common in children with severe malaria. Others, like low blood pressure, kidney failure, and a disruption of the blood clotting mechanism, occur frequently in adults with severe malaria. The extent to which TNF contributes to the pathogenesis of human clinical illness is unclear, but in a study of mice infected with a mouse malaria parasite, treatment with anti-TNF antibodies protected the animals from the cerebral complications of the disease (Grau et al., 1987), and high plasma levels of TNF in children with malaria are associated with an increased risk of dying (Grau et al., 1989; Kwiatkowski et al., 1990).

It has also been suggested that immune mechanisms may play a role in cerebral malaria. In some rodent models of malaria, cerebral lesions contain local collections of inflammatory cells. These cerebral lesions and associated neurological symptoms can be prevented by pretreatment with corticosteroids (potent anti-inflammatory agents), cyclosporin A (an inhibitor of T-lymphocyte function), or antibodies to TNF. Inflammatory lesions are not found in human cerebral malaria, however, and neither cyclosporin A nor corticosteroids have proven to be an effective treatment for human cerebral malaria, although pretreatment with these drugs has not been possible. In this respect, human *P. falciparum* malaria differs significantly from certain animal malarias, where accumulations of mononuclear cells are found in cerebral vessels (Grau et al.,

1987). At present, there is no satisfactory animal model for human cerebral malaria.

The clinical management of patients with cerebral malaria requires prompt, specific antimalarial treatment, in addition to the general supportive care required for unconscious patients. Because of the extensive spread of chloroquine-resistant *P. falciparum*, the current drugs of choice for patients with cerebral malaria are intravenous quinine and, when quinine is unavailable, quinidine (Phillips et al., 1985; Miller et al., 1989; World Health Organization, 1990). In patients who have not undergone any previous treatment, a "loading dose" should be used with each drug to produce therapeutic blood levels as quickly as possible (White et al., 1983a). The size of the loading dose may vary, depending on local parasite sensitivities and on any preadmission drug treatment.

Serious side effects include quinine- or quinidine-induced hypoglycemia (White et al., 1983b; Phillips et al., 1986b) and quinidine-related changes in the electrical conduction of the heart. Both can be mitigated by slow, controlled infusions of the medications (Phillips et al., 1985; Miller et al., 1989; Molyneux et al., 1989b). Pregnant women are particularly likely to develop hypoglycemia during the course of treatment with intravenous quinine (Looareesuwan et al., 1985). When the patient is able to eat and drink, tablets or capsules can be substituted for the intravenous medication. There is no consensus regarding the optimal duration of treatment with these two drugs. In certain parts of the world (e.g., Thailand) where the malaria parasite is less sensitive to quinine, a second drug (tetracycline) is used to eliminate parasitemia following resolution of coma (World Health Organization, 1990).

The degree of supportive care provided to patients depends on the available facilities. Very high body temperatures can be reduced with tepid sponging and fanning. Convulsions can be treated with any of a number of standard medications. For example, a recent study showed that prophylactic administration of phenobarbitone decreased the number of subsequent convulsions in a group of adults with cerebral malaria (White et al., 1988). The number of patients studied was too small, however, to allow determination of whether decreasing the number of convulsions had any effect on overall survival or the incidence of sequelae.

Exchange transfusion (replacement of a patient's blood with donor blood over a short period of time) has been used effectively to treat patients with severe malaria, especially those with high blood levels of parasites (Kurathong et al., 1979; Roncoroni and Martino, 1979; Yarrish et al., 1982; Kramer et al., 1983; Files et al., 1984; Chiodini et al., 1985; Hall et al., 1985; Miller et al., 1989). The technique is not practical in malaria-endemic areas where the prevalence of human immunodeficiency virus (HIV) seropositivity is high or in settings where close clinical monitoring of patients is not feasible. Despite optimal care, between 10 and 30 percent of children with cerebral malaria die, and a similar proportion suffer neurological damage (Molyneux et al., 1989a). In most cases, the actual cause of death is unknown (World Health Organization, 1990).

Hypoglycemia   Many illnesses cause hypoglycemia, a condition which requires immediate, specific treatment to prevent permanent brain damage and death (Kawo et al., 1990). Because its clinical presentation (confusion, coma, and convulsions) closely mimics that of cerebral malaria, the coexistence of hypoglycemia in some patients with severe malaria was not suspected until quite recently (White et al., 1983b). As a result, an unknown number of patients may have died or suffered brain damage from what is an eminently recognizable and easily treated condition. The emergency treatment of hypoglycemia is an intravenous bolus of a very concentrated sugar solution, followed by a continuous intravenous supply of glucose until the patient can take food and fluids by mouth.

Hypoglycemia is an especially common finding in pediatric malaria. In two recent studies, 23 and 32 percent of pediatric patients, respectively, were admitted with hypoglycemia (blood glucose levels less than 2.2 millimoles per liter, or 40 milligrams per deciliter) (White et al., 1983b; Taylor et al., 1988). The prognosis is particularly poor for such patients. In the Malawi study, 37 percent of those with hypoglycemia died and 26 percent were discharged with neurological sequelae (Taylor et al., 1988). These rates are six to nine times higher than those for cerebral malaria patients with normal blood sugar levels.

Studies on hypoglycemia in children suggest that the condition develops through one or more of several mechanisms. One theory suggests that malaria infection may impair the liver's capacity to produce glucose from circulating precursors. It may also be that the sequestration of parasitized red blood cells in tissue capillaries slows the circulation enough to cause a change in tissue metabolism, thereby enhancing glucose consumption.

Malarial Anemia   Red blood cells infected with malaria parasites either are destroyed outright when schizonts mature and merozoites burst from the cell or are cleared from the circulation by the spleen. In acute malarial infections, splenomegaly is often associated with mechanical destruction of normal red blood cells, perhaps because the cell architecture becomes distorted. Several studies of patients with acute malaria have shown that there is also a decrease in the bone marrow production of new red blood cells (Marchiafava and Bignami, 1894; Abdalla et al., 1980; Phillips et al., 1986a). Cytokines such as TNF may be involved in this marrow suppression and dyserythropoiesis (abnormal red blood cell production). In addition, red blood cells coated with low levels of immunoglobulin G may be removed from the circulation by the spleen more rapidly than is normally the case. The loss of red blood cells from these various mechanisms is therefore generally greater than would be expected from parasitemia alone and often causes significant anemia.

When red blood cell losses are mild, anemia is well tolerated, but anemias can quickly become life-threatening in patients with high parasitemias (Phillips et al., 1986a; Molyneux et al., 1989a). There is no consensus about what constitutes "life-threatening" anemia in a malaria patient, and the only effective treatment currently available is blood transfusion. The administration of blood carries its own inherent risks, and these are compounded by the danger of transmitting AIDS in areas where a substantial proportion of the population is HIV seropositive. Once the parasitemia has cleared, bone marrow production of red blood cells resumes, and the red blood cell mass is gradually restored to its preillness level (Phillips et al., 1986a).

While the danger of contracting AIDS is a real problem for patients with malarial anemia who undergo transfusion, there is no evidence at the present time to suggest that HIV infection places individuals at increased risk of severe malaria. The possibility of such an association, however, warrants continued surveillance.

Other Clinical Features

In areas of the world where malaria transmission fluctuates, adults do not acquire significant immunity and may be at risk for developing a severe infection involving many organ systems (World Health Organization, 1990). Women who are pregnant for the first time appear to be particularly susceptible to this form of the disease (Looareesuwan et al., 1985).

Acute Clinical Complications Adults with severe malaria often require a higher level of supportive care than do children, including mechanical ventilation for pulmonary edema and hemodialysis or peritoneal dialysis for kidney failure, the two most frequent and serious noncerebral complications of the disease (World Health Organization, 1990).

The principles of antimalarial drug therapy in these settings are the same as for treating cerebral malaria in children. Special care should be taken in treating pregnant woman with intravenous quinine, since they are more likely than other adults to develop hyperinsulinemic hypoglycemia (Looareesuwan et al., 1985).

Pulmonary edema is a serious complication of falciparum malaria and is associated with a high mortality rate (World Health Organization, 1990). Its cause is unknown. Pulmonary edema resembles adult respiratory distress syndrome, with increased pulmonary vascular permeability.

Acute renal failure in malaria has the pathological characteristics of acute tubular necrosis, but the causal mechanism remains unknown. Hypovolemia from dehydration probably contributes to the problem in some severely ill patients, but it does not appear to explain all cases (Sitprija, 1988).

There are a number of other acute but less frequent complications of malaria, which are discussed in some detail in a set of treatment guidelines recently prepared by the World Health Organization (World Health Organization, 1990). These include significant bleeding, impaired fluid balance, and impaired gastrointestinal and liver function.

Chronic Complications   Among the most frequent chronic complications of malaria are *P. malariae* glomerulopathy and hyperreactive malarial splenomegaly (HMS). *Plasmodium malariae* glomerulopathy, a nephrotic syndrome with massive proteinuria, hypoalbuminemia, and edema, results from *P. malariae* infection. Patients with renal involvement do not respond to treatment with antimalarial drugs or with corticosteroids or other antiinflammatory drugs used to treat other forms of immune complex-associated nephrotic syndrome (Houba, 1975).

HMS, previously known as tropical splenomegaly syndrome, manifests itself clinically as persistent and progressive splenic enlargement (Bryceson et al., 1983). In patients with high levels of antimalarial antibodies, spleen size and antibody levels can be reduced with long-term antimalarial treatment. The prevalence of HMS is variable, but the condition is especially common in West Africa, Indonesia, and Papua New Guinea.

Uncomplicated Malaria

The vast majority of malaria patients suffer from so-called uncomplicated disease. They may have a variety of symptoms, including fever, headache, malaise, cough, nausea, vomiting, and diarrhea, and are usually treated empirically (that is, without the benefit of a bloodfilm examination) in many malaria-endemic areas. Even if local health care systems were able to perform a diagnostic blood film on every patient suspected of having malaria, the interpretation of the smear, especially in malaria-endemic areas, would be difficult. This is because a negative blood film does not exclude malarial illness, and a positive blood film does not necessarily confirm a diagnosis of malarial illness, since many individuals with positive films may have no symptoms caused by the malaria parasites. Antimalarial drugs are usually administered orally, although intramuscular injections of quinine can be used when appropriate (Mansor et al., 1990; Waller et al., 1990).

A proportion of patients presumed to have uncomplicated malaria improve, either because the chosen drug was effective against the parasite, because they already had or rapidly developed immune responses that controlled the disease, or because they had another, self-limiting disease such as the flu rather than malaria. Some patients for various reasons do not improve, and either return for more definitive care or seek help from other sources (traditional local treatments or over-the-counter medications). Some may worsen and die, although this progression cannot be assumed, especially in a semi-immune population.

Most travelers who contract malaria initially develop the uncomplicated form of the disease. In a nonimmune patient, however, the progression to severe malaria is often very rapid. When the circumstances are appropriate, both patients and their doctors should be alert to the possibility of malaria infection and should treat the disease as a medical emergency. As is true for all malaria patients, the choice of drug treatment for travelers depends on the species of malaria parasite involved, where the infection was contracted (parasite drug sensitivities vary substantially around the world), what (if any) malaria chemoprophylaxis was used, and the pertinent details of the individual's medical history (World Health Organization, 1990).

Malaria Chemoprophylaxis and Treatment

Nonimmune visitors to malaria-endemic areas are at risk for developing severe and complicated malaria and therefore benefit from a regimen of preventive drug therapy. In the past, chloroquine chemoprophylaxis was effective and safe and was recommended for all who were at risk of acquiring the disease. The spread of chloroquine-resistant *P. falciparum* and *P. vivax* (Rieckmann et al., 1989), however, has complicated matters, particularly since each of the currently available alternatives to chloroquine has some toxicity. Mefloquine is the latest addition to the antimalarial armamentarium (Department of Health and Human Services, 1990).

There is no consensus regarding the optimal chemoprophylactic regimen for persons living in or visiting the range of locales in which malaria infection is possible (Bradley and Phillips-Howard, 1989; Department of Health and Human Services, 1990). It is important for both travelers and physicians to realize that no prophylactic regimen is completely effective in all cases and that rapid diagnosis and prompt treatment are important.

Pregnant women living in endemic areas constitute another group for which malaria chemoprophylaxis has been recommended. Babies born to first-time mothers with malaria often weigh less than babies born to uninfected mothers (Brabin, 1983; McGregor, 1984). Malaria can also cause severe anemia in women during their first pregnancy (Gilles et al., 1969; Brabin, 1983; McGregor, 1984). Although women living in malaria-endemic areas frequently receive chemoprophylaxis during pregnancy, few studies have measured the clinical value and cost-effectiveness of this practice. In one placebo-controlled trial in the Gambia, malaria chemoprophylaxis (dapsone plus pyrimethamine) administered by traditional birth attendants resulted in lower levels of parasitemia, fewer cases of anemia, and fewer low birth weight babies, but only in women experiencing their first pregnancy (Greenwood et al., 1989).

RESEARCH AGENDA

Pathogenesis

Despite a partial understanding of the host-parasite interactions in malaria, it is not known why some patients die from the disease. The remarkable recoveries enjoyed by most patients with cerebral malaria suggest that much of the pathology of this condition is reversible. If the pathogenic processes could be interrupted, or if the vulnerable organ systems could be supported until antimalarial drugs exerted their effects, the mortality rate due to serious malaria infections likely would decrease. Parasite sequestration, a characteristic of all *P. falciparum* infections, is associated with multisystem organ impairment in only a small proportion of patients. Similarly, severe malarial anemia develops in only a few of those at risk. In addressing these questions, a focus on the determinants of malaria *disease*, as distinct from the factors involved in malaria *infection*, may suggest new preventive and therapeutic options (Playfair et al., 1990).

> **RESEARCH FOCUS:** Determination of why some patient groups suffer severe disease (cerebral malaria and life-threatening anemia), while other, seemingly similar groups tolerate high parasitemia with only mild symptoms.

> **RESEARCH FOCUS:** Continuation of investigations into the pathogenesis of severe malaria (cytokines, parasite sequestration, hypoglycemia, increased intracranial pressure) and development of treatments targeted at the important mechanisms.

Treatment

Travelers to endemic areas who get malaria despite complying with a particular chemoprophylactic regimen occasionally are used as sentinels to detect the spread of drug resistance. Since their levels of exposure and degree of immunity differ significantly from those of the local population, however, this method is not particularly useful for helping formulate national treatment policies in endemic areas. The ability to determine the level of local parasite sensitivities to different drugs is important. In vitro assays, which measure the growth of parasites in increasing concentrations of a drug, are available for most of the commonly used antimalarial drugs. However, the results of in vitro assays often correlate poorly with in vivo efficacy studies in the same setting, primarily because the former cannot assess patient-specific factors, such as differences in drug metabolism and level of immunity, that can influence drug sensitivity.

> **RESEARCH FOCUS:** Development of more effective methods of tracking and assessing drug resistance in malaria-endemic countries.

> **RESEARCH FOCUS:** Development of clinically and operationally useful assays that can predict parasite sensitivity to various drugs and drug combinations.

Even in parts of the world where chloroquine resistance is widespread, the drug retains some clinical efficacy and can bring about some symptomatic improvement in many semi-immune patients, even though such patients may still harbor parasites. However, the importance of this clinical improvement with respect to assessing the effectiveness of various treatment options is unknown.

> **RESEARCH FOCUS:** Determination of the long-term effects of low-grade parasitemia on the development of anemia, on the patient's susceptibility to reinfection, and on the acquisition of antimalarial immunity.

There is a worldwide shortage of effective antimalarial drugs. Quinine is the only widely available and effective medication for the parenteral treatment of severe disease, but unfortunately quinine resistance has been documented in Thai patients (World Health Organization, 1990) (see Chapter 8).

> **RESEARCH FOCUS:** Development of new drugs and new routes of administration for existing drugs to treat patients with severe falciparum malaria infections.

Chemoprophylaxis

Plasmodium falciparum infections can progress very rapidly; the time from the first onset of symptoms to the development of coma averaged 48 hours in the Malawian children examined in one study (Molyneux et al., 1989a), and the mean duration of illness in Gambian children prior to death was three days (Greenwood et al., 1988). One preventive option is mass chemoprophylaxis for the at-risk segments of a population. Such programs have foundered in the past because of intermittent drug supplies and difficulties in ensuring proper drug use. However, if these obstacles can be overcome, there is evidence that chemoprophylaxis may be effective in young children (Greenwood et al., 1988). The relative benefits of early treatment versus mass prophylaxis will depend on the level of malaria endemicity and have yet to be clearly defined for any particular epidemiologic setting. Furthermore, the effects of sustained malaria chemosuppression on the acquisition of antimalarial immunity and on the evolution of drug resistance require further study before this approach can be recommended.

> **RESEARCH FOCUS:** Determination of the relative efficacy of mass chemoprophylaxis in reducing malaria-related morbidity and mortality in at-risk subgroups in a variety of epidemiologic settings.

> **RESEARCH FOCUS:** Evaluation of the effect of prolonged mass administration of antimalarial drugs on the acquisition of malarial immunity and the acquisition of drug resistance.

Chemoprophylaxis is recommended for pregnant women living in malaria-endemic areas, but the diminishing efficacy of chloroquine, an inexpensive, relatively safe and well-tolerated antimalarial drug, has forced a rigorous appraisal of this policy. The safety and efficacy of alternative prophylactic regimens in pregnancy is an open question (Steketee et al., 1988). The use of more toxic prophylactic drugs has to be weighed against other unknowns, such as the potential benefits of maternal chemoprophylaxis on birth weight and on neonatal and infant mortality rates.

> **RESEARCH FOCUS:** Assessment of the impact of effective prophylaxis during pregnancy on birth outcomes.

> **RESEARCH FOCUS:** Determination of the efficacy and feasibility of various chemoprophylactic regimens for pregnant women in different epidemiologic settings.

Reliable data on the efficacy of prophylactic antimalarial drugs taken by travelers and other nonimmune individuals in endemic areas have been extremely difficult to collect. Recently, a system was developed that allows health officials to monitor U.S. Peace Corps volunteers in various

West African countries for the spread of chloroquine-resistant *P. falciparum* malaria. On the basis of data collected through this surveillance system, the dosing regimen for malaria prophylaxis with mefloquine was recently revised (Department of Health and Human Services, 1991). This relatively simple surveillance network has provided up-to-date information on disease risk and should continue to serve as a model for future attempts at collecting relevant, reliable data (Moran and Bernard, 1989).

RESEARCH FOCUS: Expansion of this effort to encourage further development of rational prophylaxis regimens based on operational research and simple surveillance networks.

REFERENCES

Abdalla, S., D. J. Weatherall, S. N. Wickramasinghe, and M. Hughes. 1980. The anaemia of *P. falciparum* malaria. British Journal of Haematology 46:171-183.

Bernard, R., and J.-C. Combes. 1973. La paludisme chez l'enfant. Revue du Praticien 23:4197-4213.

Brabin, B. J. 1983. An analysis of malaria in pregnancy in Africa. Bulletin of the World Health Organization 61:1005-1016.

Bradley, D. J., and P. A. Phillips-Howard. 1989. Prophylaxis against malaria for travellers from the United Kingdom. British Medical Journal 299:1087-1089.

Brewster, D. R., D. Kwiatkowski, and N. J. White. 1990. Neurological sequelae of cerebral malaria in children. Lancet 336:1039-1043.

Bryceson, A., Y. M. Fakunle, A. F. Fleming, G. Crane, M. S. R. Hutt, K. M. de Cock, B. M. Greenwood, P. Marsden, and P. Rees. 1983. Malaria and splenomegaly [letter]. Transactions of the Royal Society of Tropical Medicine and Hygiene 77:879.

Carswell, E. A., L. J. Old, R. L. Kassel, S. Green, N. Fiore, and B. Williamson. 1975. An endotoxin-induced serum factor that causes necrosis of tumors. Proceedings of the National Academy of Sciences of the United States of America 72:3666-3670.

Chiodini, P. L., M. Somerville, I. Salam, H. R. Tubbs, M. J. Wood, and C. J. Ellis. 1985. Exchange transfusion in severe falciparum malaria. Transactions of the Royal Society of Tropical Medicine and Hygiene 79:865-866.

Cuturi, M. C., M. Murphy, M. P. Costa-Giomi, R. Weinmann, B. Perussia, and G. Trinchieri. 1987. Independent regulation of tumor necrosis factor and lymphokine production by human peripheral blood lymphocytes. Journal of Experimental Medicine 165:1581-1594.

Department of Health and Human Services. 1990. Recommendations for the prevention of malaria among travelers. Morbidity and Mortality Weekly Reports 39(RR-3):1-10.

Department of Health and Human Services. 1991. Change of dosing regimen for malaria prophylaxis with mefloquine. Morbidity and Mortality Weekly Reports 40:72-73.

Dumas, M., J. M. Leger, and M. Pestre-Alexandre. 1986. Manifestations neurologiques et psychiatriques des parasitoses [Neurological and psychiatric manifestations of parasitoses]. Pp. 143-146 in Congrès de Psychiatrie et de Neurologie de la Langue Française, LXXXIVe Session. Paris: Masson.

Field, J. W., and J. C. Niven. 1937. A note on prognosis in relation to parasite counts in acute subtertian malaria. Transactions of the Royal Society of Tropical Medicine and Hygiene 30:569-574.

Files, J. C., C. J. Case, and F. S. Morrison. 1984. Automated erythrocyte exchange in fulminant falciparum malaria. Annals of Internal Medicine 100:396.

Gilles, H. M., J. B. Lawson, M. Sibelas, A. Voller, and N. Allan. 1969. Malaria, anaemia and pregnancy. Annals of Tropical Medicine and Parasitology 63:245-263.

Grau, G. E., L. F. Fajardo, P. F. Piguet, B. Allet, P. H. Lambert, and P. Vassali. 1987. Tumor necrosis factor (cachectin) as an essential mediator in murine cerebral malaria. Science 237:1210-1212.

Grau, G. E., T. E. Taylor, M. E. Molyneux, J. J. Wirima, P. Vassalli, M. Hommel, and P. H. Lambert. 1989. Tumor necrosis factor and disease severity in children with falciparum malaria. New England Journal of Medicine 320:1586-1591.

Greenwood, B. M., A. M. Greenwood, A. K. Bradley, R. W. Snow, P. Byass, R. J. Hayes, and A. B. N'Jie. 1988. Comparison of two strategies for control of malaria within a primary health care programme in The Gambia. Lancet 1:1121-1127.

Greenwood, B. M., A. M. Greenwood, R. W. Snow, P. Byass, S. Bennett, and A. B. Natib-N'Jie. 1989. The effects of malaria chemoprophylaxis given by traditional birth attendants on the course and outcome of pregnancy. Transactions of the Royal Society of Tropical Medicine and Hygiene 83:589-594.

Guignard, J. 1965. Le paludisme pernicieux du nourrisson et de l'enfant. Considerations cliniques, pronostiques et therapeutiques. A propos de 130 cas observes en zone d'endemie palutre. Annales de Pediatrie 12:646-656.

Hall, A., A. Yardumian, and A. Marsh. 1985. Exchange transfusion and quinine concentrations in falciparum malaria. British Medical Journal 291:1169-1170.

Houba, V. 1975. Immunopathology of neuropathies associated with malaria. Bulletin of the World Health Organization 52:199-207.

Kawo, N. G., A. E. Msengi, A. B. M. Swai, L. M. Chuwa, K. G. M. M. Alberti, and D. G. McLarty. 1990. Specificity of hypoglycaemia for cerebral malaria in children. Lancet 336:454-457.

Kern, P., C. J. Hemmer, J. Van Damme, H. J. Gruss, and M. Dietrich. 1989. Elevated tumor necrosis factor alpha and interleukin-6 serum levels as markers for complicated *Plasmodium falciparum* malaria. American Journal of Medicine 87:139-143.

Kramer, S. L., C. C. Campbell, and R. E. Moncrieff. 1983. Fulminant *Plasmodium falciparum* infection treated with exchange blood transfusion. JAMA 249:244-245.

Kurathong, S., T. Srichaikul, P. Isarangkura, and S. Phanichphant. 1979. Exchange transfusion in cerebral malaria complicated by disseminated intravascular coagulation. Southeast Asian Journal of Tropical Medicine and Public Health 10:389-392.

Kwiatkowski, D., A. V. S. Hill, I. Sambou, P. Twumasi, J. Castracane, K. R. Manogue, A. Cerami, D. R. Brewster, and B. M. Greenwood. 1990. TNF concentration in fatal cerebral, non-fatal cerebral, and uncomplicated *Plasmodium falciparum* malaria. Lancet 336:1201-1204.

Looareesuwan, S., R. E. Phillips, N. J. White, S. Kietinun, J. Karbwang, C. Rackow, R. C. Turner, and D. A. Warrell. 1985. Quinine and severe falciparum malaria in late pregnancy. Lancet 2:4-8.

Mansor, S. M., T. E. Taylor, C. S. McGrath, G. Edwards, S. A. Ward, J. J. Wirima, and M. E. Molyneux. 1990. The safety and kinetics of intramuscular quinine in Malawian children with moderately severe falciparum malaria. Transactions of the Royal Society of Tropical Medicine and Hygiene 84:482-487.

Marchiafava, E., and A. Bignami. 1894. On Summer-Autumnal Fever. London: The New Syndenham Society.

McGregor, I. A. 1984. Epidemiology, malaria and pregnancy. American Journal of Tropical Medicine and Hygiene 33:517-525.

Miller, K. D., A. E. Greenberg, and C. C. Campbell. 1989. Treatment of severe malaria in the United States with a continuous infusion of quinidine gluconate and exchange transfusion. New England Journal of Medicine 321:65-70.

Molyneux, M. E., T. E. Taylor, J. J. Wirima, and A. Borgstein. 1989a. Clinical features and prognostic indicators in paediatric cerebral malaria: a study of 131 comatose Malawian children. Quarterly Journal of Medicine 71:441-459.

Molyneux, M. E., T. E. Taylor, J. J. Wirima, and G. Harper. 1989b. Effect of rate of infusion of quinine on insulin and glucose responses in Malawian children with falciparum malaria. British Medical Journal 299:602-603.

Moran, J. S., and K. W. Bernard. 1989. The spread of chloroquine-resistant malaria in Africa. Implications for travelers. JAMA 262:245-248.

Newton, C. R. J. C., F. J. Kirkham, P. A. Winstanley, G. Pasvol, N. Peshu, D. A. Warrell, and K. Marsh. 1991. Intracranial pressure in African children with cerebral malaria. Lancet 337:573-576.

Phillips, R. E., D. A. Warrell, N. J. White, S. Looareesuwan, and J. Karbwang. 1985. Intravenous quinidine for the treatment of severe falciparum malaria. Clinical and pharmacokinetic studies. New England Journal of Medicine 312:1273-1278.

Phillips, R. E., S. Looareesuwan, D. A. Warrell, S. H. Lee, J. Karbwang, M. J. Warrell, N. J. White, C. Swasdichai, and D. J. Weatherall. 1986a. The importance of anaemia in cerebral and uncomplicated falciparum malaria: role of complications, dyserythropoiesis and iron sequestration. Quarterly Journal of Medicine 58:305-323.

Phillips, R. E., S. Looareesuwan, N. J. White, P. Chanthavanich, J. Karbwang, W. Supanaranond, R. C. Turner, and D. A. Warrell. 1986b. Hypoglycaemia and antimalarial drugs: quinidine and release of insulin. British Medical Journal 292:1319-1321.

Playfair, J. H., J. Taverne, C. A. Bate, and J. B. de Souza. 1990. The malaria vaccine: anti-parasite or anti-disease? Immunology Today 11:25-27.

Posner, J. B., and F. Plum. 1967. Independence of blood and cerebrospinal fluid lactate. Archives of Neurology 16:492-496.

Rey, M., A. Nouhouayi, and D. Dio Mar. 1966. Les expressions cliniques du paladisme à *plasmodium falciparum* chez l'enfant noir Africain (d'apres une experience hospitaliere dakaroise). Bulletin de la Societe de Pathologie Exotique et de Ses Filiales 59:688-704.

Rieckmann, K. H., D. R. Davis, and D. C. Hutton. 1989. *Plasmodium vivax* resistance to chloroquine? Lancet 2:1183-1184.

Roncoroni, A. J., and O. A. Martino. 1979. Therapeutic use of exchange transfusion in malaria. American Journal of Tropical Medicine and Hygiene 28:440-444.

Sitprija, V. 1988. Nephropathy in falciparum malaria [clinical conference]. Kidney International 34:867-877.

Stace, J., P. Bilton, K. Coates, and N. Stace. 1982. Cerebral malaria in children: a retrospective study of admissions to Madang Hospital, 1980. Papua New Guinea Medical Journal 25:230-234.

Steketee, R. W., J. G. Breman, K. M. Paluku, M. Moore, J. Roy, and M. Ma-Disu. 1988. Malaria infection in pregnant women in Zaire: the effects and potential for intervention. Annals of Tropical Medicine and Parasitology 82:113-120.

Taylor, T. E., M. E. Molyneux, J. J. Wirima, K. A. Fletcher, and K. Morris. 1988. Blood glucose levels in Malawian children before and during the administration of intravenous quinine for severe falciparum malaria. New England Journal of Medicine 319:1040-1047.

Tracey, K. J., B. Beutler, S. F. Lowry, J. Merryweather, S. Wolpe, I. W. Milserk, R. J. Hariri, T. J. Fahey III, A. Zentella, J. D. Albert, G. T. Shires, and A. Cerami. 1986. Shock and tissue injury induced by recombinant human cachectin. Science 234:470-474.

Waller, D., S. Krishna, C. Craddock, D. Brewster, A. Jammeh, D. Kwiatkowski, J. Karbwang, P. Molunto, and N. J. White. 1990. The pharmacokinetic properties of intramuscular quinine in Gambian children with severe falciparum malaria. Transactions of the Royal Society of Tropical Medicine and Hygiene 84:488-491.

Warrell, D. A. 1987. Pathophysiology of severe falciparum malaria in man. Parasitology 94(Suppl.):S53-S76.

Warrell, D. A., S. Looareesuwan, M. J. Warrell, P. Kasemsarn, R. Intaraprasert, D. Bunnag, and T. Harinasuta. 1982. Dexamethasone proves deleterious in cerebral malaria. A double-blind trial in 100 comatose patients. New England Journal of Medicine 306:313-319.

White, N. J., S. Looareesuwan, D. A. Warrell, M. J. Warrell, P. Chanthavanich, D. Bunnag, and T. Harinasuta. 1983a. Quinine loading dose in cerebral malaria. American Journal of Tropical Medicine and Hygiene 32:1-5.

White, N. J., D. A. Warrell, P. Chanthavanich, S. Looareesuwan, M. J. Warrell, S. Krishna, D. H. Williamson, and R. C. Turner. 1983b. Severe hypoglycemia and hyperinsulinemia in falciparum malaria. New England Journal of Medicine 309:61-66.

White, N. J., D. A. Warrell, S. Looareesuwan, P. Chantavanich, R. C. Phillips, and P. Pongpaew. 1985. Pathophysiological and prognostic significance of cerebrospinal-fluid lactate in cerebral malaria. Lancet 1:776-778.

White, N. J., S. Looareesuwan, R. E. Phillips, P. Chanthavanich, and D. A. Warrell. 1988. Single dose phenobarbitone prevents convulsions in cerebral malaria. Lancet 2:64-66.

World Health Organization. 1990. Severe and complicated malaria, 2nd edition. Transactions of the Royal Society of Tropical Medicine and Hygiene 84(Suppl. 2):1-65.

Yarrish, R. L., J. S. Janas, J. S. Nosanchuk, R. T. Steigbigel, and J. Nusbacher. 1982. Transfusion malaria: treatment with exchange transfusion after delayed diagnosis. Archives of Internal Medicine 142:187-188.

5

Diagnostic Tests

WHERE WE WANT TO BE IN THE YEAR 2010

There will be new appreciation of the need for different malaria diagnostics at various levels of the health care system. Malaria assays will be available—each tailored to a distinct setting—that will supplement microscopy for diagnosing malaria. Microscopic examination of blood films, when used, will be simpler and more accurate as a result of improved equipment and protocols and because microscopists will be better trained. Most of the new malaria diagnostic tests will be inexpensive and simple to use, and they will provide results in less than an hour. Each will be sensitive to low parasitemias and will be able to distinguish among different parasite species. Nearly all of the assays will depend on minimally invasive specimen collection techniques (a disposable lancet for finger-prick blood sampling will be universally used in the field, greatly decreasing concerns about transmitting AIDS and hepatitis B) and will be able to be batched for high-volume diagnostic situations. Mass screening of blood slides, which often results in large backlogs of unread slides, will give way to focused and well-planned surveys of malaria prevalence. Finally, tests will soon be marketed that distinguish between the presence of parasites and the presence of disease in semi-immune individuals, and other tests will be developed that will identify those patients at risk of progressing to severe illness.

WHERE WE ARE TODAY

The most important role for malaria diagnostics is to help health care workers, whether they be in a village in Mali or in a sophisticated hospital in New York City, select the most appropriate treatment for patients whose illness may be due to infection with malaria parasites. Since the symptoms of malaria vary and can resemble those of other diseases, diagnosing malaria solely on the basis of clinical symptoms is unreliable. If evidence of malaria is found, particularly in nonimmune individuals, rapid and appropriate therapy is essential to prevent further progression of the disease. Alternatively, if parasites are absent, other explanations for the symptoms must be sought so that appropriate treatment can be started and the use of toxic antimalarial drugs can be avoided.

The simple microscopic diagnostic tests available today have two drawbacks, even when performed correctly. In patients who live in malarious areas and who are partially immune to the disease, malaria infections may be asymptomatic and of little clinical significance. The presence of parasites in such patients cannot be assumed to cause the symptoms of an illness, which may have other causes. There is currently no diagnostic to associate malaria infection with disease in such patients. In addition, repeated blood films may be necessary to detect malaria parasites in nonimmune patients, in whom symptoms can arise from very low parasitemias. Failure to detect parasites in a single blood film from such a patient (for instance, an American recently returned from a malarious area) cannot be used to exclude a diagnosis of malaria.

Diagnostic tests are also important for certain types of epidemiologic surveys. Used for this purpose, rapidity and pinpoint accuracy are not as critical as the need for the safe collection, preparation, and evaluation of a large number of samples. Because of the danger of transmitting other diseases, such as AIDS or hepatitis B, through the use of contaminated lancets, the collection of blood samples raises significant biosafety issues. In addition, the transportation and examination of blood slides for epidemiologic surveys can be both cumbersome and logistically difficult, particularly in remote areas. In many countries, there is a backlog of slides to be examined, and results may not be available for many months. The relevance of out-of-date results to the planning and evaluation of malaria field operations is questionable.

Currently, the "gold standard" for diagnosing malaria in individual patients and for epidemiologic surveys is the microscopic examination of blood smears. The presence of malaria parasites, identified by their characteristic morphology, is considered definitive proof of infection. A number of potential improvements to current microscopic methods and alternatives to microscopy for diagnosing malaria are discussed below.

Microscopy

Standard Technique

Microscopy is the most widely used laboratory-based diagnostic test for malaria, and it likely will remain the test of choice for some time. In this technique, two drops of blood, typically obtained from a finger pricked by a metal lancet, are placed on a glass microscope slide. One drop is smeared to create a thin blood film, the other drop (the thick film) is left alone, and the slide is allowed to air-dry. The cells in the thin blood smear are chemically fixed to the slide, and the slide is stained with Giemsa or some other stain formulation to facilitate detection of parasites. The water in the staining solution lyses the unfixed red blood cells in the thick blood film, removing the hemoglobin, and white blood cells and any malaria parasites are fixed to the slide.

The thick blood film allows the microscopist to look for parasites in a relatively large volume of blood, thus increasing the sensitivity of the test. The thin blood film, which better preserves parasite morphology, is used to quantify and identify parasites to the species level, if necessary. A high-power microscope (400 times to 1,000 times magnification, with an oil immersion objective) is required to read thick and thin blood films. Between 100 and 200 microscope fields must be examined to rule out the presence of parasites in a thick blood film.

The ability to detect infection by microscopy depends on the number of fields inspected and the experience of the technician reading the slide. An experienced microscopist can evaluate and make a diagnosis from a slide from a heavily parasitized individual within about a minute; additional time is required to detect parasites on a blood film from a lightly parasitized individual (Payne, 1988).

Microscopy has proved to be a tremendously resilient and useful diagnostic tool, but it is not without problems. The cost of materials (slides and staining reagents) is relatively low, but substantial investment is required to purchase microscopes and to select and train technicians; additional funds are needed for maintenance of the microscopes. Microscopy is labor-intensive, and a high level of technical skill is required for correct preparation and interpretation of slides. This means that the workload of each technician must be monitored, since fatigue or the pressure to return results can lead to a significant loss of efficiency and accuracy. In addition, many microscopes in the field, through age, deterioration, and hard use, are nearing or are at the end of their useful working lives. High-quality microscopes are expensive and often beyond the means of regional health outposts. Few if any peripheral health facilities have access to sturdy and portable microscopes required for field use.

Quantitative Buffy Coat Technique

The quantitative buffy coat (QBC) technique is a commercially available test based on fluorescence microscopy (Wardlaw and Levine, 1983). The test uses a specially made glass capillary tube of precise internal diameter containing acridine orange as a vital stain. After the tube is filled with blood, it is capped and a small plastic float is inserted. The float displaces precisely 90 percent of the interior tube space along its length, and when centrifuged, settles at the plasma-red blood cell interface, physically expanding the length of the buffy coat layer 10-fold. White blood cell components appear as discrete bands and can be accurately quantified with a specially designed optical device.

The float also extends into and expands the top portion of the red blood cell layer where the parasitized red blood cells, because of their lower density, are concentrated. The centrifuged tube is observed directly, using a fluorescence microscope. Since the contrast between stain and background is high, parasitized red blood cells are easily seen.

QBC Versus Microscopy

QBC is a relatively new technique, and the limits of its sensitivity and specificity are still being explored. In a study in Ethiopia, microscopists detected 10 percent more infections by QBC than by conventional slide methods (Spielman et al., 1988). By contrast, a similar study of QBC in Thailand found the technique to be only marginally more sensitive than conventional microscopy and of acceptable specificity (Tharavanij, 1990). Another study found QBC to be as sensitive as microscopy in experimentally infected volunteers, highly sensitive when used to diagnose malaria infection in hospital patients, but less sensitive than microscopy when used for mass screening (Rickman et al., 1989).

QBC is a quick and efficient method of processing batches of blood specimens. Its advantage in this regard is less apparent, however, when a microscopist who is an expert at interpreting blood smears for malaria infection is available. In resource-limited settings, the cost of the capillary tubes and the need for additional equipment, such as a centrifuge and fluorescence microscope, make QBC less attractive. Most facilities in malaria-endemic countries do not have access to fluorescence microscopes.

Alternatives to Microscopy

There is a recognized need for dependable alternatives to diagnostic microscopy for detecting the presence of malaria infection. Tests that are as simple and accurate as microscopy but that require less sophisticated equipment and training would be particularly valuable in field settings. In addition, the medical community's lack of experience in the use of microscopy to diagnose malaria in the United States (and other more developed countries) makes alternative tests potentially valuable for use in domestic hospitals. Research efforts to identify malaria parasite antigens and genes, which could provide the basis for such tests, have spurred the development of a number of new diagnostic methods, through the use of monoclonal antibodies and recombinant DNA techniques, which have been reviewed in detail elsewhere (Bruce-Chwatt, 1987; World Health Organization, 1988; Pammenter, 1988; Wirth et al., 1989; Tharavanij, 1990). These assays are designed to detect specific parasite antigens or nucleic acids with limits of detection equal to or better than that provided by microscopy.

The development of many initially promising assays often has languished because of the difficulty of reproducing the results of laboratory research in field trials. Development has also been slowed by the challenge of creating a simple assay and because improved diagnostic tests have not been a priority for public funding in malaria research.

Immunoassays

Immunological techniques that detect malaria parasite antigens have been described since the early 1980s. These tests would be useful in health care facilities where microscopy is not performed, and they could supplement or replace microscopy in other settings. Antigen detection techniques would also be useful epidemiologic tools, providing data for community-based public health intervention measures.

Ideal target antigens for immunological assays should not persist in the blood (or in other specimens, such as urine that might be tested) after the parasite disappears, should be abundant in blood or other clinical specimens to maximize test sensitivity, and should be genus and species specific, without cross-reactivity with host antigens or antigens from other microorganisms (World Health Organization, 1988).

Experimental tests for detecting malaria parasite antigens are based on both antigen-competition and antigen-capture formats, using both enzyme-linked immunosorbent assay (ELISA) and radioimmunoassay (RIA) methods. Researchers have described the use of both monoclonal antibodies and polyclonal antisera in assays for genus-specific antigens, such as those that cross-react with *Plasmodium berghei* (Avidor et al., 1985), undefined *P. falciparum* antigens (Mackey et al., 1982; Avraham et al., 1983; Khusmith et al., 1987), and defined malarial antigens (Fortier et al., 1987), and in idiotype-anti-idiotype detection systems (Zhou and Li, 1987).

Studies of RIA- and ELISA-based tests have demonstrated detection of very low densities of parasitized red blood cells (in the range of 0.01 to

0.001 percent, equivalent to 50 to 500 parasites per microliter of blood), with RIA techniques being slightly more sensitive on average. In general, therefore, the limits of detection of immunoassay techniques approach that of microscopy (which is able to discern 10 to 20 parasites per microliter of blood). The value of RIA methods for both immunoassays and probes (see Genetic-Probe Assays, below) has in the past been to verify that laboratory tests can be developed by using certain combinations of reagents and malarial antigens. However, because RIAs employ radioisotopes that have short shelf lives and are costly and potentially dangerous, they are impractical for routine clinical use, even at the central-hospital level in the developing world. In addition, laboratory personnel have considerably more experience and training in the application of ELISA methods, especially since the start of the AIDS epidemic. Although diagnostic ELISA kits have been used successfully at many well-equipped central health care facilities and in support of epidemiologic or vaccine programs, they are not suited for use in outlying areas where equipment is lacking. The minimum of two to four hours needed to perform an ELISA, and the desirability of testing large numbers of specimens at one time, means that same-day results may not always be available. This is not, however, a problem in large epidemiologic studies, in which same-day results are rarely required.

Antigen Inhibition and Competition   In antigen-inhibition and antigen-competition assays, parasite antigens are coated on a surface, such as a microwell plate. The test specimen is centrifuged, and the red blood cells are washed and lysed to extract parasite antigen. The specimen is then mixed with a high-titer serum or monoclonal antibody and placed in the well containing test antigen. If the specimen contains parasite antigens, they will bind to the antimalaria antibodies, thus preventing the antibodies from binding to the antigens on the plate. After rinsing, the amount of antibody bound to the plate is determined by standard RIA or ELISA techniques (Khusmith et al., 1987).

Antigen Capture   In antigen-capture (antibody-sandwich) assays, polyclonal or monoclonal antibody is adsorbed to a tube or microwell plate. The specimen is placed into the test vessel and, after washing, a second antibody source conjugated with an enzyme or radioactive label is added. If malarial antigens are present, they serve as a bridge between the antibodies in the tube or well of the plate and the labeled antibodies. The plate is then processed by RIA or ELISA as described above, and the amount of labeling is quantified. Antigen-capture assays may prove to be more practical than antigen-competition assays for diagnosing malaria. Unlike competition assays, capture methods do not require purified malarial antigens and have a greater potential for detecting a broader range of antigens. In addition, competition assays usually require centrifugation to separate red blood cells from autologous serum antibodies that can interfere with the assay and produce false-positive results. This requirement for specimen processing makes performing large numbers of competition assays time-consuming and limits the technique's usefulness in the field.

Soluble Antigens Researchers have identified soluble, parasite-specific antigens in sera from persons infected with malarial parasites (McGregor et al., 1968; Bein and Olcen, 1984; Taylor et al., 1986). Assays have been developed that target some of these antigens (Fortier et al., 1987; Parra and Taylor, 1989). The advantage of assays that detect soluble antigens is that plasma from uncoagulated whole blood can be used without extracting the red blood cells or pretreating the specimen. This type of assay system should be able to diagnosis malaria even in the absence of circulating infected red blood cells, a situation sometimes found in cerebral malaria cases.

Genetic-Probe Assays

Genetic-probe assays utilize DNA hybridization to detect parasite-specific nucleic acid sequences in red blood cell specimen extracts. Typically, red blood cells are lysed to extract nucleic acids either before or after being fixed on a filter membrane. The membrane is heated to denature the nucleic acids, blocked with nonspecific DNA, and incubated with a specific radiolabeled or biotinylated probe. Although biotinylated probes have been used most often, other modified bases are available. The membranes are then washed and developed, either by autoradiography or by enzyme-substrate labeling. Ideally, these assays could serve as single-use diagnostics and be capable of being batched for higher volume epidemiologic or public health applications.

Whole *P. falciparum* DNA derived from laboratory-cultured organisms has been radiolabeled in vitro to produce a species-specific test. The entire genome was used as a probe, and the resulting assay had a sensitivity equivalent to that of microscopy (Pollack et al., 1985). Although sensitive, such tests have a low specificity, do not allow identification of parasites to the species level, and may cross-react with human DNA. The time needed to complete the assay (usually 24 to 48 hours) and the requirement to prepare large quantities of radiolabeled probes from cultured organisms are additional drawbacks. Some researchers have used cloned DNA fragments as genetic probes (Franzen et al., 1984; Zolg et al., 1987). Others have used synthetic oligonucleotides from genomic regions containing conserved, 21-base-pair tandem repeat sequences (Barker et al., 1986; Holmberg et al., 1986; McLaughlin et al., 1987a,b; Sethabutr et al., 1988). The repeat sequences which they target are found in abundance in parasite DNA (10^4 to 10^5 copies per nucleus). Tests of the 21-oligonucleotide repeat probe in clinical trials in Thailand and Kenya revealed a sensitivity of between 82 and 89 percent and a specificity of between 99 and 94 percent, respectively, compared with microscopy (Barker et al., 1989a,b). Others, using a similar oligonucleotide probe, claim 100 percent specificity and sensitivity of 68 percent (Holmberg et al., 1987). With low levels of parasitemia, however, current DNA probes are less sensitive than microscopy (Lanar et al., 1989).

Probes using ribosomal RNA (rRNA) have been used to identify various microorganisms, including plasmodia, since each parasite species has distinct small subunit rRNA nucleotide sequences (Lal et al., 1989; Waters and McCutchan, 1989). Because rRNA constitutes between 85 and 95 percent of the total parasite complement of nucleic acid, synthetic rRNA oligonucleotide probes promise to be very sensitive. Data on rRNA probes specific for all four human *Plasmodium* species have been reported, but they have not been validated on clinical samples (Waters and McCutchan, 1989).

For all nucleic acid-based probes, radiolabeling has produced the greatest sensitivity. However, radioisotope-based assays are impractical for field use because of cost, short shelf life, hazards, and the complex equipment required. To overcome this problem, colorimetric probes are being developed and field tested (McLaughlin et al., 1987a). These probes bind enzyme-avidin conjugates and use ELISA-type enzyme-substrate systems to generate signals. Unfortunately, the hybridization procedure is complex, making it cumbersome in the field. Even the best enzyme-probe systems require equipment not often available outside of central health facilities, such as a slot-blot apparatus, vacuum pump, constant-temperature water bath or incubator, and oven, in addition to standard laboratory glassware.

Polymerase Chain Reaction

Technologies that can amplify specific sequences of DNA offer great potential when applied to the diagnosis of malaria. The polymerase chain reaction (PCR) method, for example, amplifies specific DNA segments by repeated cycles of heat denaturation, annealing with defined DNA primer pairs, and primer extension mediated by heat-resistant DNA polymerase isolated from a thermophilic bacterium. Polymerase chain reaction techniques require 25 to 30 rounds of amplification, which take three to four hours. Electrical power is needed to run a thermal cycler, and the reagents are relatively expensive. There is a recent report of an ELISA-type assay for PCR products, making the detection of PCR results at least theoretically possible in less developed settings (Nickerson et al., 1990). The technique offers a hypothetical sensitivity limit of a single malaria gene per specimen, but in practice it requires 10 to 100 gene copies.

Problems with contamination from parasite DNA that was not originally in the sample and difficulties in specimen processing need to be resolved before PCR can be used routinely as a diagnostic tool. In addition, personnel who perform the test must be highly trained, and the costs of PCR thermal cyclers and materials remain high. Improvements in PCR technology, such as rapid sample preparation, packaging of reagents to prevent cross-contamination, and the development of nonradioactive signal systems, are bringing the technique closer to the stage where it will be of practical use. The PCR technique has been used to diagnose malaria infection with DNA primers specific for *P. falciparum* and *P. vivax* (W. J. Martin, University of Southern California Medical Center, unpublished data, 1991). By sequencing the dihydrofolate reductase gene associated with pyrimethamine resistance, specific primer sequences have been identified that react with the mutant gene but not the wild-type gene. These sequences potentially could be used for clinical diagnosis, identification of the parasite to the species level, and determination of pyrimethamine resistance.

Unless results can be accurately quantified and correlated with parasitemia, PCR may not be the test of choice in areas where malaria is endemic and where the majority of inhabitants harbor low levels of parasites without disease. The optimal use of PCR may be in sophisticated clinical laboratories in developed countries that have expertise in using complex technology but are unable to maintain competency in malaria microscopy. PCR may also be useful as an epidemiologic tool. For example, the technique could be used to determine the extent of falciparum malaria in an area of mixed infection and to identify drug-resistant strains in patient specimens or in mosquitoes.

Antibody Assays

Serological assays can detect antimalarial antibodies but cannot determine whether the antibodies result from current or past infection. Therefore, such assays are not appropriate for diagnosis but can be used for certain epidemiologic applications (Voller and Draper, 1982).

Several assay methods, including indirect immunofluorescence, hemagglutination, ELISA, and avidin-biotin-peroxidase complex ELISA, have been tested for their ability to diagnose malaria. Assays have been developed to measure antibodies to crude parasite antigens (Demedts et al., 1987; Sato et al., 1990); antigamete antibodies, which may influence parasite infectivity (Mendis et al., 1987); antibodies to merozoite surface antigen 1, which may indicate acute infection (Früh et al., 1989); and antibodies to circumsporozoite proteins as a broad screen for malaria prevalence (Wirtz et al., 1987). Comparison of the sensitivities and specificities of these assays has been difficult since the various protocols and antigen extracts have not been standardized.

To overcome the difficulties associated with producing a standardized, contaminant-free supply of antigen, recombinant DNA techniques have been used to identify, clone, and express or synthesize epitopes of parasite proteins. Among these are the asparagine-alanine-asparagine-proline (NANP) repeat sequences of the *P. falciparum* circumsporozoite protein (Del Giudice et al., 1987; Knobloch et al., 1987). Synthetic peptide antigen generated by these amino acid repeat sequences was used to develop an ELISA method that identified 80 percent of the sera shown to contain *P. falciparum* antibodies by RIA (Zavala et al., 1986). A commercial ELISA kit that uses NANP as the antigen has also been developed (Esposito et al., 1990).

Other Assays

Assays that detect antibodies are generally easier to develop than those that detect antigens. There are a number of potentially simple, inexpensive antigen-based assay systems that may be used to diagnose malaria. These include latex bead agglutination, solid-phase dipstick, membrane dot-blot, and hemagglutination. At present, these tests offer generally lower sensitivity and cost in exchange for increased speed and convenience. Although in certain instances sensitivity may be less critical than speed and ease of use, a decision to use one of these tests as a replacement for microscopy should be given careful consideration.

One of the more promising rapid diagnostic methods that should be evaluated for use in malaria is the autologous red blood cell agglutination assay (Kemp et al., 1988). The technology, developed for detecting antibodies to the AIDS virus, utilizes a functionally univalent antibody reagent that binds to but does not agglutinate human red blood cells. A selected monoclonal antibody or polyclonal antiserum is then chemically conjugated to a monoclonal antibody reagent. When mixed with whole blood, the monoclonal antibody conjugates bind to the red blood cells, which then agglutinate if antigen is present. This assay, potentially rapid, simple, and inexpensive, may also be used to detect serum antibodies in whole blood by conjugating the monoclonal antibody to a specific antigen.

Specifications for Diagnostic Tests

The needs of those who use diagnostic tests must be considered when new assays are developed. Table 5-1 summarizes a set of test specifications for various categories of users. Biotechnology companies, university

TABLE 5-1 Suggested Specifications for Malaria Diagnostic Tests

	Level of Care[a]				
Desired Quality of Diagnostic Test	1	2	3	4	5
Identify specimen as positive or negative for malaria	+	+	+	+	+
Identify *Plasmodium falciparum*	+	+	+	+	+
Identify other human *Plasmodium* species	-	+	+	+	+
Estimate parasite density	-	+	+	+	-
Use whole blood	+	+	-	-	-
Use small sample volume (no venipuncture)	+	-	-	-	+
Be easily transportable	+	-	-	-	+
Not require electricity	+	+	-	-	+
Provide results in less than one hour	+	+[b]	+	+	-
Be simple to perform	+	+	+	+	-
Have long reagent shelf life at ambient temperatures	+	+	+[b]	-	+
Be sensitive	+[c]	+[c]	+[c]	+[c]	+
Be highly specific	-	+	-	-	-
Be inexpensive	+	+	+[d]	-	-
Be amenable to batch processing	-	-	-	-	+
Provide a simple means of specimen collection	-	-	-	-	+
Be easily labeled	-	-	-	-	+
Differentiate between asexual and sexual forms	-	-	-	-	+
Provide a quantitative readout (high/medium/low)	-	-	-	-	+

[a]1 = Village level; 2 = health clinic; 3 = district hospital; 4 = central hospital; 5 = epidemiologic survey.
[b]Refrigeration may be available at this level of care.
[c]Important if nonimmune populations are being tested.
[d]Of somewhat less importance at this level than at levels 1 and 2.

researchers, and others contemplating the development of new malaria diagnostics or the improvement of existing tests may find these parameters useful.

Evaluation of Diagnostic Tests

A diagnostic test should correctly differentiate between individuals who are infected and those who are not. The validity of a diagnostic test is usually determined by its sensitivity and specificity (Table 5-2). *Sensitivity* indicates the probability that a test is positive, given that the individual tested is indeed infected. As the sensitivity of a test increases, the number of false negatives (individuals who are infected but test negative) will decrease. *Specificity* indicates the probability an individual will test negative, given that he or she does not have the disease. As the specificity of a test increases, the number of false positives (individuals incorrectly classified as being infected) will decrease. In short, a highly sensitive test is very good at identifying those who are infected; a highly specific test is very good at identifying those who are not infected.

TABLE 5-2   Two-by-Two Table for Determining
Diagnostic Test Characteristics

	Disease Status		
Category	Positive	Negative	Total
Test result			
Positive	TP	FP	TP+FP
Negative	FN	TN	FN+TN
Total	TP+FN	FP+TN	N

Abbreviations: TP, true positive; FP, false positive; FN, false nega-
tive; TN, true negative.
Formulas for calculating test characteristics:
 Sensitivity (true-positive rate) = TP/(TP+FN) = $P(T^+/D^+)$
 Specificity (true-negative rate) = TN/(FP+TN) = $P(T^-/D^-)$
 Positive predictive value = PV^+ = P(disease/$test^+$) = TP/(TP+FP)
 Negative predictive value = PV^- = P(no disease/$test^-$) = TN/(FN+TN)
Multiply answers from the formulas by 100 to obtain percent.

In large epidemiologic surveys, it is more important to determine the
probability that a person who tests positive is indeed infected than it is to
know the sensitivity or specificity of an individual test. As illustrated in
Table 5-3, the positive predictive value of a diagnostic test with a fixed
sensitivity and specificity will vary according to the prevalence of a disease
in a given population.

Example: A diagnostic test with a sensitivity of 95 percent and a
specificity of 90 percent is applied to 1,000 people in each of two areas.
The prevalence of malaria infection is estimated to be 10 percent in area
A (see Table 5-3, Example 1) and 50 percent in area B (see Table 5-3,
Example 2).

As can be seen, in test area A, where the prevalence of malaria is 10
percent, the chance of correctly detecting malaria infection (positive predictive value) with the assay in question is slightly better than 50 percent,
while for area B it is over 90 percent. The probability that someone who
tests negative is indeed malaria free (negative predictive value) is high for
both areas. Clearly, knowledge of disease prevalence is crucial to assessing
the predictive value of any diagnostic technique. (It is possible to increase
a test's positive predictive value by boosting its specificity. For example,
if the specificity of the diagnostic assay in Table 5-3 were increased to 97
percent, the positive predictive value would rise to 77.8 percent.)

RESEARCH AGENDA

In situations where skilled microscopists have access to functioning microscopes and reagents for preparing and staining blood films, microscopy

TABLE 5-3 Sample Determinations of Diagnostic Test Characteristics

Category	Disease Status[a]		Total
	Positive	Negative	
Example 1[b]			
Test result			
Positive	95	90	185
Result	5	810	815
Total	100	900	1,000
Example 2[c]			
Test result			
Positive	475	50	525
Negative	25	450	475
Total	500	500	1,000

[a]Example 1—disease prevalence is 10%; Example 2—disease prevalence is 50%
[b]Sensitivity = 95/100 = 0.95 = 95%; Specificity = 810/900 = 0.90 = 90%; Positive predictive value = 95/185 = 0.514 = 51.4%; Negative predictive value = 810/815 = 0.994 = 99.4%
[c]Sensitivity = 475/500 = 0.95 = 95%; Specificity = 450/500 = 0.90 = 90%; Positive predictive value = 475/525 = 0.905 = 90.5%; Negative predictive value = 450/475 = 0.947 = 94.7%

is still the gold standard of malaria diagnosis. There are circumstances in which new diagnostic techniques would be useful, however. Health care workers in remote villages and poorly equipped clinics would benefit from simpler diagnostic tests.

RESEARCH FOCUS: Development of parasite antigen- or nucleic acid-based detection methods that use finger-prick blood samples and require no electricity and no complicated or expensive equipment.

Health care workers in nonendemic areas, where malaria occurs primarily in nonimmune individuals who become symptomatic at very low levels of parasitemia, would benefit from diagnostic methods that do not require parasites to be identified by microscopic morphology.

RESEARCH FOCUS: Development of parasite antigen- or nucleic acid-based diagnostics with limits of detection equivalent to or better than those of standard microscopy and that rely on clear-cut instrument interpretation or readouts.

Epidemiologists trying to determine the prevalence of malaria infection in a population would benefit from diagnostic tests that are less labor-intensive than standard microscopy.

RESEARCH FOCUS: Development of parasite antigen- or nucleic acid-based detection methods that collect finger-prick blood samples for later batch processing and that are inexpensive and easy to perform.

REFERENCES

Avidor, B., J. Golenser, and D. Sulitzeanu. 1985. Detection of *Plasmodium falciparum* using a radioimmunoassay based on a crossreacting, monoclonal anti-*P. berghei* antibody-*P. berghei* antigen system. Journal of Immunological Methods 82:121-129.

Avraham, H., J. Golenser, D. Bunnag, P. Suntharasamai, S. Tharavanij, K. T. Harinasuta, D. T. Spira, and D. Sulitzeanu. 1983. Preliminary field trial of a radioimmunoassay for the diagnosis of malaria. American Journal of Tropical Medicine and Hygiene 32:11-18.

Barker, R. H. Jr., L. Suebsaeng, W. Rooney, G. C. Alecrim, H. V. Duorado, and D. F. Wirth. 1986. Specific DNA probe for the diagnosis of *Plasmodium falciparum* malaria. Science 231:1434-1436.

Barker, R. H. Jr., A. D. Brandling-Bennett, D. K. Koech, M. Mugambi, B. Khan, R. David, J. R. David, and D. F. Wirth. 1989a. *Plasmodium falciparum*: DNA probe diagnosis of malaria in Kenya. Experimental Parasitology 69:226-233.

Barker, R. H. Jr., L. Suebsaeng, W. Rooney, and D. F. Wirth. 1989b. Detection of *Plasmodium falciparum* infection in human patients: a comparison of the DNA probe method to microscopic diagnosis. American Journal of Tropical Medicine and Hygiene 41:266-272.

Bein, K., and P. Olcen. 1984. Detection of malaria antigens in urine using a solid-phase radioimmunoassay: preliminary study. Ethiopian Medical Journal 22:119-127.

Bruce-Chwatt, L. J. 1987. From Laveran's discovery to DNA probes: new trends in diagnosis of malaria. Lancet 2:1509-1511.

Del Giudice, G., A. S. Verdini, M. Pinori, A. Pessi, J.-P. Verhave, C. Tougne, B. Ivanoff, P.-H. Lambert, and H. D. Engers. 1987. Detection of human antibodies against *Plasmodium falciparum* sporozoites using synthetic peptides. Journal of Clinical Microbiology 25:91-96.

Demedts, P., C. Vermuelen-Van Overmeir, and M. Wery. 1987. Simultaneous use of *Plasmodium falciparum* crude antigen and red blood cell control antigen in the enzyme-linked immunosorbent assay for malaria. American Journal of Tropical Medicine and Hygiene 36:257-263.

Esposito, F., P. Fabrizi, A. Provvedi, P. Tarli, A. Habluetzel, and S. Lombardi. 1990. Evaluation of an ELISA kit for epidemiological detection of antibodies to *Plasmodium falciparum* sporozoites in human sera and bloodspot eluates. Acta Tropica 47:1-10.

Fortier, B., P. Delplace, J. F. Dubremetz, F. Ajana, and A. Vernes. 1987. Enzyme immunoassay for detection of antigen in acute *Plasmodium falciparum* malaria. European Journal of Clinical Microbiology 6:596-598.

Franzen, L., G. Westin, R. Shabo, L. Aslund, H. Perlmann, T. Persson, H. Wigzell, and U. Petterson. 1984. Analysis of clinical specimens by hybridisation with probe containing repetitive DNA from *Plasmodium falciparum*: a novel approach to malaria diagnosis. Lancet 1:525-527.

Früh, K., H.-M. Muller, H. Bujard, and A. Crisanti. 1989. A new tool for the serodiagnosis of acute *Plasmodium falciparum* malaria in individuals with primary infection. Journal of Immunological Methods 122:25-32.

Holmberg, M., A. Bjorkman, L. Franzen, L. Aslund, M. Lebbad, U. Pettersson, and H. Wiggzell. 1986. Diagnosis of *Plasmodium falciparum* infection by spot hybridization assay: specificity, sensitivity, and field applicability. Bulletin of the World Health Organization 64:579-585.

Holmberg, M., F. C. Shenton, L. Franzen, K. Janneh, R. W. Snow, U. Pettersson, H. Wigzell, and B. M. Greenwood. 1987. Use of a DNA hybridization assay for the detection of *Plasmodium falciparum* in field trials. American Journal of Tropical Medicine and Hygiene 37:230-234.

Kemp, B. E., D. B. Rylatt, P. G. Bundesen, R. R. Doherty, D. A. McPhee, D. Stapleton, L. E. Cottis, K. Wilson, M. A. John, J. M. Khan, D. P. Dinh, S. Miles, and C. J. Hillyard. 1988. Autologous red cell agglutination assay for HIV-1 antibodies: simplified test with whole blood. Science 241:1352-1354.

Khusmith, S., S. Tharavanij, R. Kasemsuth, C. Vejvongvarn, and D. Bunnag. 1987. Two-site immunoradiometric assay for detection of *Plasmodium falciparum* antigen in blood using monoclonal and polyclonal antibodies. Journal of Clinical Microbiology 25:1467-1471.

Knobloch, J., M. Schreiber, S. Grokhovsky, and A. Scherrf. 1987. Specific and nonspecific immunodiagnostic properties of recombinant and synthetic *Plasmodium falciparum* antigens. European Journal of Clinical Microbiology 6:547-551.

Lal, A. A., S. Changkasiri, M. R. Hollingdale, and T. F. McCutchan. 1989. Ribosomal RNA-based diagnosis of *Plasmodium falciparum* malaria. Molecular and Biochemical Parasitology 36:67-72.

Lanar, D. E., G. L. McLaughlin, D. F. Wirth, R. J. Barker, J. W. Zolg, and J. D. Chulay. 1989. Comparison of thick films, in vitro culture and DNA hybridization probes for detecting *Plasmodium falciparum* malaria. American Journal of Tropical Medicine and Hygiene 40:3-6.

Mackey, L. J., I. A. McGregor, N. Paounova, and P. H. Lambert. 1982. Diagnosis of *Plasmodium falciparum* infection in man: detection of parasite antigens by ELISA. Bulletin of the World Health Organization 60:69-75.

McGregor, I. A., M. W. Turner, K. Williams, and P. Hall. 1968. Soluble antigens in the blood of African patients with severe *Plasmodium falciparum* malaria. Lancet 1:881-884.

McLaughlin, G. L., W. E. Collins, and G. H. Campbell. 1987a. Comparison of genomic, plasmid, synthetic, and combined DNA probes for detecting *Plasmodium falciparum* DNA. Journal of Clinical Microbiology 25:791-795.

McLaughlin, G. L., J. L. Ruth, E. Jablonski, R. Steketee, and G. H. Campbell.

1987b. Use of enzyme-linked synthetic DNA in diagnosis of falciparum malaria. Lancet 1:714-716.

Mendis, K. N., Y. D. Munesinghe, Y. N. Y. deSilva, I. Keragalla, and R. Carter. 1987. Malaria transmission-blocking immunity induced by natural infections of *Plasmodium vivax* in humans. Infection and Immunity 55:369-372.

Nickerson, D. A., R. Kaiser, S. Lappin, J. Stewart, L. Hood, and U. Landergen. 1990. Automated DNA diagnostics using an ELISA-based oligonucleotide ligation assay. Proceedings of the National Academy of Sciences of the United States of America 87:8923-8927.

Pammenter, M. D. 1988. Techniques for the diagnosis of malaria. South African Medical Journal 74(2):55-57.

Parra, M. E., and D. W. Taylor. 1989. Presence of histidine-rich protein 2 (Pf HRP-2) in the sera of people infected with *Plasmodium falciparum*. Abstract 262 from the program of the 38th Annual Meeting of the American Society of Tropical Medicine and Hygiene, Honolulu, Hawaii.

Payne, D. 1988. Use and limitations of light microscopy for diagnosing malaria at the primary health care level. Bulletin of the World Health Organization 66:621-626.

Pollack, Y., S. Metzger, R. Shemer, D. Landau, D. T. Spira, and J. Golenser. 1985. Detection of *Plasmodium falciparum* in blood using DNA hybridization. American Journal of Tropical Medicine and Hygiene 34:663-667.

Rickman, L. S., G. W. Long, R. Oberst, A. Cabanban, R. Sangalang, J. I. Smith, J. D. Chulay, and S. L. Hoffman. 1989. Rapid diagnosis of malaria by acridine orange staining of centrifuged parasites. Lancet 1:68-71.

Sato, K., S. Kano, H. Yamaguchi, F. M. Omer, S. H. El Safi, A. A. El Gaddal, and M. Suzuki. 1990. An ABC-ELISA for malaria serology in the field. American Journal of Tropical Medicine and Hygiene 42:24-27.

Sethabutr, O., A. E. Brown, J. Gingrich, H. K. Webster, N. Pooyindee, D. N. Taylor, and P. Echeverria. 1988. A comparative field study of radiolabeled and enzyme-conjugated synthetic DNA probes for the diagnosis of falciparum malaria. American Journal of Tropical Medicine and Hygiene 39:227-231.

Spielman, A., J. B. Perrone, A. Teklehaimanot, F. Balcha, S. C. Wardlaw, and R. A. Levine. 1988. Malaria diagnosis by direct observation of centrifuged samples of blood. American Journal of Tropical Medicine and Hygiene 39:337-342.

Taylor, D. W., C. B. Evans, G. W. Hennessy, and S. B. Aley. 1986. Use of a two-sited antibody assay to detect a heat-stable malarial antigen in the sera of mice infected with *Plasmodium yoelii*. Infection and Immunity 51:884-890.

Tharavanij, S. 1990. New developments in malaria diagnostic techniques. Southeast Asian Journal of Tropical Medicine and Public Health 21:3-16.

Voller, A., and C. C. Draper. 1982. Immunodiagnosis and seroepidemiology of malaria. British Medical Bulletin 38:173-177.

Wardlaw, S. C., and R. A. Levine. 1983. Quantitative buffy coat analysis: a new laboratory tool functioning as a screening complete blood cell count. JAMA 249:617-620.

Waters, A. P., and T. F. McCutchan. 1989. Rapid, sensitive diagnosis of malaria based on ribosomal RNA. Lancet 1:1343-1346.

Wirth, D. W., W. O. Rogers, R. Barker, H. Dourado, L. Suesebang, and B. Albuquerque. 1989. Leishmaniasis and malaria: DNA probes for diagnosis and epidemiologic analysis. Annals of the New York Academy of Sciences 569:183-192.

Wirtz, R. A., F. Zavala, Y. Charoenvit, G. H. Campbell, T. R. Burkot, I. Schneider, K. M. Esser, R. L. Beaudoin, and R. G. Andre. 1987. Comparative testing of monoclonal antibodies against *Plasmodium falciparum* sporozoites for ELISA development. Bulletin of the World Health Organization 65:39-45.

World Health Organization. 1988. Malaria diagnosis: memorandum from a WHO meeting. Bulletin of the World Health Organization 66:575-594.

Zavala, F., J. P. Tam, and A. Masuda. 1986. Synthetic peptides as antigens for the detection of humoral immunity to *Plasmodium falciparum* sporozoites. Journal of Immunological Methods 93:55-61.

Zhou, W., and Y. Li. 1987. Anti-idiotypic antibodies: preparation and identification; application to the detection of antigens of *Plasmodium falciparum*. Parasite Immunology 9:747-755.

Zolg, J. W., L. E. Andrade, and E. D. Scott. 1987. Detection of *Plasmodium falciparum* DNA using repetitive DNA clones as species specific probes. Molecular and Biochemical Parasitology 22:145-151.

6

Parasite Biology

WHERE WE WANT TO BE IN THE YEAR 2010

For centuries, malaria parasites have successfully evaded the biological defenses of their human hosts. Researchers are perplexed by the complexity of these organisms, and many questions remain unanswered. By the year 2010, advances in the field of parasite biology will have exposed many of the complex biochemical mechanisms that allow this evasion to occur. A detailed understanding of how malaria parasites recognize and invade human liver and red blood cells, for example, how their multistage life cycle is regulated and how they rapidly become drug resistant will have provided a major boost to efforts to develop malaria vaccines and will have resulted in innovative approaches to more durable antimalarial drugs.

WHERE WE ARE TODAY

The Parasite

The human malaria parasite—actually four species of the genus *Plasmodium*—undergoes over a dozen distinguishable stages of development as it moves from the mosquito vector to the human host and back again. One way to conceptualize this complex life cycle is to consider it in three distinct parts: the liver phase, the blood phase, and the mosquito phase.

90

Depending on the developmental stage and species, malaria parasites can be spherical, ring shaped, elongated, or crescent shaped, and can range in size from 1 to 20 microns in diameter (1 micron equals 1 millionth of a meter or approximately 125,000 of an inch). By comparison, a normal red blood cell has a diameter of about 7 microns.

Although the four species of human malaria parasites are closely related, there are major differences among them. *Plasmodium falciparum*, the most pathogenic of the four species, has been found to be more closely related to avian and rodent species of *Plasmodium* than to the other primate and human species (McCutchan et al., 1984). The following sections of this chapter discuss general aspects of malaria parasite biology, with a focus on *P. falciparum*. Interspecies differences are noted where appropriate.

Parasite-Host Interactions

Liver Phase

The liver phase of malaria begins when the female anopheline mosquito injects the sporozoite stage of the parasite into the human host during a blood meal (see Chapter 2, Figure 2-3). After just a few minutes, the sporozoites arrive at the liver and invade the liver cells (hepatocytes). Over the course of 5 to 15 days, depending on the species, the sporozoites undergo a process of asexual reproduction (known as schizogony, the "splitting process") that results in the production of as many as 30,000 "daughter" parasites, called merozoites. It is the merozoites that, once released from the liver, carry the malaria infection into the red blood cells (erythrocytes).

The surface of the sporozoite is coated with many copies of a protein that is thought to play a key role in host cell recognition and perhaps cell invasion. Antibodies to certain portions of this circumsporozoite protein can prevent sporozoites from entering liver cells in culture and may play an important role in protecting against infection. People exposed to irradiated sporozoites are protected against infection by unaltered sporozoites. This level of immunity has not yet been obtained with use of subunit, synthetic, or gene-cloned vaccines (see Chapter 9).

The circumsporozoite protein can be detected throughout the parasite's development in the liver and may also be associated with liver-stage merozoites. The circumsporozoite protein has a unique structure of immunodominant, highly repetitive complexes of amino acids (Santoro et al., 1983). Although different *Plasmodium* species have distinct antigenic properties, the repetitive complexes seen in *P. falciparum* sporozoites are also seen in *P. vivax* and other parasite species, although the actual makeup of these proteins is species specific.

It is not clear how the parasite arrives at the surface of the hepatocytes, since liver cells are not in direct contact with the blood. Also, although many mechanisms have been postulated, details of how the parasites invade liver cells remain obscure (Miller, 1977). The physiological changes that the sporozoite undergoes during the shift from a cold-blooded mosquito host to a warm-blooded human host are not well understood, nor is it understood how the parasite manages the reverse situation, as the sexual stage precursor—the gametocyte—travels from human to mosquito. In the latter case, there is evidence suggesting that changes in temperature and pH help stimulate the emergence of the gametes in the insect midgut. Schizogony in the liver had been thought to proceed without pathological manifestations, but recent evidence points to the existence of inflammatory mechanisms and cellular infiltration, including cytotoxic T cells, all of which may be immunologically important.

It has been known for many years that the symptoms of malaria can recur without reexposure to the parasite, but the biological mechanisms underlying this phenomenon have only recently been determined. The reappearance of symptoms may either be due to relapse, i.e., the development of latent sporozoites, called hypnozoites, in the liver following a period during which the blood itself was parasite free, or recrudescence, a sudden upsurge of blood-stage parasites after a protracted period of very low parasite density (Krotoski et al., 1982). Relapses occur only in *P. vivax* and *P. ovale* infections, while recrudescence generally occurs in *P. falciparum* and *P. malariae*. Although the hypnozoite does not appear to undergo development during its dormant state, the fact that hypnozoites are readily eliminated by the action of the drug primaquine implies some level of metabolic activity.

Blood Phase

When merozoites are released from the liver into the bloodstream, asexual blood-stage reproduction, or erythrocytic schizogony, has begun. Parasite invasion of red blood cells unfolds in four steps: attachment of the merozoite to the erythrocyte, rapid deformation of the red blood cell, invagination of the erythrocyte membrane where the parasite is attached and subsequent envelopment of the merozoite, and the resealing of the erythrocyte membrane around the parasite (Aikawa et al., 1978; Hadley et al., 1986; Perkins, 1989; Bannister and Dluzewski, 1990; Wilson, 1990).

Attachment, an event separate from invasion, may occur without endocytosis. There is indirect evidence that organelles at the tip of the parasite, the apical complex, are involved in invasion. For example, only invasive stages have apical organelles, and the organelles rapidly disappear after invasion. Although little is known about the biochemical functions associated with these organelles, efforts to clone proteins found in them may provide some insight into their roles (Coppel et al., 1987). The attachment phase is a potential target for vaccine developers, since antibody that interferes with this process may prevent parasite invasion of red blood cells. Red blood cells have receptors for malaria parasites on their surfaces, although these receptors may be different for different parasite species. The best example of a parasite receptor on a red blood cell is the Duffy antigen, which is recognized by *P. vivax*; this parasite cannot invade Duffy-negative cells. Of considerable interest is the recent cloning and characterization of the *P. vivax* (and *P. knowlesi*) gene encoding the parasite protein which binds to the Duffy antigen (Adams et al., 1990; Fang et al., 1991). This protein is located in one of the apical organelles (micronemes) thought to play a role in the invasion process. Unfortunately, our understanding of the attachment process for *P. falciparum* is less sophisticated.

Although the exact mechanism of invasion is still unresolved (see reviews cited above), it is likely that specific parasite proteases are involved (Perkins, 1989). Suggested candidates include a neutral endopeptidase (Bernard and Schrevel, 1987; Braun-Breton et al., 1988) and a chymotrypsin-like enzyme (Dejkriengkraikhul and Wilairat, 1983); selective protease inhibitors could thus be of potential interest as chemotherapeutic agents which prevent invasion.

After invasion, the parasite lies within a membranous parasitophorus vacuole, where it synthesizes nucleic acids, proteins, lipids, mitochondria, and ribosomes and assembles these components into new merozoites (Ginsburg, 1990b). The entire erythrocytic asexual cycle takes between two and three days to run its course, depending on the species.

Once merozoite assembly is completed, the erythrocyte ruptures and merozoites are released into the plasma, where they attach to other erythrocytes and begin the process anew. Some merozoites, for reasons not well understood, differentiate into the sexual forms of the parasite, the gametocytes. The factors that determine the sex of the gametocyte are unknown. Gametocyte development takes between 2 days (for *P. vivax*) and 10 days (for *P. falciparum*). The release of merozoites precipitates malaria's classical paroxysms of fever, chills, headache, myalgia, and malaise. Although the cause of the fevers is unknown, one theory is that endotoxin-like substances may be released during schizont rupture. The paroxysm itself may be due to transient increases in cytokines, such as interleukin-1 and tumor necrosis factor (Kwiatkowski et al., 1990). Children living in highly endemic areas often have significant parasitemias without symptoms, leading researchers to suspect the presence of "antitoxic" immunity.

Mosquito Phase

When gametocytes are taken up during a mosquito's blood meal, a number of factors, including temperature, concentrations of oxygen and carbon dioxide, pH, and a mosquito exflagellation factor, are thought to contribute to the maturation of gametocytes. Male microgametes are released during a process called exflagellation. Fusion of the female macrogamete with a single microgamete results in fertilization and the formation of the ookinete. The ookinete migrates to the wall of the mosquito midgut, where it penetrates the peritrophic membrane and epithelium and comes to rest on the external surface of the stomach. Over a period of days, this stage of the parasite matures into an oocyst containing up to 10,000 motile sporozoites. When the oocyst ruptures, the sporozoites enter the mosquito circulation and travel to the salivary glands, where they are injected into the human host when the mosquito feeds. The number of sporozoites that enter the human host during a single blood meal is thought to be highly variable.

Parasite Physiology and Biochemistry

Feeding

Malaria parasites feed by ingesting intact erythrocyte cytosol, the internal fluid portion of the cell, through an organelle, the cytostome. This process has been reconstructed recently in three dimensions from micrographs (Slomianny, 1990). When the cytostome closes around cytosol, it creates a membrane-bound vacuole. In *P. falciparum*, the ingested host cytosol is then exposed to a mixture of potent digestive enzymes. That digestion of hemoglobin is required for parasite survival was shown in experiments in which hemoglobin was chemically cross-linked, making it resistant to degradation by *P. falciparum* proteases and cathepsin D; parasites which invaded red blood cells with cross-linked hemoglobin failed to develop to trophozoites and eventually died (Geary et al., 1983). Recently, two proteases important for hemoglobin digestion in *P. falciparum* have been characterized. One is a cysteinyl proteinase (Rosenthal et al., 1988) and the other, which apparently initiates digestion, is an aspartyl proteinase (Goldberg et al., 1991). Reversible inhibitors of the cysteinyl protease (such as leupeptin) block hemoglobin digestion and suspend parasite growth. However, growth resumes even after prolonged incubations when the inhibitor is removed. Irreversible protease inhibitors, on the other hand, killed the parasites (Rosenthal et al., 1988). Selective protease inhibitors which block either of these two enzymes would be of considerable interest as potential antimalarial drugs. As the process of hemoglobin digestion becomes better understood (Goldberg et al., 1990), additional sites for chemotherapeutic intervention should be uncovered.

During digestion, about three-fourths of the host cell hemoglobin is destroyed. The residue left from this process is an insoluble particulate complex call hemozoin; this complex contains, among other material, the heme derived from hemoglobin. Although the chemistry of this complex is becoming better understood (Goldie et al., 1990; Slater et al., 1991), its role in pathogenesis, drug action, or immunology remains undocumented.

Permeability Changes in Erythrocyte Membranes

Following parasite invasion, the intracellular metabolism of infected erythrocytes increases significantly. Nutrients must be brought in from outside, and waste products must be disposed of expeditiously. The cell membrane responds by increasing its capacity to transport a variety of substrates in and out of the erythrocyte, including essential amino acids, nucleosides, lactate, and fatty acids. The changes in membrane permeability allow a number of substrates, that otherwise would not be let in at all or would be let in to a limited degree, to enter the infected red blood cell. These substrates include hexitols, acidic and neutral amino acids, several small inorganic ions, and organic acids.

The appearance of new erythrocyte membrane transport pathways is the result of host cell "remodeling" by the intracellular malaria parasites. It is thought that in remodeling, proteins of parasite origin become associated with host membrane components, either by adhering to the inner aspects of the membrane or by inserting themselves directly into the membrane. The experimental data strongly support this hypothesis (Haldar et al., 1986; Ginsburg and Stein, 1987; Cabantchik, 1989, 1990; Ginsburg, 1990a; Tanabe, 1990a,b).

Other Parasite-Directed Changes in Erythrocyte-Membrane Structure

In *P. falciparum*, the trophozoite stage inserts new molecules into the host erythrocyte plasma membrane. These new membrane components are responsible for the sequestration of mature parasite stages in capillaries by the process of cytoadherence. Although among the human malaria parasites only *P. falciparum* exhibits cytoadherence, *P. vivax* also induces alterations in the infected erythrocyte membrane. Ultrastructure studies have shown that the membranes of erythrocytes infected with *P. vivax* contain caveolar structures that appear to be connected to vesicles (Atkinson and Aikawa, 1990; Barnwell, 1990). These caveolae-vesicle complexes appear to play a role in parasite interaction with the extracellular environment. They induce antibody production and are antigenically highly variable.

Nutrition and Metabolism

A malaria infection initiated by a single malaria parasite may produce as many as 10 billion new organisms. Nearly all the metabolic processes of the parasite are focused on supporting this enormous reproductive effort. The relatively recently acquired ability to cultivate *P. falciparum* in vitro has greatly expanded biochemists' ability to study parasite nutrition and metabolism.

In *P. falciparum*, glucose can be replaced by fructose, but the parasite will not develop in vitro when another sugar, such as galactose, mannose, maltose, or ribose is substituted (Geary et al., 1985a). Although malaria parasites are capable of synthesizing the amino acids glutamate, aspartate, alanine, and leucine from glucose, they probably acquire them either through digestion of hemoglobin or from sources outside the red blood cell. Most early studies on the uptake of amino acids by malaria parasites utilized the animal parasites *P. berghei*, *P. lophurae*, *P. gallinaceum*, and *P. knowlesi* either in vivo, an approach in which experimental parameters are difficult to control, or in vitro, using less than ideal culture procedures. Observations on parasite biochemistry using cultures of *P. falciparum* have not always supported conclusions drawn from these flawed models.

In experiments using cultured *P. falciparum*, it has been shown that 13 of the 20 amino acids can be obtained from the digested erythrocyte cytosol; the parasite must receive the other seven amino acids from sources outside the erythrocyte. Selective transport facilities may exist for any or all of these amino acids in *P. falciparum*, but evidence from other *Plasmodium* species suggests that this is not the case for all amino acids. Attempts to supplement glutamine, one of the amino acids, with other metabolites have been unsuccessful. Both glutamate and glutamine are required for continuous cultivation, indicating that interconversion is limited at best.

There appears to be only one vitamin, calcium pantothenate, that is not provided by the erythrocyte but is needed by the parasite for survival. Evidence for this comes from in vitro studies using culture medium containing this vitamin (Divo et al., 1985a). The malaria parasite's requirement for *para*-aminobenzoic acid and folic acid is well documented. The requirement for these vitamins, found in red blood cells, is probably strain specific. Sulfonamides, which inhibit folic acid synthesis, have been used as antimalarial drugs for years. The story of folic acid metabolism is complicated, however, and not all sulfonamides are equally potent as antimalarials. Surprisingly, unlike most organisms, *P. falciparum* does not seem to require biotin. The ability to develop in the absence of this vitamin was demonstrated by growing the parasites in the presence of several biotin antagonists, including avidin (Geary et al., 1985b).

Pyrimidines and purines are the two main building blocks of DNA. Malaria parasites can synthesize the former de novo, but purines are a required nutrient (Gero and O'Sullivan, 1990). Hypoxanthine is the preferred purine source, but other purines readily substitute for hypoxanthine. Studies of the kinetics of DNA synthesis in *P. falciparum* have revealed that incorporation of labeled purines into DNA begins approximately 30 hours after merozoite invasion and increases logarithmically for another 14 to 18 hours, when schizogony is completed.

Because erythrocytes contain considerable concentrations of amino acids and vitamins that may be important to parasite development, it is difficult to determine in experimental settings whether decreased parasite viability due to nutritional factors is a result of effects on the parasite itself or on the red blood cell. Thus, it is not known whether nutrients identified as crucial for malaria parasite cultivation are required for erythrocytes only, parasites only, or both. For example, the amino acids glutamine, glycine, and cysteine, while necessary for long-term survival of erythrocytes in culture, may not be required parasite nutrients.

Energy Transformations and Mitochondria

There has been considerable debate about whether the erythrocytic stages of mammalian malaria parasites possess mitochondria, the energy-producing organelles essential for all life forms. The falciparum parasite uses glucose as its primary energy source. In fact, glucose utilization is significantly greater in the infected erythrocyte than in the uninfected cell. Progress is being made in the characterization of the enzymes involved in glycolysis in *P. falciparum* (Roth et al., 1988; Roth, 1990). However, there is no evidence supporting the presence of a Krebs cycle, a key energy-producing process of the mitochondria.

The presence of mitochondria in the erythrocytic asexual stages of *P. falciparum* has recently been shown, but their actual function is not well understood (Divo et al., 1985b). Recent advances in the molecular biology of the mitochondrial DNA of malaria parasites may help to unravel the role of the mitochondrion (Gardner et al., 1988). The importance of this organelle to the parasite is underscored by the fact that mitochondrial toxins are highly lethal. Antibiotics used to treat falciparum infection, such as the tetracyclines, clindamycin, and erythromycin, appear to work by blocking the development of parasite mitochondria (Prapunwattana et al., 1988). Of great interest in this regard is the recent finding that mitochondrial DNA of *P. falciparum* encodes an RNA polymerase which is closely related to prokaryotic polymerases and is sensitive to rifampicin, potentially explaining the antimalarial activity of this drug (Gardner et al., 1991).

The erythrocytic stages of many mammalian malaria parasites appear not to derive their metabolic energy through classical electron transport. The mitochondria may participate in ion transport, but the role this plays in metabolism is unclear. It is not known whether components analogous to those present in the mammalian terminal electron transport system function in the malaria parasite, and for what purpose, since the organism, like many other parasitic protozoans and all parasitic worms so far studied, has rather limited terminal respiration (Scheibel, 1988). Mammalian malaria parasites are aerobic fermenters, capable of partially decomposing metabolic substrates to fermentation products but unable to oxidize them completely to carbon dioxide and water. Since the substrates are not completely metabolized, it would appear that terminal respiration is either absent or rate limiting in the parasite. Available evidence supports the view that malaria parasites are microaerophilic, homolactate fermenters (Scheibel et al., 1979).

Parasite Lipids

Bloodstage malaria parasites contain no lipid reserves (all lipids of intracellular plasmodia are membrane associated), and they lack the means for degrading lipids. Plasmodia also appear to lack the capacity to synthesize fatty acids de novo from acetate, but they can and do incorporate exogenous fatty acids into their phospholipids, thereby maintaining a lipid-fatty acid composition distinct from that of the host cell (Vial et al., 1990).

Because malaria parasites lack lipid reserves, they are incapable of fabricating fatty acids and cholesterol, and they have limited capacity for saturation and desaturation as well as for chain-elongating and chain-shortening reactions. The blood stages of *Plasmodium* species must satisfy their lipid requirements by relying on dynamic exchanges with plasma, an activity akin to that of the red blood cell itself but at a much higher rate (Scheibel and Sherman, 1988).

Evasion of Host Defenses

Cytoadherence

The greater virulence of *P. falciparum* than of other human malaria parasites is due to the sequestration of parasitized erythrocytes into the deep vasculature. The attachment of infected red blood cells to the vascular endothelium in *P. falciparum* malaria occludes capillaries in the brain, heart, and other vital organs and causes tissue anoxia. Cerebral malaria, the most serious and often fatal consequence of falciparum malaria, is thought to be caused in part by the cytoadherence of infected erythrocytes, although changes in vascular permeability and cytokine-related cerebral inflammation may also be important (MacPherson et al., 1985). Cytoadherence in other tissues causes serious, but rarely fatal, anoxia. Recent evidence suggests that the cytoadherence properties of parasite strains is correlated with the severity of disease but not with cerebral malaria (Ho et al., 1991).

Cytoadherence sequesters infected red blood cells in the venous circulation's lower oxygen environment, an important consideration for an organism known to be microaerophilic and highly susceptible to oxidant stress, and prevents the cells from circulating through the spleen, where they would be destroyed. Infections with *P. falciparum* parasites that have lost the ability to cytoadhere are invariably attenuated, and parasite reproduction rates are readily controlled by the spleen (Langreth and Peterson, 1985). One reason *P. falciparum* has such an explosive reproduction rate may be due in part to the fact that it escapes the role that the spleen seems to play in limiting infections by other malaria species.

The ability to cytoadhere is tied to the appearance of knobs, conical protrusions about 100 nanometers by 30 nanometers, on the host erythrocyte membrane. A considerable understanding of the biochemistry of knobs has been gained, extending to the cloning of the most important protein associated with them (Sharma and Kilejian, 1987; Ellis et al., 1987; Pologe et al., 1987; Triglia et al., 1987). Although some parasite-infected red blood cells that form knobs do not adhere, all natural infections with *P. falciparum* are both K+ (indicating knob formation) and C+ (indicating cytoadherence). When parasites have been cultured for a period of time, they lose their ability to produce knobs and to cytoadhere (K-,C-). Some cultured parasites form knobs but do not adhere (K+,C-). When clones of K-,C- parasites (which have never been found in natural infections) are injected into aotus monkeys, the resulting infections are mild with low parasite densities. Cultured parasites without knobs but with cytoadherent capability (K-,C+) have been observed, which raises questions about the relationship between knob formation and cytoadherence (Udomsangpetch et al., 1989). Whether K-,C+ parasites occur naturally or are simply an artifact of in vitro experimental manipulations is unknown (Trager, 1989).

Just as there is an incomplete picture of the parasite-derived molecules necessary for cytoadherence, so too are the relevant receptors on endothelial cells incompletely defined. One cell surface protein that appears to have a role in cytoadherence is an 88 kilodalton antigen known as CD-36. This glycoprotein is expressed on the surface of cells that mediate cytoadherence, such as endothelial cells, monocytes, and C32 melanoma cells, but not on related cells to which infected erythrocytes do not adhere. Antibody to CD-36 readily reverses cytoadherence. Other proteins thought to serve as cell surface receptors during cytoadherence are thrombospondin and ICAM-1 (CD-54) (Howard and Gilladoga, 1989; Chulay and Ockenhouse, 1990).

Neoantigens

There are several additional parasite-induced antigens that appear on the surface of infected red blood cells and may be immunologically important. Some of these "neoantigens" appear to be linked to knob formation and are responsible for cytoadherence, while for others no clear role has

TABLE 6-1 Well-Characterized *P. falciparum* Proteins Associated with Infected Erythrocyte Membranes

Name	Synonym(s)	MW (kDa)	Comments
PfEMP-1	IP	265-285[a]	Believed to mediate cytoadherence; trypsin sensitive; antigenically variable; selection for cytoadherence selects for larger PfEMP-1
MESA[b,c]	PfEMP-2	250-300[a]	Phosphoprotein; binds to band 4.1; located at knobs
KAHRP[b,c] KP	PfHRP-I,	80-109[a]	Present at knobs; isolates lacking this protein do not have knob structures detectable by electron microscopy
PfHRP-II[b,c]			Secreted from intact red blood cells
11-1[b,c]		>1,200	Associated with knobs
41-2[b]		29	
RESA[b,c]	Pf155	155	Phosphoprotein; present in ring stage; minor variability; binds to spectrin
TR		105	Putative receptor for transferrin

[a]Varies in size between isolates.
[b]Nucleotide sequence data available.
[c]Blocks of tandem repeats in protein.
Abbreviations: PfEMP-1, *P. falciparum* erythrocyte membrane protein-1; PfEMP-2, *P. falciparum* erythrocyte membrane protein 2; IP, iodinatable protein; MESA, mature-parasite-infected erythrocyte surface antigen; KAHRP, knob-associated histidine-rich protein; PfHRP-I, *P. falciparum* histidine-rich protein I; PfHRP-II, *P. falciparum* histidine-rich protein II; KP, knob protein; 11-1 and 41-2, individual recombinant clones; RESA, ring-infected erythrocyte surface antigen; TR, transferrin receptor; MW, molecular weight; kDa, kilodaltons.

been determined. Table 6-1 outlines several important erythrocyte membrane alterations caused by parasite-derived antigens (Howard, 1988; Petersen et al., 1990).

Molecular Biology

Most work on malaria parasite molecular biology has been devoted to the identification and cloning of genes which encode potentially protective antigens. As noted above, however, the use of molecular biology techniques has opened new avenues for research on the basic biology of these organisms. This section describes advances in other areas of parasite molecular biology which indicate the enormous potential of the technology in pursuing questions of fundamental relevance. Several recent reviews can be consulted for more detail (Walliker et al., 1987; Braun, 1988; Weber et al., 1988). It should be noted that the unusual codon bias found in *P. falciparum*, which is highly skewed toward adenine-thymidine richness, generates some fundamental difficulties for the use of typical gene expression systems (Saul and Battistutta, 1988).

Parasite Genetic Diversity

There is considerable genetic diversity among malaria parasite populations (Fenton and Walliker, 1990; Kemp et al., 1990). An analysis of 60 *P. falciparum* isolates collected from three continents found that all were different (Creasey et al., 1990). This heterogeneity reflects the extreme "plasticity" of the falciparum genome and is a major reason the parasite is so able to evade host immune responses. Diversity has been observed in isoenzyme patterns, drug resistance, morphology, two-dimensional electrophoretic protein patterns, karyotype, and significantly for the host, antigenic repertoire.

Karyotype

The genome of *P. falciparum* (and probably of all other *Plasmodium* species) contains 14 chromosomes. Parasite chromosomes cannot be seen by conventional light microscopy. The kinetochores, structures involved in the attachment of chromosomes to spindle microtubules, can be identified by electron microscopy. In recent years, the technique of pulse field-gradient gel electrophoresis has allowed researchers to visualize the chromosomes, which range in length from 800 to 3,500 kilobases. Genes for various parasite proteins have been located on individual chromosomes (Kemp et al., 1985, 1987b).

A striking feature of *P. falciparum* chromosomes from different isolates is their size variation (Kemp et al., 1985). While the details of chromosome structure have not yet been determined, mapping studies indicate that such variations are the result of deletions occurring at various chromosomal locations (Corcoran et al., 1986, 1988; Pologe and Ravetch, 1988; Biggs et al., 1989; Pologe et al., 1990). Occasionally these deletions result in the loss of a particular protein (Pologe and Ravetch, 1986; Cappai et al., 1989; Ravetch, 1989). Since most genetic studies are performed on parasites grown in vitro, it is not clear whether these mutations exist commonly in nature.

Protein Expression

Considerable diversity is found in the proteins of the asexual stages from different isolates of *P. falciparum*. This diversity exists at four levels: minor antigenic change (gene mutation), nonexpression (gene deletion), allelic variants of a single gene (through recombination or gene conversion), and antigenic variation of unknown cause.

Mutations In *P. falciparum*, as in any organism, occasional genetic mutations occur and may be retained if they are not harmful to the parasite. Different isolates of several parasite proteins have been shown to have minor sequence differences (Coppel et al., 1985; Hope et al., 1985; Stahl et al., 1986; Simmons et al., 1987; Weber et al., 1988; Thomas et al., 1990). In the case of one protein, Exp-1/CRA, the substitution of a single amino acid, aspartic acid, by glycine affected the binding of a monoclonal antibody to the parasite and changed its antigenicity (Simmons et al., 1987).

Gene Deletions   Certain gene deletions occasionally result in the loss of protein coding sequences. This phenomenon has been described for RESA, MESA, PfHRP-I, and PfHRP-II (see Table 6-1 for definitions), all proteins that interact with the erythrocyte membrane and whose presence apparently is not essential for parasite survival in vitro (Stahl et al., 1985; Pologe and Ravetch, 1986; Culvenor et al., 1987; Cappai et al., 1989; Petersen et al., 1989).

Allelic Variants   By far the most common cause of antigenic diversity is the existence of alleles. The best examples are the heat-stable S antigens, although MSA-1 and MSA-2 (see Table 6-1) are two other well-studied examples (Kemp et al., 1990).

A prominent structural feature of many *P. falciparum* antigenic proteins is blocks of tandemly repeated peptide sequences (Kemp et al., 1987a). The repeats can be extremely well conserved, as in S antigens (Brown et al., 1987) and MSA-2 (Smythe et al., 1990), or highly variable, as for FIRA (Stahl et al., 1987). These repeat sequences often serve as the predominant B-cell epitope on the protein; in proteins such as S antigens, it is not possible to detect naturally occurring antibody responses to other regions. Although immunologically interesting, the biological functions of the S and FIRA proteins remain unknown.

Antigenically diverse forms of both S antigens and MSA-2 have extensive repeat blocks that differ in length, number of copies, and sequence. It is possible to discern a relationship between repeat sequences of different S antigens; the diversity is probably the result of DNA insertions, deletions, mutations, and alterations in reading frame.

For MSA-1, a major vaccine candidate protein, the basis of diversity is somewhat different. Analysis of the sequence of multiple alleles suggests that repeat blocks may be conserved, semiconserved, or variable. The variable blocks occur in two forms, and antigenic diversity results from reassortment of these blocks, probably through intragenic recombination between two parental alleles (Tanabe et al., 1987; M. Peterson et al., 1988a). There is a short region of repetitive sequence at the aminoterminus of MSA-1, and a further level of diversity is generated by differences in repeat sequences at that locus (Certa et al., 1987; M. Peterson et al., 1988b).

Antigenic Variation   Antigenic variation is the ability of a cloned line of parasites to alter its antigenic repertoire. Although there is some evidence suggestive of antigenic variation in *P. falciparum*, it is not known how important this mechanism may be to malaria infections and disease. For example, recent research has shown that the protein implicated in cytoadherence, PfEMP-1, may undergo antigenic variation, but the extent of the variation is unclear.

Other Mechanisms of Genetic Variability

Because a single malaria infection can generate a huge reservoir of asexual-stage parasites, the possibility of point mutations, upon which selection could act, is quite high. Genetic recombination during the sexual phase of reproduction offers further opportunities for genetic diversity (Walliker, 1989a,b).

Drug Resistance

Drug resistance is due to genetic mutations that allow the parasite to avoid damage from a previously lethal antimalarial agent. With pyrimethamine resistance in *P. falciparum*, for example, a mutation in the gene for the enzyme dihydrofolate reductase confers resistance. In all pyrimethamine-resistant parasites examined to date, this enzyme possesses the amino acid asparagine at position 108, while parasites still sensitive to the drug have serine or threonine (Cowman et al., 1988; D. Peterson et al., 1988).

The situation for chloroquine resistance is more complicated. This antimalarial drug is thought to act by accumulating in and interfering with the function of *P. falciparum* acid vesicles, such as the food vacuole. Parasites resistant to chloroquine expel the drug rapidly in an unaltered form before it accumulates. The discovery that verapamil partially reverses resistance to chloroquine in vitro led to the proposal that chloroquine efflux may involve a mechanism similar to that found in mammalian multidrug resistant tumor cell lines. At least two genes have been proposed to be involved, one of which is PfMDR-1, a homologue of the P-glycoprotein gene in multidrug resistant mammalian tumor cells (Foote et al., 1989; Wellems et al., 1990). In some resistant parasites, these genes are either mutated or amplified (Foote et al., 1989, 1990). However, recent molecular genetic evidence suggests that these genes are not linked to chloroquine efflux and resistance (Wellems, 1991). Thus, the mechanism of chloroquine resistance in *P. falciparum* remains unknown.

Cloning of Genes for Functional Proteins

A small but significant number of genes that encode proteins with known functions have been cloned. Examples include enzymes involved in carbohydrate metabolism, including lactate dehydrogenase (Simmons et al., 1985) and aldolase, which is of interest also as a potentially protective antigen (Certa et al., 1988; Dobeli et al., 1990); enzymes involved in purine metabolism, including adenine phosphoribosyltransferase (Pollack et al., 1985) and hypoxanthine-guanine phosphoribosyltransferase (King and Melton, 1987); and alpha- and beta-tubulins (Delves et al., 1989, 1990; Holloway et al., 1989, 1990; Wesseling et al., 1989; Sen and Godsen, 1990). Some of these genes encode proteins that are intriguing targets for drug discovery, and their cloning should help elucidate host-parasite differences in their sequences that provide an opportunity for selective inhibition. Of considerable interest in this regard is the functional expression of active thymidylate synthase-dihydrofolate reductase from *P. falciparum* (Sirawaraporn et al., 1990; Hall et al., 1991), which can provide large amounts of the critical enzyme for drug studies.

Differential Gene Expression

The timing and execution of the developmental program in intracellular parasites is undoubtedly of critical importance. Little is known about these processes, yet they are likely to be of considerable interest as targets for drug intervention. Despite a poor understanding of the cellular biology of development in malaria parasites, recent advances in molecular biology may provide the tools to analyze the genetic mechanisms involved in the switch from one stage to another. The types of actin (Wesseling et al., 1989) and tubulin (Delves et al., 1990) differ between the sexual and asexual stages of *P. falciparum*. Analysis of the factors that regulate the transcription of the genes encoding these proteins could provide clues about the molecular switches that govern development. Furthermore, it has been recently shown that both ribosomes (Gunderson et al., 1987; Waters et al., 1989) and ribosomal RNA (Zhu et al., 1990) vary between the sporozoite and hepatocyte stages of this organism. The processes governing the switch between the mosquito and host stages are of obvious interest as indicators of potential sites for drug intervention. Finally, the cloning of genes that encode proteins related to heat-shock proteins (Bianco et al., 1986; Yang et al., 1987) and stress proteins (Kumar et al., 1988) is important in this regard because such proteins are often critical to temperature-dependent adaptations in other organisms.

Research Training

Only through a significant improvement in our understanding of malaria parasite biology can new and more efficient drugs, potential vaccines, and novel approaches to malaria control be developed. Many of the research bottlenecks that hinder efforts to control malaria result from a lack of basic information on the biology, physiology, and biochemistry of the parasite itself.

If true progress is to be made in understanding and controlling malaria, more scientists who appreciate and are interested in the biology of the malaria parasite need to be trained. The availability of money to conduct malaria research is presently attracting talent from other scientific disciplines. However, many of these investigators are research opportunists whose talents go to the highest bidder. Developing a solid core of scientists dedicated to the field of parasitology in general, and malaria in particular, is of paramount importance. There is also a need for scientists who appreciate the difficult problems one encounters with malaria research strategies—investigators who are dedicated to the discipline of malaria rather than driven by technology.

RESEARCH AGENDA

Sporogonic Phase

No gaps in our knowledge of malaria parasite biology are greater than those associated with the mosquito phase. For example, the enzymes that control the numerous metabolic pathways of the parasite during human infection must function at or near 37°C. Conversely, metabolic processes in the mosquito phase must occur at ambient temperatures. Morever, the entire environment, with regard to availability of oxygen and nutrients, differs significantly between the two hosts. The details of such characteristics as gamete maturation, fertilization, reduction division, mosquito midgut penetration, parasite nutritional needs during sporogony, maturation of sporozoites, and penetration into salivary glands are known only in the crudest sense.

Liver Phase

As with sporogony, the biology of the liver stage of the parasite is poorly understood. Although irradiated sporozoites invade liver cells and induce a protective immune response, for unknown reasons they do not develop fully. Inoculation with living, radiation-damaged sporozoites produces a greater immune response than does immunization with subunit or killed immunogens, but the biological mechanisms underlying such protection are unclear. Virtually nothing is known about the dormant hypnozoite stage of the parasite, which is responsible for malaria relapse. Furthermore, the nutritional and biochemical dependence of the parasite on the hepatocyte remains unknown.

RESEARCH FOCUS: The genetic control of metabolic switches that allow the parasite to rapidly adapt from warm-blooded to cold-blooded hosts. The nutritional biochemistry and developmental events of sporogony are areas of study that could prove useful in new control strategies aimed at the mosquito host.

RESEARCH FOCUS: The biology of the parasite's liver stages in general, and hypnozoites in particular, with the goal of developing better antirelapse therapies.

Blood Phase

Parasite-erythrocyte interaction appears to be mediated by specific recognition sites, which probably do not undergo much, if any, alteration. Parasite invasion of erythrocytes and hepatocytes also is linked to the special organelles of the merozoite and sporozoite stages. Little is know about these organelles, which disappear rapidly after the parasite enters the host cell. Interventions aimed at these aspects of malaria infection could halt parasite development.

RESEARCH FOCUS: Hepatocyte and erythrocyte recognition sites that facilitate parasite invasion and the role of parasite organelles involved in this process.

Since the erythrocyte surface contains parasite receptors, it makes sense that there may be erythrocyte ligands associated with merozoites, but this has not yet been demonstrated. Such receptors, if found, might offer another useful target for antimalarial drug therapy, as well as important vaccine candidates.

RESEARCH FOCUS: The presence and function of erythrocyte receptors on the surface of merozoite-stage malaria parasites.

Much attention has centered on controlling parasite reproduction by using chemotherapy or antibodies generated by immunization. The fact that many individuals function normally while infected with the parasite, however, suggests an antitoxic immunity, of which nothing is known. A vaccine or therapy that could duplicate this asymptomatic immunity would be a tremendous achievement.

RESEARCH FOCUS: The immunological basis of asymptomatic malaria infections, including the role of cytokines in disease as well as immunity.

Physiology and Biochemistry

The mitochondrion, an organelle essential to parasite survival, is the target of a number of antimalarial antibiotics. These antibiotics, while clinically useful, were formulated for use against bacterial infections but could be better focused to kill malaria parasites if more were known about the biochemistry of the parasite mitochondrion. Drugs that impede mitochondrial function and that work more rapidly than the presently used antibacterial antibiotics would be a useful addition to the current chemotherapeutic armamentarium.

RESEARCH FOCUS: Mitochondrial biochemistry, with the goal of better targeting malaria antibiotics.

Malaria parasites have an absolute requirement for purines, one of the principal building blocks of DNA. The purine salvage pathways used by the parasite appear to be distinct from those of the erythrocyte.

RESEARCH FOCUS: Parasite enzymes in the purine salvage pathway that could serve as targets for drug therapy.

Developmental Biology

A remarkable progression of development is observed in nearly all stages of the malaria parasite, but we know almost nothing of the bases for the unfolding of these programmed changes. A greater understanding of the mechanisms that control the developmental progression of sporozoites to exoerythrocytic schizonts and of ring stages to trophozoites and erythrocytic schizonts, of the developmental regulation of gametocytogenesis, and of fertilization and development in the mosquito is expected to lead to the identification of a number of attractive targets for chemotherapeutic intervention.

RESEARCH FOCUS: The cell biology of development in the various stages of the life cycle of malaria parasites. With the availability of a convenient culture system, the blood stage parasites represent a useful subject for initial studies.

Drug Action and Resistance

Little is known about the mode of action of chloroquine and other quinoline-containing antimalarial drugs. This lack of knowledge has hindered rational drug design. In addition, studies of apparent resistance genes, and of chloroquine resistance genes in particular, do not explain the apparent lack of resistance seen with many other quinoline-containing antimalarial drugs. The danger is that newly developed antimalarial drugs may be clinically useless by the time their mechanism of action is discovered.

> **RESEARCH FOCUS:** The mode of action of antimalarial drugs, especially chloroquine, and the genetic and biological components of antimalarial drug resistance.

Clinical Immunity

In the optimistic rush to develop a malaria vaccine, the concept of clinical immunity (premunition or concomitant immunity) has received little attention. Clinically immune individuals are believed by some investigators to be protected from disease because they maintain a low-grade infection that continually stimulates an otherwise lethargic immune response, thereby preventing a serious rise in parasite numbers. This phenomenon is different from sterilizing immunity, which controls infection by eliminating parasitemia or by preventing infection altogether.

> **RESEARCH FOCUS:** Factors that determine clinical immunity.

Cytoadherence

Parasite cytoadherence antigens on the surface of infected erythrocytes may be the most important antigens associated with the immunological clearance of a natural infection. Antibodies to these cytoadherence antigens free schizont-infected erythrocytes from the vascular endothelium and release them into the general circulation, where they are removed by the spleen. This mechanism of parasite destruction is probably more efficient than any other and may be the most important means of controlling infections in clinically immune adults.

> **RESEARCH FOCUS:** The identification and characterization of parasite cytoadherence antigens, with the aim of understanding their role in parasite development and pathogenesis.

Parasite Genes

The DNA of malaria parasites is very difficult to clone into stable vector systems, making construction of an ordered parasite gene library in *Escherichia coli* virtually impossible. Knowing the number and location of genes within the parasite DNA, and the proteins produced by each, would greatly aid efforts at understanding parasite function.

RESEARCH FOCUS: A complete genomic library for *P. falciparum* and *P. vivax* and an in vitro system for translating genes into their protein products.

RESEARCH FOCUS: The construction of complementary DNA libraries specific for the many stages of parasite development. Such a library would be a powerful tool for unfolding the mysteries of specific parasite developmental processes such as pre-erythrocytic and erythrocytic schizogony, gametogeny, and sporogeny.

RESEARCH FOCUS: The identification of a system for the transformation of *P. falciparum* that would be of tremendous benefit in defining the roles of parasite genes.

In Vitro Cultivation

Perhaps no research tool has promoted research in malaria more thoroughly during the past 50 years than the continuous cultivation of *P. falciparum*. Although other *Plasmodium* species have been successfully propagated in vitro, no other species that infects humans can be cultured.

RESEARCH FOCUS: The development of an in vitro system for the continuous cultivation of *P. vivax* and the other species that cause disease in humans.

REFERENCES

Adams, J. H., D. E. Hudson, M. Torii, G. E. Ward, T. E. Wellems, M. Aikawa, and L. H. Miller. 1990. The Duffy receptor family of *Plasmodium knowlesi* is located within the micronemes of invasive malaria merozoites. Cell 63:141-153.

Aikawa, M., L. H. Miller, J. Johnson, and J. Rabbege. 1978. Erythrocyte entry by malaria parasites: a moving junction between erythrocyte and parasite. Journal of Cell Biology 77:72-82.

Atkinson, C. T., and M. Aikawa. 1990. Ultrastructure of malaria-infected erythrocytes. Blood Cells 16:351-368.

Bannister, L. H., and A. R. Dluzewski. 1990. The ultrastructure of red cell invasion in malaria infections: a review. Blood Cells 16:257-292.

Barnwell, J. W. 1990. Vesicle-mediated transport of membrane and proteins in malaria-infected erythrocytes. Blood Cells 16:379-395.

Bernard, F., and J. Schrevel. 1987. Purification of a *Plasmodium berghei* neutral endopeptidase and its localization in merozoites. Molecular and Biochemical Parasitology 26:167-173.

Bianco, A. E., J. M. Favaloro, T. R. Burkot, J. G. Culvenor, P. E. Crewther, G. V. Brown, R. F. Anders, R. L. Coppel, and D. J. Kemp. 1986. A repetitive antigen of *Plasmodium falciparum* that is homologous to heat shock protein 70 of *Drosophila melanogaster*. Proceedings of the National Academy of Sciences of the United States of America 83:8713-8717.

Biggs, B. A., D. J. Kemp, and G. V. Brown. 1989. Subtelomeric chromosome deletions in field isolates of *Plasmodium falciparum* and their relationship to loss of cytoadherence in vitro. Proceedings of the National Academy of Sciences of the United States of America 86:2428-2432.

Braun, R. 1988. Molecular and cellular biology of malaria. Bioessays 8:194-199.

Braun-Breton, C., T. L. Rosenberry, and L. P. da Silva. 1988. Induction of the proteolytic activity of a membrane protein in *Plasmodium falciparum* by phosphatidyl inositol-specific phospholipase C. Nature 332:457-459.

Brown, H., D. J. Kemp, N. Barzaga, G. V. Brown, R. F. Anders, and R. L. Coppel. 1987. Sequence variation in S-antigen genes of *Plasmodium falciparum*. Molecular and Biological Medicine 4:365-376.

Cabantchik, Z. I. 1989. Altered membrane transport of malaria-infected erythrocytes: a possible pharmacologic target. Blood 74:1464-1471.

Cabantchik, Z. I. 1990. Properties of permeation pathways induced in the human red cell membrane by malaria parasites. Blood Cells 16:421-432.

Cappai, R., M.-R. van Schravendijk, R. F. Anders, M. G. Peterson, L. M. Thomas, A. F. Cowman, and D. J. Kemp. 1989. Expression of the RESA gene in *Plasmodium falciparum* isolate FCR3 is prevented by a subtelomeric deletion. Molecular and Cellular Biology 9:3584-3587.

Certa, U., D. Rotmann, H. Matile, and R. Reber-Liske. 1987. A naturally occurring gene encoding the major surface antigen precursor p190 of *Plasmodium falciparum* lacks tripeptide repeats. EMBO Journal 6:4137-4142.

Certa, U., P. Ghersa, H. Dobeli, H. Matile, H. P. Kocher, I. K. Shrivastava, A. R. Shaw, and L. H. Perrin. 1988. Aldolase activity of a *Plasmodium falciparum* protein with protective properties. Science 240:1036-1038.

Chulay, J. D., and C. F. Ockenhouse. 1990. Host receptors for malaria-infected erythrocytes. American Journal of Tropical Medicine and Hygiene 43(Suppl. 2):6-14.

Coppel, R. L., J. M. Favaloro, P. E. Crewther, T. R. Burkot, A. E. Bianco, H. D. Stahl, D. J. Kemp, R. F. Anders, and G. V. Brown. 1985. A blood stage antigen of *Plasmodium falciparum* shares determinants with the sporozoite coat protein. Proceedings of the National Academy of Sciences of the United States of America 82:5121-5125.

Coppel, R. L., A. E. Bianco, J. G. Culvenor, P. E. Crewther, G. V. Brown, R. F. Anders, and D. J. Kemp. 1987. A cDNA clone expressing a rhoptry protein of *Plasmodium falciparum*. Molecular and Biochemical Parasitology 25:73-81.

Corcoran, L. M., K. P. Forsyth, A. E. Bianco, G. V. Brown, and D. J. Kemp. 1986. Chromosome size polymorphisms in *Plasmodium falciparum* can involve deletions and are frequent in natural parasite populations. Cell 44:87-95.

Corcoran, L. M., J. K. Thompson, D. Walliker, and D. J. Kemp. 1988. Homologous recombination within subtelomeric repeat sequences generates chromosome size polymorphisms in *P. falciparum*. Cell 53:807-813.

Cowman, A. F., M. J. Morry, B. A. Biggs, G. A. M. Cross, and S. J. Foote. 1988. Amino acid changes linked to pyrimethamine resistance in the dihydrofolate reductase-thymidylate synthase gene of *Plasmodium falciparum*. Proceedings of the National Academy of Sciences of the United States of America 85:9109-9113.

Creasey, A., B. Fenton, A. Walker, S. Thaithong, S. Oliveira, S. Mutambu, and D. Walliker. 1990. Genetic diversity of *Plasmodium falciparum* shows geographical variation. American Journal of Tropical Medicine and Hygiene 42:403-413.

Culvenor, J. G., C. J. Langford, P. E. Crewther, R. B. Saint, R. L. Coppel, D. J. Kemp, R. F. Anders, and G. V. Brown. 1987. *Plasmodium falciparum*: identification and localization of a knob protein antigen expressed by a cDNA clone. Experimental Parasitology 63:58-67.

Dejkriengkraikhul, P.-n, and P. Wilairat. 1983. Requirement of malarial protease in the invasion of human red cells by merozoites of *Plasmodium falciparum*. Zeitschrift für Parasitenkunde 69:313-317.

Delves, C. J., R. G. Ridley, M. Goman, S. P. Holloway, J. E. Hyde, and J. G. Scaife. 1989. Cloning of a beta-tubulin gene from *Plasmodium falciparum*. Molecular Microbiology 3:1511-1519.

Delves, C. J., P. Alano, R. G. Ridley, M. Goman, S. P. Holloway, J. E. Hyde, and J. G. Scaife. 1990. Expression of gamma and beta tubulin genes during the asexual and sexual blood stages of *Plasmodium falciparum*. Molecular and Biochemical Parasitology 43:271-278.

Divo, A. A., T. G. Geary, N. L. Davis, and J. B. Jensen. 1985a. Nutritional requirements of *Plasmodium falciparum* in culture. I. Exogenously supplied dialyzable components necessary for continuous growth. Journal of Protozoology 32:59-64.

Divo, A. A., T. G. Geary, and J. B. Jensen. 1985b. The mitochondrion of *Plasmodium falciparum* visualized by rhodamine 123 fluorescence. Journal of Protozoology 32:442-446.

Dobeli, H., A. Trzeciak, D. Gillessen, H. Matile, I. K. Srivastava, L. H. Perrin, P. E. Jakob, and U. Certa. 1990. Expression, purification, biochemical characterization and inhibition of recombinant *Plasmodium falciparum* aldolase. Molecular and Biochemical Parasitology 41:259-268.

Ellis, J., D. O. Irving, T. E. Wellems, R. J. Howard, and G. A. M. Cross. 1987. Structure and expression of the knob-associated histidine-rich protein of *Plasmodium falciparum*. Molecular and Biochemical Parasitology 26:203-214.

Fang, X., D. C. Kaslow, J. H. Adams, and L. H. Miller. 1991. Cloning of the *Plasmodium vivax* Duffy receptor. Molecular and Biochemical Parasitology 44:125-132.

Fenton, B., and D. Walliker. 1990. Genetic analysis of polymorphic proteins of the human malaria parasite *Plasmodium falciparum*. Genetical Research 55:81-86.

Foote, S. J., J. K. Thompson, A. F. Cowman, and D. J. Kemp. 1989. Amplification of the multidrug resistance gene in some chloroquine-resistant isolates of *P. falciparum*. Cell 57:921-930.

Foote, S. J., D. E. Kyle, R. K. Martin, A. M. J. Oduola, K. Forsyth, D. J. Kemp, and A.

F. Cowman. 1990. Several alleles of the multidrug-resistance gene are closely linked to chloroquine resistance in *Plasmodium falciparum.* Nature 345:255-258.

Gardner, M. J., P. A. Bates, I. T. Ling, D. J. Moore, S. McCready, M. B. R. Gunasekera, R. J. M. Wilson, and D. H. Williamson. 1988. Mitochondrial DNA of the human malarial parasite *Plasmodium falciparum.* Molecular and Biochemical Parasitology 31:11-18.

Gardner, M. J., D. H. Williamson, and R. J. M. Wilson. 1991. A circular DNA in malaria parasites encodes an RNA polymerase like that of prokaryotes and chloroplasts. Molecular and Biochemical Parasitology 44:115-124.

Geary, T. G., E. J. Delaney, I. M. Klotz, and J. B. Jensen. 1983. Inhibition of the growth of *Plasmodium falciparum* in vitro by covalent modification of hemoglobin. Molecular and Biochemical Parasitology 9:59-72.

Geary, T. G., A. A. Divo, D. C. Bonanni, and J. B. Jensen. 1985a. Nutritional requirements of *Plasmodium falciparum* in culture. III. Further observations on essential nutrients and anti-metabolites. Journal of Protozoology 32:608-613.

Geary, T. G., A. A. Divo, and J. B. Jensen. 1985b. Nutritional requirements of *Plasmodium falciparum* in culture. II. Effects of anti-metabolites in a semi-defined medium. Journal of Protozoology 32:65-69.

Gero, A. M., and W. J. O'Sullivan. 1990. Purines and pyrimidines in malarial parasites. Blood Cells 16:467-484.

Ginsburg, H. 1990a. Alterations caused by the intraerythrocytic malaria parasite in the permeability of its host cell membrane. Comparative Biochemistry and Physiology 95A:31-39.

Ginsburg, H. 1990b. Some reflections concerning host erythrocyte-malarial parasite interrelationships. Blood Cells 16:225-235.

Ginsburg, H., and W. D. Stein. 1987. New permeability pathways induced by the malaria parasite in the membrane of its host erythrocyte: potential routes for targeting of drugs into infected cells. Bioscience Reports 7:455-463.

Goldberg, D. E., A. F. G. Slater, A. Cerami, and G. B. Henderson. 1990. Hemoglobin degradation in the malaria parasite *Plasmodium falciparum*: an ordered process in a unique organelle. Proceedings of the National Academy of Sciences of the United States of America 87:2931-2935.

Goldberg, D. E., A. F. G. Slater, R. Beavis, B. Chait, A. Cerami, and G. B. Henderson. 1991. Hemoglobin degradation in the human malaria pathogen *Plasmodium falciparum*: catabolic pathway initiated by a specific aspartate protease. Journal of Experimental Medicine 173:961-969.

Goldie, P., E. F. Roth Jr., J. Oppenheim, and J. P. Vanderberg. 1990. Biochemical characterization of *Plasmodium falciparum* hemozoin. American Journal of Tropical Medicine and Hygiene 43:584-596.

Gunderson, J. H., M. L. Sogin, G. Woollett, M. Hollingdale, V. F. de la Cruz, A. P. Waters, and T. F. McCutchan. 1987. Structurally distinct, stage-specific ribosomes occur in *Plasmodium.* Science 238:933-937.

Hadley, T. J., F. W. Klotz, and L. H. Miller. 1986. Invasion of erythrocytes by malaria parasites: a cellular and molecular overview. Pp. 451-477 in Annual Review of Microbiology, Ornston, L. N., A. Balows, and P. Baumann, eds. Palo Alto: Annual Reviews, Inc.

Haldar, K., C. L. Henderson, and G. A. M. Cross. 1986. Identification of the parasite transferrin receptor of *Plasmodium falciparum*-infected erythrocytes and its acylation via 1,2-diacyl-sn-glycerol. Proceedings of the National Academy of Sciences of the United States of America 83:8565-8569.

Hall, S. J., P. F. G. Sims, and J. E. Hyde. 1991. Functional expression of the dihydrofolate reductase and thymidylate synthetase activities of the human malaria parasite *Plasmodium falciparum* in *Escherichia coli*. Molecular and Biochemical Parasitology 45:317-330.

Ho, M., B. Singh, S. Looareesuwan, T. M. E. Davis, D. Bunnag, and N. J. White. 1991. Clinical correlates of in vitro *Plasmodium falciparum* cytoadherence. Infection and Immunity 59:873-878.

Holloway, S. P., P. F. G. Sims, C. J. Delves, J. G. Scaife, and J. E. Hyde. 1989. Isolation of alpha-tubulin genes from the human malaria parasite, *Plasmodium falciparum*: sequence analysis of alpha-tubulin I. Molecular Microbiology 3:1501-1510.

Holloway, S. P., M. Gerousis, C. J. Delves, P. F. G. Sims, J. G. Scaife, and J. E. Hyde. 1990. The tubulin genes of the human malaria parasite *Plasmodium falciparum*, their chromosomal location and sequence analysis of the alpha-tubulin II gene. Molecular and Biochemical Parasitology 43:257-270.

Hope, I. A., M. Mackay, J. E. Hyde, M. Goman, and J. Scaife. 1985. The gene for an exported antigen of the malaria parasite *Plasmodium falciparum* cloned and expressed in *Escherichia coli*. Nucleic Acids Research 13:369-379.

Howard, R. J. 1988. Malarial proteins at the membrane of *Plasmodium falciparum*-infected erythrocytes and their involvement in cytoadherence to endothelial cells. Progress in Allergy 41:98-147.

Howard, R. J., and A. D. Gilladoga. 1989. Molecular studies related to the pathogenesis of cerebral malaria. Blood 74:2603-2618.

Kemp, D. J., L. M. Corcoran, R. L. Coppel, H. D. Stahl, A. E. Bianco, and G. V. Brown. 1985. Size variation in chromosomes from independent cultured isolates of *Plasmodium falciparum*. Nature 315:347-350.

Kemp, D. J., R. L. Coppel, and R. F. Anders. 1987a. Repetitive proteins and genes of malaria. Pp. 181-208 in Annual Review of Microbiology, Ornston, L. N., A. Balows, and P. Baumann, eds. Palo Alto: Annual Reviews, Inc.

Kemp, D. J., J. K. Thompson, D. Walliker, and L. M. Corcoran. 1987b. Molecular karyotype of *Plasmodium falciparum*: conserved linkage groups and expendable histidine-rich protein genes. Proceedings of the National Academy of Sciences of the United States of America 84:7672-7676.

Kemp, D. J., A. F. Cowman, and D. Walliker. 1990. Genetic diversity in *Plasmodium falciparum*. Advances in Parasitology 29:75-149.

King, A., and D. W. Melton. 1987. Characterization of cDNA clones for hypoxanthine-guanine phosphoribosyltransferase from the human malarial parasite, *Plasmodium falciparum*: comparisons to the mammalian gene and protein. Nucleic Acids Research 15:10469-10481.

Krotoski, W. A., W. E. Collins, R. S. Bray, P. C. C. Garnham, F. B. Cogswell, R. W. Gwadz, R. Killick-Kendrick, R. Wolf, R. Sinden, L. C. Koontz, and P. S. Stanfill. 1982. Demonstration of hypnozoites in sporozoite-transmitted *Plasmodium vivax* infection. American Journal of Tropical Medicine and Hygiene 31:1291-1293.

Kumar, N., C. Syin, R. Carter, I. Quakyi, and L. H. Miller. 1988. *Plasmodium falciparum* gene encoding a protein similar to the 78-kDa rat glucose-regulated stress protein. Proceedings of the National Academy of Sciences of the United States of America 85:6277-6281.

Kwiatkowski, D., A. V. S. Hill, I. Sambou, P. Twumasi, J. Castracane, K. R. Manogue, A. Cerami, D. R. Brewster, and B. M. Greenwood. 1990. TNF concentration in fatal cerebral, non-fatal cerebral, and uncomplicated *Plasmodium falciparum* malaria. Lancet 336:1201-1204 .

Langreth, S. G., and E. Peterson. 1985. Pathogenicity, stability, and immunogenicity of a knobless clone of *Plasmodium falciparum* in Colombian owl monkeys. Infection and Immunity 47:760-766.

MacPherson, G. G., M. J. Warrell, N. J. White, S. Looareesuwan, and D. A. Warrell. 1985. Human cerebral malaria: a quantitative ultrastructural analysis of parasitized erythrocyte sequestration. American Journal of Pathology 119:385-401.

McCutchan, T. F., J. B. Dame, L. H. Miller, and J. Barnwell. 1984. Evolutionary relatedness of *Plasmodium* species as determined by the structure of DNA. Science 225:808-811.

Miller, L. H. 1977. Hypothesis on the mechanism of erythrocyte invasion by malaria merozoites. Bulletin of the World Health Organization 55:157-162.

Perkins, M. E. 1989. Erythrocyte invasion by the malarial merozoite: recent advances. Experimental Parasitology 69:94-99.

Petersen, C., R. Nelson, C. Magowan, W. Wollish, J. Jensen, and J. Leech. 1989. The mature erythrocyte surface antigen of *Plasmodium falciparum* is not required for knobs or cytoadherence. Molecular and Biochemical Parasitology 36:61-66.

Petersen, C., R. Nelson, J. Leech, J. Jensen, W. Wollish, and A. Scherf. 1990. The gene product of the *Plasmodium falciparum* 11.1 locus is a protein larger than one megadalton. Molecular and Biochemical Parasitology 42:189-196.

Peterson, D. S., D. Walliker, and T. E. Wellems. 1988. Evidence that a point mutation in dihydrofolate reductase-thymidylate synthase confers resistance to pyrimethamine in falciparum malaria. Proceedings of the National Academy of Sciences of the United States of America 85:9114-9118.

Peterson, M. G., R. L. Coppel, P. McIntyre, C. J. Langford, G. Woodrow, G. V. Brown, R. F. Anders, and D. J. Kemp. 1988a. Variation in the precursor to the major merozoite surface antigens of *Plasmodium falciparum*. Molecular and Biochemical Parasitology 27:291-302.

Peterson, M. G., R. L. Coppel, M. B. Moloney, and D. J. Kemp. 1988b. Third form of the precursor to the major merozoite surface antigens of *Plasmodium falciparum*. Molecular and Cellular Biology 8:2664-2667.

Pollack, Y., R. Shemer, S. Metzger, D. T. Spira, and J. Golenser. 1985. *Plasmodium falciparum*: expression of the adenine phosphoribosyltransferase gene in mouse L cells. Experimental Parasitology 60:270-275.

Pologe, L. G., and J. V. Ravetch. 1986. A chromosomal rearrangement in a *P. falciparum* histidine-rich protein gene is associated with the knobless phenotype. Nature 322:474-477.

Pologe, L. G., and J. V. Ravetch. 1988. Large deletions result from breakage and healing of *P. falciparum* chromosomes. Cell 55:869-874.

Pologe, L. G., A. Pavlovec, H. Shio, and J. V. Ravetch. 1987. Primary structure and subcellular localization of the knob-associated histidine-rich protein of *Plasmodium falciparum.* Proceedings of the National Academy of Sciences of the United States of America 84:7139-7143.

Pologe, L. G., D. de Bruin, and J. V. Ravetch. 1990. A and T homopolymeric stretches mediate a DNA inversion in *Plasmodium falciparum* which results in loss of gene expression. Molecular and Cellular Biology 10:3243-3246.

Prapunwattana, P., W. J. O'Sullivan, and Y. Yuthavong. 1988. Depression of *Plasmodium falciparum* dihydroorotate dehydrogenase activity in in vitro culture by tetracycline. Molecular and Biochemical Parasitology 27:119-124.

Ravetch, J. V. 1989. Chromosomal polymorphisms and gene expression in *Plasmodium falciparum.* Experimental Parasitology 68:121-125.

Rosenthal, P. J., J. H. McKerrow, M. Aikawa, H. Nagasawa, and J. H. Leech. 1988. A malarial cysteine protease is necessary for hemoglobin degradation by *Plasmodium falciparum.* Journal of Clinical Investigation 82:1560-1566.

Roth, E. Jr. 1990. *Plasmodium falciparum* carbohydrate metabolism: a connection between host cell and parasite. Blood Cells 16:453-460.

Roth, E. F. Jr., M.-C. Calvin, I. Max-Audit, J. Rosa, and R. Rosa. 1988. The enzymes of the glycolytic pathway in erythrocytes infected with *Plasmodium falciparum* malaria parasites. Blood 72:1922-1925.

Santoro, F., A. H. Cochrane, V. Nussenzweig, E. H. Nardin, R. S. Nussenzweig, R. W. Gwadz, and A. Ferreira. 1983. Structural similarities among the protective antigens of sporozoites from different species of malaria parasites. Journal of Biological Chemistry 258:3341-3345.

Saul, A., and D. Battistutta. 1988. Codon usage in *Plasmodium falciparum.* Molecular and Biochemical Parasitology 27:35-42.

Scheibel, L. W. 1988. Plasmodial metabolism and related organellar function during various stages of the life-cycle: carbohydrates. Pp. 219-252 in Principles and Practice of Malariology, Wernsdorfer, W., and I. McGregor, eds. New York: Churchill Livingstone.

Scheibel, L. W., and I. W. Sherman. 1988. Plasmodial metabolism and related organellar function during various stages of the life-cycle: proteins, lipids, nucleic acids and vitamins. Pp. 219-252 in Principles and Practice of Malariology, Wernsdorfer, W., and I. McGregor, eds. New York: Churchill Livingstone.

Scheibel, L. W., S. H. Ashton, and W. Trager. 1979. *Plasmodium falciparum*: microaerophilic requirements in human red blood cells. Experimental Parasitology 47:410-418.

Sen, K., and G. N. Godsen. 1990. Isolation of alpha- and beta-tubulin genes of *Plasmodium falciparum* using a single oligonucleotide probe. Molecular and Biochemical Parasitology 39:173-182.

Sharma, Y. D., and A. Kilejian. 1987. Structure of the knob protein (KP) gene of *Plasmodium falciparum.* Molecular and Biochemical Parasitology 26:11-16.

Simmons, D., G. Woollett, M. Bergin-Cartwright, D. Kay, and J. Scaife. 1987. A malaria protein exported into a new compartment within the host erythrocyte. EMBO Journal 6:485-491.

Simmons, D. L., J. E. Hyde, M. Mackay, M. Goman, and J. Scaife. 1985. Cloning studies on the gene coding for L-(+)-lactate dehydrogenase of *Plasmodium falciparum.* Molecular and Biochemical Parasitology 15:231-243.

Sirawaraporn, W., R. Sirawaraporn, A. F. Cowman, Y. Yuthavong, and D. V. Santi.

1990. Heterologous expression of active thymidylate synthase-dihydrofolate reductase from *Plasmodium falciparum*. Biochemistry 29:10779-10785.

Slater, A. F. G., W. J. Swiggard, B. R. Orton, W. D. Flitter, D. E. Goldberg, A. Cerami, and G. B. Henderson. 1991. An iron-carboxylate bond links the heme units of malaria pigment. Proceedings of the National Academy of Sciences of the United States of America 88:325-329.

Slomianny, C. 1990. Commentary: three-dimensional reconstruction of the feeding process of the malaria parasite. Blood Cells 16:369-378.

Smythe, J. A., M. G. Peterson, R. L. Coppel, A. J. Saul, D. J. Kemp, and R. F. Anders. 1990. Structural diversity in the 45-kilodalton merozoite surface antigen of *Plasmodium falciparum*. Molecular and Biochemical Parasitology 39:227-234.

Stahl, H. D., D. J. Kemp, P. E. Crewther, D. B. Scanlon, G. Woodrow, G. V. Brown, A. E. Bianco, R. F. Anders, and R. L. Coppel. 1985. Sequence of a cDNA encoding a small polymorphic histidine- and alanine-rich protein from *Plasmodium falciparum*. Nucleic Acids Research 13:7837-7846.

Stahl, H. D., A. E. Bianco, P. E. Crewther, R. F. Anders, A. P. Kyne, R. L. Coppel, G. F. Mitchell, D. J. Kemp, and G. V. Brown. 1986. Sorting large numbers of clones expressing *Plasmodium falciparum* antigens in *Escherichia coli* by differential antibody screening. Molecular and Biological Medicine 3:351-368.

Stahl, H.-D., P. E. Crewther, R. F. Anders, and D. J. Kemp. 1987. Structure of the FIRA gene of *Plasmodium falciparum*. Molecular and Biological Medicine 4:199-211.

Tanabe, K. 1990a. Glucose transport in malaria infected erythrocytes. Parasitology Today 6:225-229.

Tanabe, K. 1990b. Ion metabolism in malaria-infected erythrocytes. Blood Cells 16:437-449.

Tanabe, K., M. Mackay, M. Goman, and J. G. Scaife. 1987. Allelic dimorphism in a surface antigen gene of the malaria parasite *Plasmodium falciparum*. Journal of Molecular Biology 195:273-287.

Thomas, A. W., A. P. Waters, and D. Carr. 1990. Analysis of variation in PF83, an erythrocytic merozoite vaccine candidate antigen of *Plasmodium falciparum*. Molecular and Biochemical Parasitology 42:285-288.

Trager, W. 1989. Erythrocyte knobs and malaria [letter]. Nature 304:352.

Triglia, T., H. D. Stahl, P. E. Crewther, D. Scanlon, G. V. Brown, R. F. Anders, and D. J. Kemp. 1987. The complete sequence of the gene for the knob-associated histidine-rich protein from *Plasmodium falciparum*. EMBO Journal 6:1413-1419.

Udomsangpetch, R., M. Aikawa, K. Berzins, M. Wahlgren, and P. Perlmann. 1989. Cytoadherence of knobless *Plasmodium falciparum*-infected erythrocytes and its inhibition by a human monoclonal antibody. Nature 338:763-765.

Vial, H. J., M.-L. Ancelin, J. R. Philippot, and M. J. Thuet. 1990. Biosynthesis and dynamics of lipids in *Plasmodium*-infected mature mammalian erythrocytes. Blood Cells 16:531-555.

Walliker, D. 1989a. Genetic recombination in malaria parasites. Experimental Parasitology 69:303-309.

Walliker, D. 1989b. Implications of genetic exchange in the study of protozoan infections. Parasitology 99:S49-S58.

Walliker, D., I. A. Quakyi, T. E. Wellems, T. F. McCutchan, A. Szarfman, W. T. London, L. M. Corcoran, T. R. Burkot, and R. Carter. 1987. Genetic analysis of the human malaria parasite *Plasmodium falciparum*. Science 236:1661-1666.

Waters, A. P., C. Syin, and T. F. McCutchan. 1989. Developmental regulation of stage-specific ribosome populations in *Plasmodium*. Nature 342:438-440.

Weber, J. L., J. A. Lyon, R. H. Wolff, T. Hall, G. H. Lowell, and J. D. Chulay. 1988. Primary structure of a *Plasmodium falciparum* malaria antigen located at the merozoite surface and within the parasitophorous vacuole. Journal of Biological Chemistry 263:11421-11425.

Wellems, T. E. 1991. Molecular genetics of drug resistance in *Plasmodium falciparum* malaria. Parasitology Today 7:110-112.

Wellems, T. E., L. J. Panton, I. Y. Gluzman, V. E. do Rosario, R. W. Gwadz, A. Walker-Jonah, and D. J. Krogstad. 1990. Chloroquine resistance not linked to mdr-like genes in a *Plasmodium falciparum* cross. Nature 345:253-255.

Wesseling, J. G., R. Dirks, M. A. Smits, and J. G. G. Schoenmakers. 1989. Nucleotide sequence and expression of a beta-tubulin gene from *Plasmodium falciparum*, a malarial parasite of man. Gene 83:301-309.

Wilson, R. J. M. 1990. Biochemistry of red cell invasion. Blood Cells 16:237-252.

Yang, Y.-F., P. Tan-ariya, Y. D. Sharma, and A. Kilejian. 1987. The primary structure of a *Plasmodium falciparum* polypeptide related to heat shock proteins. Molecular and Biochemical Parasitology 26:61-68.

Zhu, J., A. P. Waters, A. Appiah, T. F. McCutchan, A. A. Lal, and M. R. Hollingdale. 1990. Stage-specific ribosomal RNA expression switches during sporozoite invasion of hepatocytes. Journal of Biological Chemistry 265:12740-12744.

7

Vector Biology, Ecology, and Control

WHERE WE WANT TO BE IN THE YEAR 2010

Vector biology will play a major role in the battle against malaria. Improved vector surveillance networks will allow most countries, particularly those in Africa, to mount effective control efforts and to predict outbreaks of disease. Researchers will be able to conduct epidemiologic surveys and track drug resistance simply by analyzing mosquito populations. Simple techniques will be used in the field to identify morphologically indistinguishable mosquitoes that have different capabilities to transmit malaria parasites, leading to more effective application of vector control measures. The entomological risk factors for severe disease and death will be identified, and interventions will be implemented. The development of environmentally safe antimosquito compounds will complement traditional residual insecticide spraying, and genetically engineered microbial agents will be used to kill mosquito larvae. An antimosquito vaccine will add to the growing arsenal of malaria control weapons. Feasibility studies will be carried out to replace populations of malaria vectors with natural or genetically altered forms that cannot transmit human malaria.

WHERE WE ARE TODAY

Vector biology, broadly defined, is the science devoted to studying insects that transmit pathogens, their contact with humans, and their interaction with the disease-causing organisms. In the case of malaria, the vector is the anopheline mosquito and the disease-causing organism is the malaria parasite. Humans and anopheline mosquitoes are both considered to be the parasite's hosts.

One of the primary goals of vector biology in malaria research is to promote a better understanding of the disease cycle that will facilitate more effectively targeted control strategies. The vast majority of successful antimalaria campaigns have relied heavily on vector control.

The distribution of malaria within human populations is linked closely to site-specific characteristics of vector populations. Within any given area, there are usually fewer than five vector species, although the biology of each species is unique in many respects, including the sites where larvae develop, adult mosquito behavior (especially human-biting behavior), susceptibility to *Plasmodium* parasites, and the ability to transmit these parasites.

Not all mosquitoes can transmit human malarial parasites. Of the thousands of described mosquito species, only a fraction of those in the genus *Anopheles* serve as vectors. Some anopheline species do not feed on humans, others are not susceptible to human malaria parasites, and a number have life spans too short to allow the parasite to fully mature. Vector species that pose the greatest threat are abundant, long-lived, commonly feed on humans, and typically dwell in proximity to people. Their role in malaria transmission depends largely on the presence of a favorable environment for larval development and adult survival, and the ability to feed on humans. Transmission also depends significantly on human habits that promote host-vector contact.

Perhaps the least understood process in malaria transmission is the development of the parasite in the vector. To transmit malaria, vectors must be able to support parasite development through several key stages over 8 to 15 days. Only then are the sporozoite-stage parasites present and ready for transmission to new human hosts. Thus, from the standpoint of vector biology, there are three main points of attack for controlling malaria: the environment, human habits, and parasite development in the vector.

In cases in which the impact and feasibility of vector control are questioned, the result is often an overwhelming reliance on chemotherapy-based measures for reducing malaria-related mortality and morbidity. In countries with the most severe malaria problems, there are seldom funds for anything but antimalarial drugs and, in some cases, for limited vector control activities (mostly in urban areas). Such approaches usually do little to prevent malaria transmission, however. The continuous need for adequate drug supplies to treat clinically ill residents of endemic areas severely limits progress toward malaria prevention. In most malarious regions of the world, there is little baseline information on vector populations and variation in the intensity of malaria transmission. Thus, it is exceedingly difficult, and often unrealistic, for developing countries to formulate malaria control strategies aimed at prevention.

As in other areas of tropical health, distinctions between field and laboratory research in vector biology are sometimes blurred, since basic research problems often require use of field-collected specimens to explore natural phenomena. Similarly, even the least sophisticated laboratories are now using modern techniques. The distinction between basic and applied research in vector biology is difficult to make, because most research topics have long-term applied or operational applications.

Throughout the world, vector biology field studies generally use a common set of techniques for collecting vectors and processing field-collected specimens. The same general methods used to study malaria transmission and vector behavior are used to evaluate new vector control strategies. As new vector-related techniques are developed for investigating the biology of anopheline mosquitoes, they are quickly adopted by field-based malaria control programs. Thus, developments in malaria vector control are highly dependent on basic research.

Vector-Parasite Interactions

Sporogonic Development in Anopheles *Mosquitoes*

The four human malarial parasites—*Plasmodium falciparum, P. vivax, P. malariae,* and *P. ovale*—all undergo a similar process of sporogonic development in the mosquito host (Garnham, 1966). Development begins when a susceptible female mosquito ingests microgametocytes (male forms) and macrogametocytes (female forms) during blood feeding on an infected human. Sexual reproduction (and, importantly, genetic recombination) occurs in the mosquito host as microgametocytes quickly exflagellate, producing microgametes that fuse with macrogametes to form zygotes. Zygotes develop into ookinetes, which penetrate the midgut epithelial cells and mature into oocysts. These in turn mature and release thousands of sporozoites into the mosquito hemolymph system. A mosquito is considered infective as soon as sporozoites invade the salivary glands. Transmission to humans occurs when sporozoites are injected with salivary fluids during a blood meal.

The time needed for sporozoites to reach the salivary glands of the mosquito depends on both the species of parasite and the ambient temperature. For example, *P. falciparum* takes 9 days at 30°C, 10 days at 25°C,

11 days at 24°C, and 23 days at 20°C, a difference of 14 days over a range of 10°C. At 25°C, the process is completed in 9 days for *P. vivax*, compared with 15 to 20 days for *P. malariae* and 16 days for *P. ovale*. The relatively short extrinsic incubation periods of *P. falciparum* and *P. vivax* are among the several reasons why these parasite species are more common than either *P. malariae* or *P. ovale*.

Once a female mosquito is infective, she remains so for life. Generally, mosquitoes are capable of transmitting sporozoites during each blood-feeding episode, sometimes to multiple individuals during each feeding cycle. Boyd and Stratman-Thomas (1934) demonstrated that *P. vivax*-infected mosquitoes could infect 90 percent of patients during the first three weeks, 66 percent by the fifth week, and only 20 percent by the seventh week. Although old infective mosquitoes that have fed 5 to 10 times can still transmit malaria sporozoites, over time these sporozoites tend to lose infectivity.

Factors Affecting Susceptibility

Factors that affect the susceptibility of anopheline mosquitoes to human malaria parasites are poorly understood. Mosquitoes of the genera *Culex* and *Aedes* contain numerous species that feed on humans and transmit a number of infectious diseases. However, none of these species transmit human malarias. The physiological and genetic basis of this insusceptibility to the human malaria parasite is unknown, just as are the differences in susceptibility among various *Anopheles* species.

The inability of malaria parasites to develop in some mosquito species may be due to the absence of some critical factor in the mosquito required for normal parasite development, or it could be due to the presence of a toxin that actively inhibits or aborts parasite development (Weathersby, 1952). One mechanism that may make mosquitoes susceptible to parasites is species-specific stimulation of exflagellation (Micks, 1949; Nijhout, 1979), while encapsulation of ookinetes and oocysts (Collins et al., 1986) and the failure of sporozoites to penetrate salivary glands (Rosenberg, 1985) may help explain mosquito resistance to malaria parasites.

The genetic basis for mosquito susceptibility or refractoriness to malaria is extremely complex (Curtis and Graves, 1983). Using laboratory-reared vectors and malaria parasites from animals, it is possible to select for highly susceptible and highly refractory strains of mosquitoes. In most cases, several genes and often complicated modes of inheritance appear to be involved.

Factors Affecting Transmission

The basic process of sporogonic development in susceptible vector species is poorly understood. The numbers of gametocytes ingested, ookinetes and oocysts that develop, sporozoites in the hemolymph and in the salivary glands, and sporozoites transmitted during a blood meal have not been well quantified. Most studies of vector competence count only oocysts on the midgut wall and crudely estimate salivary gland sporozoites. Thus, there is little information on this very important process for any vector species, and there is no basis for comparison among vector species.

Studies of sporogonic development in the vector and vector-parasite relationships for human malaria parasites are largely restricted to *P. falciparum*, the only species that can be grown in vitro. The extent to which similar vector-related studies, using animal model systems (Mons and Sinden, 1990), are relevant to human malaria is unknown.

Malaria Transmission

Most vector biology field studies focus on determining human-vector contact, feeding and resting habits, survival, and other life history parameters of vector populations. Usually, the vector status of populations is defined by determining sporozoite and oocyst rates (the proportion of infective mosquitoes in a vector population and the proportion of mosquitoes with oocysts, respectively). This approach provides essential but not sufficient information about vectorial systems (all anopheline species in a given area that transmit malaria).

Field studies of malaria transmission need to be reoriented toward quantifying other important epidemiologic parameters of anopheline populations. For example, little is known about the variation in the number of sporozoites in mosquito salivary glands (sporozoite loads), nor is there much information on the numbers of sporozoites transmitted per feeding and whether this parameter is affected by sporozoite loads. Globally, the diversity of vectorial systems should allow for great heterogeneity in the ability of vectors to transmit sporozoites; this has significant implications for malaria control. For example, a sporozoite vaccine may be effective in one country where a certain *Anopheles* species transmits an average of 5 sporozoites per bite, but not in another country where a different *Anopheles* species transmits 500 sporozoites per bite.

Factors influencing variation in sporozoite rates and in sporozoite loads, within geographic zones, are equally important. Life stages of *Plasmodium* in the vector, other than oocysts and sporozoites, have never been studied in nature. Lack of information about the early stages of sporogonic development, from the point of ingestion of gametocytes to ookinetes to the appearance of oocysts, is critical because these stages influence the development of sporozoites. It is also likely that the life history parameters of vector populations, such as vector size, feeding habits, frequency of feeding, age, and reproductive state, can influence the mosquito's susceptibility to parasites and the probability it will survive long enough for the parasite to fully develop.

Vector biologists know very little about vector-related factors that affect sporozoite viability in nature. Epidemiologic studies indicate that, at most, between 1 and 20 percent of sporozoite inoculations produce infections in nature (Pull and Grab, 1974). Effective, direct assays for determining sporozoite viability for individual, field-collected mosquitoes do not exist. Human antibodies ingested by mosquitoes may play some role in regulating sporozoite infectivity. In one study, human immunoglobulin G antibody was found on sporozoites in over 80 percent of infected mosquitoes sampled in Kenya (Beier et al., 1989); the significance in terms of sporozoite infectivity is unknown.

Regulation of Vector Populations—Larval Ecology

The mechanisms that regulate vector populations are poorly understood but are of great importance for malaria control (Molineaux, 1988). For example, there is limited information on the biology of aquatic stages of malaria vectors. The factors affecting larval survival and the mechanisms controlling adult production are largely unknown for even the most important vector species. The basic concept of density-dependent regulation has never been studied for populations in nature. It is extremely important to know whether populations are regulated through competition (intra- and/or interspecific) and predation in the aquatic habitat. Furthermore, there is no baseline information on the foraging habits and strategies of larval-stage vector populations. The study of larval biology is complicated further by inadequate techniques for the identification of larvae belonging to species complexes. Consequently, few entomologists seek to tackle this important area of anopheline biology.

A basic understanding of the aquatic stages of vectors is extremely relevant to malaria control. Source reduction through the modification of larval habitats was the key to malaria eradication efforts in the United States, Israel, and Italy (Kitron and Spielman, 1989). In these countries, a variety of measures directed against the aquatic stages of important vectors reduced cases of malaria and eliminated parasite transmission.

Vector Incrimination

The identification of anopheline mosquitoes responsible for malaria transmission is known as vector incrimination, and the approach is the same for any given area. Mosquitoes, preferably those coming to feed on humans, are collected, identified, and dissected to determine the presence of sporozoites in the salivary glands. Immunological techniques can be used to identify particular *Plasmodium* species. This is important since sporozoites of all *Plasmodium* species that infect humans are morphologically similar, and sporozoites of most animal malarias cannot be distinguished morphologically from those that infect humans.

Species are sometimes referred to as primary and secondary vectors. The incrimination of primary vectors is usually clear-cut; they are often abundant, commonly feed on humans, and have measurable sporozoite rates. Incrimination of secondary vectors is more complicated, because these species may be uncommon and have low sporozoite rates. However, they may be seasonally abundant and, at times, play a major role in transmission. Adult mosquito behavior and larval ecology may be significantly different in primary versus secondary vectors, and measures taken to control primary vectors may not have an impact on secondary vectors.

Gathering site-specific information about vectors is an important first step in planning vector control measures. It is sometimes necessary to extrapolate vector-related data from areas where actual vector identification has been performed. Such an approach is not without problems, since epidemiologically significant shifts in primary vector species can occur due to changes in the environment, such as urbanization, deforestation, and irrigation.

Vector Species and Distributions

Haworth (1988) provides a detailed review of the global distribution of human malaria and, for each geographic zone, lists the primary and secondary vectors. In general, malaria in each zone is transmitted by a specific set of *Anopheles* species. Distribution patterns for mosquito species are fairly stable. Vector species rarely completely disappear from a region, and in no case have indigenous vectors been deliberately eradicated. The introduction of malaria vectors into nonindigenous areas is a serious public health concern. For example, the introduction of *Anopheles gambiae* to Brazil and Egypt in the 1940s caused devastating epidemics and required unparalleled efforts to eliminate the newly arrived vector (Duffy, 1977).

The natural distribution patterns of anophelines are largely determined by environmental conditions. Each species has unique environmental tolerance limits. The same is true for malarial parasites. For example, the distributions of *P. vivax* and *P. falciparum* are theoretically limited by summer isotherms of 15°C and 18°C, respectively, the temperatures required for the completion of the sporogonic cycle in the mosquito host (Boyd, 1949).

Mosquito Taxonomy and Species Complexes

In malaria entomology, anopheline species are grouped according to morphological criteria and related taxonomic information. Much of modern-day taxonomy addresses problems associated with species complexes, that is groups of morphologically indistinguishable species that are genetically different and that may differ greatly in vectorial potential. The limits of the traditional morphological approaches to species identification became apparent in Europe with the puzzling observation of "anophelism without malaria": certain areas with low densities of *An. maculipennis* had malaria transmission, while other areas with an abundance of *An. maculipennis* had no malaria transmission at all. This observation subsequently led to the discovery of the *An. maculipennis* complex.

There are more than 20 recognized species complexes in the genus *Anopheles*, many of which include malaria vectors (Coluzzi, 1988). A variety of methods are available for discriminating among species—the gold standard relies on cytogenetics—but none are simple or as yet, practical for routine use in the field.

The identification of vectors that belong to species complexes has long been a stumbling block in malaria epidemiology and control. The failure to recognize sibling species can mean that vector species are mistaken for nonvector species, and vice versa. The results of field studies that evaluate larval ecology, seasonal biting rates, host preference, infection rates, resting habits, and malaria control efforts may be misleading if morphologically defined "species" actually are a mixture of two or three species. In Africa, for example, sibling mosquito species living in the same area respond differently to insecticides, presenting formidable obstacles to vector control operations.

Parasite Transmission

There are distinct groups of mosquito vectors associated with almost every major type of malaria (see Chapter 10). Very often, the single greatest source of variation within these regions is the mosquito itself. The variation among species, feeding habits, seasonality, abundance, and vectorial capacity all help determine how malaria is transmitted to and expressed in individuals and populations.

Field Studies

The principles and methods used for sampling anopheline mosquitoes have been the same for the past 25 years, and are described in detail by the

World Health Organization (1975). Methods include collecting mosquitoes that come to feed on humans or animals and collecting resting vectors in houses, in animal shelters, outdoors, or in traps. In general, these methods can be adapted to any geographic location or malaria situation.

Once collected, mosquitoes can be identified by external morphology and dissected for malaria oocysts and salivary gland sporozoites, and ovaries can be examined to determine parity and egg-stage development. Further analysis can reveal blood meal contents, insecticide susceptibility, chromosomal patterns for species identification, and the presence of nonmalaria parasites (World Health Organization, 1975).

Immunological methods for detecting species-specific malaria sporozoites in mosquitoes have been developed (Zavala et al., 1982; Wirtz et al., 1987). In malaria field studies, these methods are useful for estimating sporozoite rates and for identifying the species of *Plasmodium* detected by dissection (Beier et al., 1990a). Advances in methods used to analyze blood meals (Beier et al., 1988; Tempelis, 1989) and to determine insecticide resistance (Brown and Brogdon, 1987) have been made. Major advances in the genetic analysis of vector populations using DNA-based technologies also have been made (Collins et al., 1990). A combination of traditional methods and a battery of newer immunological or molecular assays can now be performed on single specimens of anopheline mosquitoes to yield critical biological and epidemiologic information.

Indices of Malaria Transmission

Determining the intensity of malaria transmission by mosquito populations is a key component of epidemiologic studies of malaria. Two important dimensions of malaria transmission are the entomological inoculation rate (EIR) and vectorial capacity (VC). The EIR is a measure of the number of infective bites each person receives per night, and is a direct measure of the risk of human exposure to the bites of infective mosquitoes. The VC measures the potential for malaria transmission, based on several key parameters of vector populations. It is important to realize how these measurements differ and how each is important for describing malaria situations.

The EIR is the product of the human-biting rate and the sporozoite rate. Human-biting rates are best estimated by all-night collections of mosquitoes that come to feed on humans. The sporozoite rate is determined by dissection and examination of mosquito salivary glands or by immunological methods. Measurement of EIRs during longitudinal studies provides information on seasonal variations in transmission. The EIR is the only direct measure of malaria transmission and the only useful index for predicting malaria epidemics (Onori and Grab, 1980).

Vectorial capacity is based on several key parameters of vector populations. The equation used to calculate VC is $C = ma^2p^n/-log_e p$, where $C =$ vectorial capacity, m = density of vectors in relation to humans, a = number of blood meals taken on humans per vector per day, p = daily survival probability of vectors (measured in days), and n = incubation period in the vector (measured in days). The formula expresses the capacity of a vector population to transmit malaria based on the potential number of secondary inoculations originating per day from an infective person. The formula is specific for a given species of vector, because different species vary with respect to m, a, and p. If several vector species coexist, the VC is the sum of the vectorial capacities of each of the individual vector species. Vectorial capacity is an essential component of mathematical models of malaria transmission. There are a number of assumptions that must be taken into account when VC is used to either assess the status of a malarious situation or predict its evolution (Molineaux, 1988).

Theoretically, VC can predict the extent to which mosquito populations must be reduced to affect the intensity of malaria transmission. For example, according to the formula, the mosquito population would have to be reduced by 99 percent in a holoendemic area before any change in transmission would occur. Such predictions are difficult to verify in natural situations, however. Indeed, there is a need to determine how reductions in vectorial capacity affect patterns of disease in human populations.

Surveillance Strategies

Malaria surveillance may be the most important first step for endemic countries hoping to understand and manage their malaria problems. Surveillance networks must be able to monitor the disease in human populations, track patterns of parasite drug resistance, and monitor transmission by vector populations.

The geographic variation in the intensity of malaria transmission is of prime importance for development of appropriate control measures. Few endemic countries have useful information on the patterns and intensities of transmission. This is in marked contrast to small, size-limited studies, in which information has been collected over many years. For example, investigators have studied malaria in the Kisumu area of Kenya for 60 years, but relatively little is known about vectors and transmission anywhere else in the country.

Recently developed immunoassays that detect sporozoites in mosquitoes make vector surveillance more feasible, especially in areas where vectors prefer indoor environments and can be easily sampled, as in parts of Africa. The ability to dry and store mosquitoes for later processing by enzyme-linked immunosorbent assay will facilitate the collection of mosquitoes from multiple sites for testing in central facilities. Indices of transmission intensity, derived from measurements of vector densities and sporozoite rates (analogous to the EIR), can provide useful information about patterns of endemicity in human populations. For the purposes of malaria management, it is useful to know whether individuals receive 5, 50, or 500 infective bites per year, as well as when the transmission occurs. Vector-derived EIR estimates are highly correlated with measurements of malaria incidence. In this respect, EIRs provide stronger predictive capabilities than do estimates of prevalence.

Analysis of fresh blood meals of human-fed anophelines for the presence of antimalarial antibodies represents a possible alternative approach to serosurveys. Human antiparasite antibodies remain intact, undigested, for about 24 hours. Even though anophelines ingest only 1 to 2 microliters of blood, stage-specific antibodies can be detected by simple immunoassays (Beier et al., 1989). Although molecular probes do not appear to be sensitive enough to detect the presence of parasites in this small volume of blood, polymerase chain reaction methods could be used in the future to detect low numbers of parasites in mosquito blood meals. If sufficient epidemiologic information can be extracted from analyzing the blood meals of mosquitoes, there may be less need to draw blood from residents of endemic communities. As a replacement for traditional surveys, then, the effectiveness of such an approach deserves consideration.

Entomological Components of Malaria Vaccine Development

The development and testing of P. *falciparum* sporozoite vaccines depend on the availability of sporozoites from experimentally infected mosquitoes. Sporozoites are in great demand for use in antibody assays and in the characterization and evaluation of candidate vaccines. Studies testing the efficacy of vaccines against sporozoite challenge have used infective mosquitoes to feed on volunteers.

This methodology raises a number of vector-related questions. For example, since the number of sporozoites transmitted by infective mosquitoes is unknown, vaccines are being tested without reference to levels of sporozoite inocula. There is also the concern that laboratory infected mosquitoes may have a greater sporozoite transmission potential than do those in nature, since sporozoite loads are generally 10 to 200 times higher in the former (Davis et al., 1989). These entomological concerns are of equal importance when one is testing vaccines against blood stages of the malaria parasites.

Vector-related issues will become even more important as vaccines move from laboratory testing to field evaluation. Some of the concerns have already been outlined (World Health Organization, 1986). A prerequisite for vaccine field trials is the long-term characterization of malaria transmission by vector populations in prospective study sites. Baseline information on both the intensity and seasonality of transmission is necessary for planning vaccine trials. For phase IIb, III, and IV trials, concurrent measurements of sporozoite challenge (EIR) will be extremely useful to gauge vaccine efficacy. The supporting role of vector studies in malaria vaccine field trials has received little attention. There is a need to define strategies for measuring entomological variables to assist in the design, implementation, and evaluation of such trials. The differing objectives and methods used in phase IIb, III, and IV trials will require different entomological approaches (Beier et al., 1990b).

Vector Control

Like many vector-borne diseases, variations in malaria transmission are linked closely to the ecologic conditions in which the vectors exist. Rather than planning malaria control for broad geographic areas, consideration must be given to differences in transmission within specific ecologic zones (e.g., forest, savannas, and coastal areas) within countries, as well as variations that occur at the district and village level (see Chapter 10).

Prevention and Control of Transmission

There are two distinct approaches to preventing malaria transmission: treating infected individuals to kill or reduce the number of gametocytes, the stage of the parasite that initiates infections in mosquitoes; and vector control.

In areas of heavy transmission, clinical treatment of malaria cases does not necessarily have any impact on transmission (Breman and Campbell, 1988). Standard therapies that use schizonticidal drugs, such as chloroquine, do not kill or even affect the infectivity of mature gametocytes. Thus, treated individuals harboring infectious gametocytes continue to contribute to the transmission cycle. Many individuals also become reinfected soon after treatment. Another consideration is that asymptomatic infections, which are usually difficult and expensive to detect, contribute significantly to the maintenance of transmission.

If drug treatment is to have an impact on transmission, the primary reservoir of infection, usually children under the age of 12 (Muirhead-Thomson, 1954), who have not acquired significant clinical immunity, must be targeted. In areas of low to moderate endemicity, mass administration of schizonticidal and gametocidal drugs can reduce the parasite reservoir enough to lower the level of transmission. Except in special circumstances, however, such as actual or potential epidemics, this approach cannot be recommended because of significant safety and operational limitations.

Antivector measures are the most effective tools for preventing and controlling malaria transmission. Common measures include indoor and outdoor insecticide spraying; the use of insecticide-impregnated bednets and curtains; the treatment of larval development sites with chemical or microbiological larvicides or with biological control agents such as larvivorous fishes; and environmental measures, such as reducing or managing aquatic larval sites, and designing and locating houses and animal shelters in areas with the least possible exposure to malaria transmission.

Application of these measures can, alone or in combination, reduce vector abundance, human-vector contact, and vector infectivity. Steps taken to disrupt the mosquito larval cycle, by larviciding, the use of biological control agents, and environmental modification, will reduce vector abundance. Reduction of human-vector contact is typically achieved by insecticide spraying, by some environmental measures such as mosquito-proofing dwellings, and by personal protective measures such as bednets. The spraying of pesticides also reduces vector infectivity by reducing the vector survival rate and increasing the length of the sporogonic cycle (when indoor-resting mosquitoes are forced to rest outside, where ambient temperatures are suboptimal for parasite maturation). Reducing vector abundance has a comparatively lower impact on malaria transmission than does reducing human-vector contact. The greatest impact, however, is seen with a reduction in vector infectivity.

Selection of Antivector Measures

Theoretically, in view of its ability to reduce vector abundance, human-vector contact, and vector infectivity, insecticide spraying aimed at killing adult mosquitoes is the antivector measure of choice in malaria control. In fact, however, spraying is effective, acceptable, and sustainable only under certain circumstances. Residually acting insecticides sprayed on the interior walls of houses and, in some areas, on cattle sheds plays a key role in interrupting malaria transmission where the stability of the parasite cycle depends on the endophilic behavior of both vector and human host. This spraying tactic makes the domestic environment inhospitable to both mosquitoes and malaria parasites developing within them.

Residual spraying is particularly effective for situations in tropical and subtropical areas, including some highlands, where vectors feed on humans and rest inside houses. In situations where mosquitoes both feed and rest outdoors, residual insecticides applied indoors will have little or no impact on malaria transmission. Insecticide spraying outside is seldom effective, and being justified only under certain epidemic conditions. Overall, the effectiveness of properly applied insecticides depends on mosquito susceptibility to the insecticide, the timing of spraying, achievement of adequate contact between the vector and the insecticide, and the degree or intensity of malaria transmission. In many areas of heavy transmission, reducing transmission by even 99 percent may not produce significant decreases in infection rates.

Insecticide spraying for limited or intermittent vector control might be considered appropriate in urban or semiurban settings where a significant proportion of nonimmune people live in crowded conditions and are surrounded by a variety of larval development sites in large-scale population settlements in endemic areas (e.g., refugee and military camps); in agro-industrial development projects, such as cotton or sugarcane plantations and rice-growing regions that employ workers from nonendemic regions; and in areas threatened by malaria epidemics.

The use of larvicides is warranted only in certain urban malaria situations or to control larval development in discrete and readily accessible habitats. In many such cases, water management by drainage, intermittent flushing, aquatic plant control, introduction of larvivorous fishes, and covering of wells is a cost-effective option.

Personal Protection Measures

There are numerous, simple measures that can be used by individuals to decrease their exposure to infective mosquitoes. Farid (1988) discusses the optimal application of repellents (e.g., skin lotions, applications for clothing, and mosquito coils which are burned to release insecticide), bednets and screens, housing design and siting, and chemical and mechanical measures to repel or kill mosquitoes.

Personal protection measures are definitely an appropriate form of malaria control for the individual. Even if they are not 100 percent effective in preventing exposure to all infective mosquito bites, they do reduce the overall risk of infection. This is an important concern for individuals living in endemic areas, where it is not possible or even advisable for everyone to maintain long-term prophylaxis with drugs. For short-term travelers, personal protection measures should be considered as a supplement to chemoprophylaxis. The challenge for the future will be to promote the concept of individual responsibility for malaria prevention, to promote the use of existing measures for personal protection, and to develop new and appropriate methods to protect individuals.

Insecticide-impregnated bednets are increasingly being promoted as a relatively inexpensive and often culturally acceptable method for reducing human-mosquito contact. There is little doubt that insecticide-treated bednets are a useful form of protection for the individual. Whether community-wide use of bednets has a significant impact on malaria transmission, morbidity, and mortality remains to be determined, however.

Over the last several years, field trials in several endemic areas have evaluated the effectiveness of insecticide-treated bednets and curtains (reviewed by Rozendaal, 1989). Some of the largest trials with the most dramatic results have been in China, where a decline in malaria incidence has been noted over several years. Most of the trials in Africa, Asia and the Pacific, and South America have noted significant reductions in key parameters of malaria transmission by vector populations (e.g., human-vector contact, sporozoite rates, and vector survival). Corresponding reductions in malaria prevalence, malaria incidence, severe infections and death have been more difficult to document, since they depend on local factors such as vector behavior, seasonality of transmission, levels of endemicity, and the immune status of populations. It is unclear whether wide-scale community use of insecticide-treated bednets alone can confer substantial benefit to populations living in areas of low to moderate endemicity or seasonal transmission. Further, the degree of protection that bednets can provide in areas of high, year-round transmission is unknown.

Insecticide-treated bednets are gaining in popularity, but many significant questions remain regarding their effectiveness, acceptability, and sustainability. Now in progress are large-scale trials that are attempting to measure the overall impact, acceptance, and future role of bednets in malaria control efforts.

Insecticide Resistance

Insecticide resistance in mosquitoes is a major obstacle to malaria control. Resistance is usually the result of agricultural rather than public health use of pesticides. The World Health Organization (WHO) has simple test kits to determine the susceptibility levels and discriminating doses of insecticides required at the field level. At least 50 mosquito species have developed resistance to one or more insecticides since 1947 (Brown, 1983). Many species also develop "irritability" (a behavior to avoid treated surfaces) toward DDT and other insecticides. The increasingly high cost of insecticides is a major disincentive for their use in developing countries.

Ecological and Public Health Impacts of Pesticides

Worldwide, the annual impact of pesticide use for environmental and public health purposes causes $100 billion to $200 billion worth of unintended damage (Pimentel, 1990a,b). Irrespective of the particular ecosystem affected, the environmental and public health impacts of using insecticides for malaria control should be weighed against the potential benefit of improving and sustaining public health.

WHO (1986) emphasizes that DDT is still the insecticide of choice for use in indoor residual spraying, provided that the vector is susceptible. This chlorinated hydrocarbon remains one of the most effective insecticides for malaria control efforts in endemic countries. Compared with other available insecticides, it is inexpensive and, importantly, is nontoxic to humans. Few of the accidental poisonings each year can be attributed to DDT use in public health disease control programs. Parenthetically, the use of DDT as a residual indoor spray does not introduce DDT into the environment in amounts sufficient to enter the food chain, and thus this usage does not have adverse ecological consequences.

Innovative Vector Control Measures

Antimosquito Vaccines The idea that blood-feeding vectors may be damaged by mammalian antibodies directed against insect tissues is not new. Recently, scientists developed an antitick vaccine that protects cattle against tick infestations (Willadsen et al., 1989). The antibodies induced by this vaccine are directed against "concealed antigens" on tick gut cells that are not exposed during the blood-feeding process.

Preliminary studies using homogenized mosquito tissues or whole mosquitoes as the immunogen have demonstrated significant effects on mosquito survival, fecundity, and egg viability (see Chapter 9). The direct effects of antibodies produced by these methods on the sporogonic development of *P. falciparum* and other human malaria parasites are unknown, however, as are the mosquito antigens that might elicit the most effective human antibody response. Modern tools of immunology and molecular biology offer hope for the development of mosquito-derived antigens that could serve as candidate vaccines for malaria control.

Genetic Modification of Mosquito Vectors It is theoretically possible to replace populations of malaria-transmitting mosquitoes with genetically altered forms that cannot transmit the malaria parasite. The foundation for vector replacement strategies is based on continued progress and major advances in critical areas of vector biology. Already there have been successful attempts to insert foreign genes into the mosquito genome (Miller et al., 1987), and molecular probes for species identification have been developed and field tested (Collins et al., 1988).

Much research remains to be done before genetically engineered mosquitoes can be used for malaria control. Regardless of the long-term outcome of such research, however, valuable new techniques and approaches for identifying the genetic basis of malaria transmission will be developed along the way.

Environmentally Safe Biological Control Agents Natural predators and pathogens, ranging from viruses to nematodes, help regulate populations of both immature and adult-stage mosquitoes. A number of studies are looking at candidate biological control agents. Although some appear to have an impact on mosquito populations, none have a primary role in current antimalaria control operations (Service, 1983).

The most promising avenue in biological control is focusing on the larval ecology of major vector species to determine which organisms serve as food resources in the aquatic environment. Modern genetic engineering methods may eventually be used to insert genes that would promote the release of substances that would kill or disable mosquito larvae.

Training in Vector Biology

The contributions of vector biology to infectious disease research are diminishing around the world because of a lack of trained personnel, training resources, career opportunities in academia and the government, and financial support (Reeves, 1989; Moore, 1990). From 1970 to 1982, at 24 leading training institutions in the United States, 144 doctoral degrees were awarded in vector biology and 88 postdoctoral fellows were trained in the field (National Research Council, 1983). Slightly more than a fifth of these doctoral and postdoctoral scientists received their training at medical schools or schools of public health. Each year, only 10 new doctoral candidates can be expected to enter vector biology training programs in the United States. A workshop sponsored by the National Research Council developed recommendations to prevent or delay the expected national shortage of vector biologists, but these recommendations have so far not been implemented.

Although there have been no assessments since 1982, there appear to be fewer and fewer students receiving training in vector biology. Many of the outstanding educators in the field have retired and have not been replaced. Several vector biology training programs have simply closed down. None of the six textbooks on medical entomology published since 1970 are still in print, and there are no replacements in sight (Reeves, 1989).

The declining number of students trained in vector biology is related to a general trend in infectious disease research. The emphasis on biochemical- and molecular-level investigations of pathogens has superseded the biological studies of vectors, vector-pathogen interactions, and the specialty areas of medical entomology and disease ecology. The vector biologist in academia has limited access to research grant funding; work in this area is generally not considered to be at the cutting edge of science. In the immediate future, the need for vector biologists will be tied closely to increases in malaria and other vector-borne diseases expected to result from the repercussions of population growth over the next 25 years. It may be that special programs will need to be developed to fund those scientists willing to devote years to working in relative isolation in the field.

RESEARCH AGENDA

Over the next 15 to 20 years, malaria research in the area of vector biology should focus concurrently on four areas: field investigations, laboratory-based research in support of field investigations, innovative methods for malaria control, and vector control evaluation in endemic areas.

Field Investigations

Patterns of Transmission

Each type of malaria (see Chapter 10) is associated with a distinct group of mosquito vectors that vary greatly in their potential to transmit malaria parasites. An understanding of patterns of malaria transmission depends on vector field studies focused on defining ecological interactions among mosquito vector populations, malaria parasites, and humans. The identification of key points at which transmission can be interrupted will provide clues for malaria control in areas of high transmission and will lead to new strategies for malaria eradication in areas of low transmission.

> **RESEARCH FOCUS:** The dynamics of malaria transmission by vector populations and the risk of exposure for human populations in various ecosystems.

Microepidemiology

A critical question is why some individuals living in areas of stable malaria transmission develop severe and life-threatening disease. The incidence of severe malaria may depend, among other things, on the local patterns (microdistribution) of malaria transmission and on the intensity of sporozoite inoculation. Identifying vector-related determinants of severe malaria requires new approaches for measuring house-by-house variations in malaria transmission.

> **RESEARCH FOCUS:** Characterization of "microepidemiologic" patterns of malaria transmission, including the identification of vector-related and environmental risk factors for the development of severe malaria.

Regulation of Anopheline Populations

Factors affecting larval survival and mechanisms controlling adult production in aquatic habitats are largely unknown, even for the most important vector species. There is limited information on the foraging habits of larvae (what they eat), and the extent to which natural populations are limited by intra- and/or interspecific competition and predation is unknown. The failure to understand population survival strategies and natural mechanisms of competitive exclusion among *Anopheles* taxa presents obstacles for the development of population replacement strategies, whereby attempts could be made to replace a vector species with introduced non-vector mosquitoes. Another obstacle involves difficulties in identifying larvae belonging to species complexes. Lack of knowledge in all of these areas hinders malaria control efforts.

> **RESEARCH FOCUS:** The foraging habits of larvae and the role of intra- and/or interspecific competition and predation in regulating vector populations.

Country-Wide Vector Surveillance

Geographic variation in the intensity of malaria transmission is of prime importance for the development and stratification of control measures. In most endemic countries, there is little or no information on patterns and intensities of transmission on a national scale. Efficient new surveillance techniques are needed to establish country-wide networks for monitoring the disease in human populations, patterns of drug resistance in parasites, and transmission intensity by vector populations. In areas of tropical Africa, where vectors are highly anthropophilic and endophilic, vector sampling inside houses and corresponding evaluation of sporozoite rates by immunoassay would provide sensitive indicators of transmission intensity (estimates of EIR). There are unexplored possibilities for assaying human blood meals of mosquitoes for the presence of stage-specific malaria antibodies (objective: analogous to serosurveys), malaria parasite antigens (objective: analogous to prevalence surveys), antimalarial drugs (objective: monitor drug use by humans), and even drug-resistant parasites (objective: monitor drug resistance). Progress in the area of vector surveillance for monitoring malaria on a national scale will minimize the need of traditional mass blood surveys and would promote more effective measures for predicting epidemics and allocating resources for malaria control.

> **RESEARCH FOCUS:** Innovative vector surveillance strategies for assessing malaria transmission by vector popu-

lations, for measuring the risk of exposure for human populations, and for monitoring epidemiologic parameters in human populations (e.g., malaria antibodies, malaria antigens, and drug use) in country-wide efforts to improve malaria management capabilities.

Vaccine Field Trials

Vector-related issues assume great importance as candidate vaccines move from laboratory testing to field evaluation. Baseline information on both the intensity and seasonality of transmission is necessary for planning vaccine trials. During vaccine field trials, concurrent measurements of sporozoite challenge (EIR) will be useful for gauging vaccine efficacy, especially in large trials conducted at sites with different transmission intensities.

> **RESEARCH FOCUS:** Site-specific characterization of malaria transmission by vector populations before vaccine field trials and concurrent efforts to monitor transmission intensity during field trials.

Transmission-blocking vaccines are being developed to elicit human antigametocyte antibodies that block early stages of parasite development in the mosquito. Such vaccines, when used in a mixture with other vaccines, may extend their effective life by reducing the rate at which variant forms of parasites appear. Both naturally occurring and laboratory-generated transmission-blocking antibodies are usually tested by mixing sera containing antibodies with malaria parasites and assessing the development of oocysts in the vector. It is difficult to predict the potential efficacy of transmission-blocking vaccines because the extent to which antigametocyte antibodies regulate vector infectivity in nature has never been determined in focused studies on vector populations.

> **RESEARCH FOCUS:** Field studies to assess natural effects of transmission-blocking antibodies on the early stages of parasite development in vector populations.

Laboratory-Based Research

Malaria Parasite Development in Mosquitoes

Malaria parasite development in anopheline vectors is a complex process that takes 8 to 15 days from the ingestion of gametocytes to the appearance of sporozoites in the salivary glands of the mosquito. Regulatory mechanisms affecting sporogonic development in susceptible anopheline species are largely unknown. A greater understanding of the differences in sporogonic development and transmission potential among vector species may provide important clues about malaria epidemiology and establish new directions for blocking the transmission cycle in nature. In marked contrast to parasite stages in the human host (see Chapter 6), there have been relatively few attempts to understand the behavior, physiology, and biochemistry of parasite stages in the definitive host, the mosquito.

> **RESEARCH FOCUS:** Basic mechanisms of malaria parasite development in anopheline species and vector-parasite interactions that affect sporozoite transmission potential.

> **RESEARCH FOCUS:** Development of in vitro culture systems for stages of the malaria parasite that occur in the mosquito host.

The fact that most anopheline mosquitoes cannot transmit malaria indicates the presence of one or more refractory mechanisms that inhibit parasite development. The problems of maintaining colonies of anopheline species and cultures of human malaria parasites in the laboratory make the study of these mechanisms difficult.

> **RESEARCH FOCUS:** The genetic, physiological, and biochemical basis for mechanisms of mosquito refractoriness to malaria parasites, with the goal of developing novel approaches for blocking or interrupting sporogonic development in the vectors.

Technique Development for Field Studies

Given advances in biotechnology, there are a number of field-test systems that would be extremely useful to vector biologists. The most immediate need is for simple and inexpensive methods to differentiate among anopheline species in areas where morphologically indistinguishable vector and nonvector species exist. Field researchers also require better methods to identify genetic variants within anopheline species, as well as new techniques for assessing the chronological age of vectors and for characterizing parasites in vectors according to drug resistance and genetic diversity. The ideal assay system would be capable of simultaneously analyzing individual mosquitoes for multiple epidemiologic variables, including sporozoites, blood meals, insecticide resistance, and species identification.

RESEARCH FOCUS: Development and field testing of immunological and molecular assay systems, in conjunction with studies of natural malaria transmission and malaria control efforts for determining vector-related parameters.

Innovative Methods for Malaria Control

Antimosquito Vaccines

Unlike vaccines directed against the malaria parasite, an antimosquito vaccine would be effective against all *Plasmodium* species carried by a common vector. A successful vaccine would not necessarily have to kill the mosquito immediately after it feeds on humans to be effective. Vaccine-induced effects on mosquito survival, blood meal digestion, feeding frequency, reproduction, or physiological processes may have profound effects on the sporogonic development of the parasites and, ultimately, vector transmission potential.

RESEARCH FOCUS: Development of candidate anti-mosquito vaccines that produce host antibodies with an immunopathological impact on the vector or that disrupt parasite development in the vector.

Genetic Modification of the Mosquito Vector

An interesting future possibility for malaria control involves the replacement of vector mosquitoes by genetically altered mosquitoes that cannot transmit malaria. To progress beyond the theoretical, simultaneous advances are needed in key areas of vector biology, including the identification of factors regulating parasite development in vectors; the identification, genetics, and movement of refractory genes; the development of molecular probes for identifying members of species complexes; and various other aspects of mosquito molecular biology. A long-term goal would be to use techniques and findings from molecular-level studies to explore mechanisms operating in nature, with the ultimate hope of genetically engineering mosquitoes for release in endemic areas for malaria control.

RESEARCH FOCUS: Further development of molecular-level approaches for understanding the genetics of vector populations and their natural abilities to transmit malaria parasites.

Drug Development

A potentially promising area for malaria prevention is the use of antimalarial drugs to reduce the intensity of parasite transmission by vectors. There is a continuing need for new drugs that kill or reduce the infectivity of gametocytes in the human bloodstream. At the same time, a number of already available drugs may prove effective against parasite stages that occur in the vector. The identification and evaluation of these compounds may be one of the best hopes for preventing malaria in endemic countries. Determining the ability of these drugs to affect malaria transmission will require field studies in endemic areas, probably in conjunction with trials of schizonticidal drugs.

> **RESEARCH FOCUS:** New or existing drugs that kill or reduce the infectivity of gametocytes or reduce the transmission potential of vectors through disrupting normal sporogonic development.

> **RESEARCH FOCUS:** Vector-based field evaluation of transmission-blocking drugs in endemic areas.

Evaluation of Vector Control Methods

Every effort at malaria control should be evaluated for its impact on the intensity of transmission and the incidence of disease. It is equally important to assess how the control measures are received at the community level and whether they have any adverse effects on humans or the environment. Continuous evaluations of control activities will ensure that the methods used are appropriate for the particular epidemiologic situation.

> **RESEARCH FOCUS:** The impact of existing and future vector control interventions on the intensity of malaria transmission and patterns of disease.

REFERENCES

Beier, J. C., P. V. Perkins, R. A. Wirtz, J. Koros, D. Diggs, T. P. Gargan II, and D. K. Koech. 1988. Bloodmeal identification by direct enzyme-linked immunosorbent assay (ELISA), tested on *Anopheles* (Diptera: Culicidae) in Kenya. Journal of Medical Entomology 25:9-16.

Beier, J. C., C. N. Oster, J. K. Koros, F. K. Onyango, A. K. Githeko, E. Rowton, D. K. Keoch, and C. R. Roberts. 1989. Effect of human circumsporozoite antibodies in *Plasmodium*-infected *Anopheles* (Diptera: Culicidae). Journal of Medical Entomology 26:547-553.

Beier, J. C., P. V. Perkins, J. K. Koros, F. K. Onyango, T. P. Gargan, R. A. Wirtz, D. K. Keoch, and C. R. Roberts. 1990a. Malaria sporozoite detection by dissection and ELISA to assess infectivity of Afrotropical *Anopheles* (Diptera: Culicidae). Journal of Medical Entomology 27:377-384.

Beier, J. C., P. V. Perkins, F. Onyango, T. P. Gargan, C. N. Oster, R. E. Whitmire, D. K. Keoch, and C. R. Roberts. 1990b. Characterization of malaria transmission by *Anopheles* (Diptera: Culicidae) in western Kenya in preparation for malaria vaccine trials. Journal of Medical Entomology 27:570-577.

Boyd, M. F. 1949. Malariology: A Comprehensive Survey of All Aspects of This Group of Diseases from a Global Standpoint. Philadelphia: Saunders.

Boyd, M. F., and W. K. Stratman-Thomas. 1934. On the duration of infectiousness in anophelines harbouring *Plasmodium vivax*. American Journal of Hygiene 19:539-540.

Breman, J. G., and C. C. Campbell. 1988. Combating severe malaria in African children. Bulletin of the World Health Organization 66:611-620.

Brown, A. W. A. 1983. Insecticide resistance as a factor in the integrated control of Culicidae. Pp. 161-235 in Integrated Mosquito Control Methodologies, Laird, M., and J. W. Miles, eds. New York: Academic Press.

Brown, T. M., and W. G. Brogdon. 1987. Improved detection of insecticide resistance through conventional and molecular techniques. Pp. 145-162 in Annual Review of Entomology, Mittler, T. E., F. J. Radovsky, and V. H. Resh, eds. Palo Alto: Annual Reviews, Inc.

Collins, F. H., R. K. Sakai, K. D. Vernick, S. Paskewitz, D. C. Seeley, L. H. Miller, W. E. Collins, C. C. Campbell, and R. W. Gwadz. 1986. Genetic selection of a *Plasmodium*-refractory strain of the malaria vector *Anopheles gambiae*. Science 234:607-610.

Collins, F. H., P. C. Mehaffey, M. O. Rasmussen, A. D. Brandling-Bennett, J. S. Odera, and V. Finnerty. 1988. Comparison of DNA-probe and isoenzyme methods for differentiating *Anopheles gambiae* and *Anopheles arabiensis* (Diptera: Culicidae). Journal of Medical Entomology 25:116-120.

Collins, F. H., S. M. Paskewitz, and V. Finnerty. 1990. Ribosomal RNA genes of the *Anopheles gambiae* species complex. Pp. 1-28 in Advances in Disease Vector Research, Vol. 6, Harris, K. F., ed. New York: Springer-Verlag.

Coluzzi, M. 1988. Anopheline mosquitoes: genetic methods for species differentiation. Pp. 411-485 in Malaria: Principles and Practice of Malariology, Wernsdorfer, W. H., and I. McGregor, eds. Edinburgh: Churchill Livingstone.

Curtis, C. F., and P. M. Graves. 1983. Genetic variation in the ability of insects to transmit filariae, trypanosomes and malarial parasites. Pp. 31-62 in Current Topics in Vector Research, Harris, K. F., ed. New York: Praeger.

Davis, J. R., J. R. Murphy, D. F. Clyde, S. Baqar, A. H. Cochrane, F. Zavala, and R. S. Nussenzweig. 1989. Estimate of *Plasmodium falciparum* sporozoite content of *Anopheles stephensi* used to challenge human volunteers. American Journal of Tropical Medicine and Hygiene 40:128-130.

Duffy, J. 1977. Ventures in World Health. The Memoirs of Fred Lowe Soper. Washington, D.C.: Pan American Health Organization.

Farid, M. A. 1988. Simple measures for interrupting man-vector contact. Pp. 1251-

1261 in Malaria: Principles and Practice of Malariology, Wernsdorfer, W. H., and I. McGregor, eds. Edinburgh: Churchill Livingstone.

Garnham, P. C. C. 1966. Malaria Parasites and Other Haemosporidia. Oxford: Blackwell Scientific Publications.

Haworth, J. 1988. The global distribution of malaria and the present control effort. Pp. 1379-1420 in Principles and Practice of Malariology, Wernsdorfer, W. H., and I. McGregor, eds. Edinburgh: Churchill Livingstone.

Kitron, U., and A. Spielman. 1989. Suppression of transmission of malaria through source reduction: antianopheline measures applied in Israel, the United States, and Italy. Reviews of Infectious Diseases 11:391-406.

Micks, D. W. 1949. Investigations on the malaria transmission of *Plasmodium elongatum* Huff. Journal of the National Malaria Society 8:206-218.

Miller, L. H., R. K. Sakai, P. Romans, R. W. Gwadz, P. Kantoff, and H. G. Coon. 1987. Stable integration and expression of a bacterial gene in the mosquito *Anopheles gambiae*. Science 237:779-781.

Molineaux, L. 1988. The epidemiology of human malaria as an explanation of its distribution, including some implications for its control. Pp. 913-998 in Malaria: Principles and Practice of Malariology, Wernsdorfer, W. H., and I. McGregor, eds. Edinburgh: Churchill Livingstone.

Mons, B., and R. E. Sinden. 1990. Laboratory models for research in vivo and in vitro on malaria parasites of mammals: current status. Parasitology Today 6:3-7.

Moore, C. G. 1990. The future of vector-borne disease control: needs and directions. Bulletin of the Society for Vector Ecology 15:1-4.

Muirhead-Thomson, R. C. 1954. Factors determining the true reservoir of infection of *Plasmodium falciparum* and *Wuchereria bancrofti* in a West African village. Transactions of the Royal Society of Tropical Medicine and Hygiene 48:208-225.

National Research Council. 1983. Manpower Needs and Career Opportunities in the Field Aspects of Vector Biology. Report of a Workshop. Washington, D.C.: National Academy Press.

Nijhout, M. M. 1979. *Plasmodium gallinaceum*: exflagellation stimulated by a mosquito factor. Experimental Parasitology 48:75-80.

Onori, E., and B. Grab. 1980. Indicators for the forecasting of malaria epidemics. Bulletin of the World Health Organization 58:91-98.

Pimentel, D. 1990a. Environmental and social implications of waste in U.S. agriculture and food sectors. Journal of Agricultural Ethics 3:5-20.

Pimentel, D. 1990b. Estimated annual worldwide pesticide use. Pp. 54 in Facts and Figures: International Agricultural Research. New York: The Rockefeller Foundation.

Pull, J. H., and B. Grab. 1974. A simple epidemiological model for evaluating the malaria inoculation rate and the risk of infection in infants. Bulletin of the World Health Organization 51:507-516.

Reeves, W. C. 1989. Concerns about the future of medical entomology in tropical medicine research [editorial]. American Journal of Tropical Medicine and Hygiene 40:569-570.

Rosenberg, R. 1985. Inability of *Plasmodium knowlesi* sporozoites to invade *Anoph-*

eles freeborni salivary glands. American Journal of Tropical Medicine and Hygiene 34:687-691.

Rozendaal, J. A. 1989. Impregnated mosquito nets and curtains for self-protection and vector control. Tropical Diseases Bulletin 86(7):R1-R66.

Service, M. W. 1983. Biological control of mosquitoes—has it a future? Mosquito News 43:113-120.

Tempelis, C. H. 1989. Estimation of vectorial capacity: mosquito host selection. Bulletin of the Society for Vector Ecology 14:55-59.

Weathersby, A. B. 1952. The role of the stomach wall in the exogenous development of *Plasmodium gallinaceum* as studied by means of haemocoel injections of susceptible and refractory mosquitoes. Journal of Infectious Diseases 91:198-205.

Willadsen, P., G. A. Riding, R. V. McKenna, D. H. Kemp, R. L. Tellam, J. N. Nielsen, J. Lahnstein, G. S. Cobon, and J. M. Gough. 1989. Immunologic control of a parasitic arthropod. Identification of a protective antigen from *Boophilus microplus*. Journal of Immunology 143:1346-1351.

Wirtz, R. A., F. Zavala, Y. Charoenvit, G. H. Campbell, T. R. Burkot, I. Schneider, K. M. Esser, R. L. Beaudoin, and R. G. Andre. 1987. Comparative testing of monoclonal antibodies against *Plasmodium falciparum* sporozoites for ELISA development. Bulletin of the World Health Organization 65:39-45.

World Health Organization. 1975. Manual On Practical Entomology in Malaria. Geneva: World Health Organization.

World Health Organization. 1986. Principles of malaria vaccine trials: memorandum from a WHO meeting. Bulletin of the World Health Organization 64:185-204.

Zavala, F., R. W. Gwadz, F. H. Collins, R. S. Nussenzweig, and V. Nussenzweig. 1982. Monoclonal antibodies to circumsporozoite proteins identify the species of malaria parasite in infected mosquitoes. Nature 299:737-738.

8

Drug Discovery and Development

WHERE WE WANT TO BE IN THE YEAR 2010

The ready availability of relatively low-cost prophylactic and thera-peutic antimalarial drugs will dramatically reverse rising malaria morbidity and mortality evident throughout much of the world. Co-operative efforts among academic, government, and industry researchers will lead to the discovery and development of these new drugs, which will be available in several formulations, effective against all devel-opmental stages of the four human malaria parasites, stable without refrigeration for extended periods, and have few unacceptable side effects. These drugs will include compounds that reverse resistance to chloroquine (thereby restoring its utility), others that act quickly (and thus will be of great benefit in treating severe falciparum ma-laria), and still others that can be administered to severely ill pa-tients by methods other than injection (reducing the risk of acquiring other infections through contaminated needles). Finally, an enhanced understanding of basic host-parasite differences will lead to the cre-ation of sophisticated new drug discovery strategies that will pro-vide a continual stream of novel antimalarial drugs for human testing.

WHERE WE ARE TODAY

Principles of Prophylaxis and Treatment

There is ample evidence documenting the increasing incidence of malaria worldwide, due in large part to the spread of *Plasmodium falciparum*. The deteriorating efficacy of existing antimalarial drugs, because of increasing numbers of drug-resistant parasite strains, makes routine prophylaxis and treatment of the disease a therapeutic challenge.

Deciding which drug to use depends on a number of factors, including the patient's age and his or her clinical and immune status. Other important considerations are the type of malaria (vivax, falciparum, ovale, or malariae), outcome desired, drug availability and costs, side effects and degree of compliance expected with the prescribed regimen, drug sensitivity of the parasite strain in the area in which the infection was acquired, and the most appropriate route of administration.

Antimalarial drugs are used for five basic purposes (Webster, 1990): to prevent infection from establishing itself in the body (causal prophylaxis); to prevent an established infection from manifesting itself clinically (suppressive prophylaxis); to treat an acute attack of malaria in order to relieve symptoms, eliminate asexual stages of the parasite, or completely eliminate malaria parasites from the body (treatment therapy); to eliminate parasites, whether or not they are causing symptoms (curative therapy); and to eliminate persisting liver forms of the parasite (antirelapse treatment). A sixth use of antimalarial drugs, not now employed, relies on mass distribution of compounds that eliminate gametocytes in infected individuals to reduce parasite transmission in human populations.

Since causal prophylactic agents are few, logistically difficult to administer (daily doses are required), and often toxic, this approach to preventing malaria is seldom practical. Additionally, there is parasite resistance to one of the major causal prophylactics, pyrimethamine. Most prophylactic drugs suppress parasitemia and clinical disease. Antirelapse or radical curative treatment may be given either after clinical treatment of a relapsing malaria (caused by *P. vivax* or *P. ovale*) or following suppressive prophylaxis when exposure to either of these parasites has occurred.

The goals of treating an established infection can also vary. In people who have no natural immunity and are only temporarily exposed to the parasite (e.g., migrants, travelers, military personnel, and temporary laborers), infections must be treated vigorously to eliminate all malaria parasites from the body, since parasitemia may reach life-threatening levels in a short period of time. Children up to the age of four living in endemic regions are at serious risk of severe and even fatal infection. Prompt treatment and, in some instances, prophylaxis of these children can be life-saving.

In other situations, however, completely eradicating parasitemia may not be necessary or even desirable. For example, older children and adults living in areas where exposure to *P. falciparum* malaria is constant and uncontrolled derive more protection from their own immunity than from antimalarial drugs. In such settings, medications that help control clinical attacks of malaria and prevent an uncontrolled rise in parasitemia are sufficient, since they prevent death and allow for the gradual acquisition of immunity.

It is not the intention of this report to provide current treatment guidelines. Those who are interested in this aspect of malaria are urged to consult recent documents that describe treatment options in detail (World Health Organization, 1990).

Status of Prophylaxis and Treatment

There are three distinct population groups for whom antimalarial drugs are important: indigenous inhabitants of malarious areas, temporary (nonindigenous) inhabitants of malarious areas, and individuals who become ill with malaria or are diagnosed with the disease in nonmalarious regions of the world. The status of drug treatment and prophylaxis for each of the four malaria parasites is presented below.

Plasmodium malariae *and* P. ovale

Drugs used for prophylaxis and treatment of infections caused by *P. ovale* or *P. malariae* seem satisfactory. There are no reports of resistance in these species. In terms of both disease severity and numbers of cases, these parasites are of less concern than *P. vivax* and *P. falciparum*.

Plasmodium vivax

Drug treatment and prophylaxis of *P. vivax* malaria is far less than satisfactory. Most significantly, there are serious side effects with primaquine, a causal prophylactic used to eliminate latent liver-stage parasites. Recently, there have also been problems with drug supplies. Without primaquine, curative therapy or prevention of relapses is not currently possible. Although chloroquine has been used to eliminate blood-stage parasites, and is thus used to treat the symptoms of vivax malaria, there are strains of *P. vivax* resistant to this drug (Rieckmann et al., 1989). Fresh therapeutic approaches must be developed.

Plasmodium falciparum

The situation for drug treatment and prophylaxis of *P. falciparum* malaria is desperate (Payne, 1987; Moran and Bernard, 1989). Given the toxicity and scarcity of primaquine, causal prophylaxis is not a viable option. Daily doses of proguanil provide causal prophylaxis in areas where resistance to this drug is not present, but the compound is not marketed in the United States.

Since this species of parasite does not cause relapse, suppressive prophylaxis should be able to prevent the disease. However, strains of *P. falciparum* resistant to one or more of the available antimalarial drugs have been documented throughout the world. Resistance to the dihydrofolate reductase inhibitors pyrimethamine and proguanil is widespread, and the potential for serious toxicity with the *para*-aminobenzoic acid (PABA) antimetabolites sulfadoxine, sulfalene, and dapsone has limited their use in combination with reductase inhibitors for this purpose.

The nearly global spread of chloroquine resistance precludes its routine use for suppressive prophylaxis. In the worst situations, such as along the Thailand-Cambodia border, parasite strains resistant to mefloquine and/or quinine are also disturbingly common, and few viable prophylactic regimens exist.

Among the antibiotics with antimalarial activity, most attention is currently focused on doxycycline, a tetracycline derivative suitable for once-daily dosing (Pang et al., 1987, 1988). Concerns about the widespread use of doxycycline or other tetracyclines for prophylaxis of malaria include the emergence of drug-resistant strains of *P. falciparum*, potentially eroding the clinical utility of these drugs in combination with quinine for the treatment of severe malaria (Bruce-Chwatt, 1987). In addition, there are concerns that doxycycline prophylaxis could select drug-resistant strains of pathogenic bacteria (Peters, 1990a,b). Tetracyclines are broadly available in many malarious areas, however, and the impact on resistance patterns from the use of tetracyclines for malaria prophylaxis is unclear. A recent report suggests that the use of doxycycline for malaria prophylaxis in Thailand was not associated with an increased risk of diarrhea from drug-resistant strains of enteric pathogens (Arthur et al., 1990). Furthermore, tetracyclines are often taken as prophylaxis against "travelers' diarrhea" by visitors to less-developed countries. The safety of these drugs is remarkable. Given these considerations, it is appropriate to use doxycycline, at least for travelers in regions where chloroquine resistance is a problem, for malaria prophylaxis.

That there are more treatment options for falciparum malaria than prophylactic regimens is not cause for optimism. The problem of drug resistance seriously compromises the therapeutic options for malaria infections acquired in many parts of the world. The choice of a drug should be guided at least in part by an understanding of the drug sensitivities of the parasites in the locality in which the infection originated. Typically, quinine, mefloquine, or halofantrine can be used to cure falciparum malaria that is resistant to pyrimethamine and chloroquine. In areas where artemisinin or artemether is available, these drugs generally seem to be effective. As a last line of defense, prolonged courses of tetracyclines can be useful. However, these antibiotics are slower acting than other antimalarial drugs and, when used alone, are not satisfactory for treating severe disease. For the several areas of the world plagued by strains of multidrug-resistant *P. falciparum*, only very restricted treatment options exist. As these strains spread, the effectiveness of antimalarial drugs will continue to erode.

Available Antimalarial Drugs

Causal Prophylactics

Primaquine   The 8-aminoquinoline class of antimalarial drugs, of which primaquine is the most studied, were derived from methylene blue in one of the earliest efforts in medicinal chemistry. The discovery of methylene blue's antimalarial activity by Guttman and Ehrlich in 1891 is sometimes considered to mark the advent of modern chemotherapy (Carson, 1984).

In 1926, the world's first synthetic antimalarial agent, pamaquine, was produced in Germany. A close structural analog of primaquine, this compound proved too toxic for clinical use. Primaquine was subsequently developed during a massive screening program for new antimalarial drugs instituted by the U.S. Army during World War II.

The use of primaquine was somewhat hampered by its limited supply, but this situation has been resolved. The utility of primaquine therapy is also limited because it has a relatively low therapeutic index. That is, the dose required to produced a cure is only slightly lower than the amount considered toxic in humans. Prominent side effects include gastrointestinal distress, methemoglobinemia, and in patients with a genetic deficiency in the enzyme glucose-6-phosphate dehydrogenase, oxidant stress-induced hemolytic anemia. Changes in the drug's formulation may reduce the incidence or severity of these reactions.

The mechanism of action of primaquine against malaria liver-stage parasites and gametocytes has not been determined. Metabolism of primaquine by the host is thought to be necessary for drug activity, and most investigations have focused on the ability of primaquine metabolites to generate active oxygen species that kill the parasite (Bates et al., 1990). Though this is an attractive hypothesis, more research is needed to specify the molecular events that underlie the antimalarial activity of primaquine.

In addition to its use as a causal prophylactic, primaquine has on occasion been used as a gametocytocidal drug. Alone among available antimalarial drugs, primaquine has significant activity against these sexual stages. Since by destroying the gametocyte stages primaquine can theoretically reduce malaria transmission, mass treatment of infected individuals could be of potential benefit. Given the drug's toxicity, however, and the fact that such therapy offers no immediate benefit to the patient, this usage is not generally recommended.

No efforts are now being devoted to the discovery of compounds that act specifically against gametocytes. Use of gametocytocidal drugs as part of a malaria control strategy would require wide distribution, repeated dosing, and a high rate of compliance. Since no drug is entirely without side effects and the target population would acquire no short-term therapeutic benefits, the development of such a drug, in the absence of activity against liver- or blood-stage malaria parasites, is not attractive. The need for wide drug distribution and a high compliance rate also reduce the likelihood that gametocytocidal therapy will play a role in future malaria control operations.

Schizonticidal Drugs Several compounds demonstrate activity against both liver- and blood-stage malaria parasites. These drugs, including pyrimethamine, proguanil, and doxycycline, are described in the next section.

Drugs Used for Treatment

Quinine The antifever properties of Peruvian cinchona bark were revealed to Europeans in the early 1600s. More than 200 years later, the structure of the cinchona alkaloids was determined. Quinine is just one of a number of active constituents in this botanical preparation.

Quinine remains an important therapeutic agent, especially for drug-resistant *P. falciparum* infections. As a front-line antimalarial drug, however, quinine is restricted by a short half-life, side effects at therapeutic blood concentrations, and the need to reserve its usage for certain situations, such as treatment of drug-resistant falciparum malaria. There is also some disagreement about the proper route of administration for quinine, although the problems associated with intramuscular use of the drug appear to be less severe than originally thought. Quinine's role in causing hypoglycemia when used to treat severe malaria has been questioned (White et al., 1983a,b; Taylor et al., 1988). The occurrence of the constellation of symptoms termed "cinchonism," described during routine antimalarial therapy, requires further evaluation.

The mechanism of action of quinine is not known, nor is it known whether this drug, and others that contain a quinoline nucleus, share a common mechanism. This topic is discussed in more detail for chloroquine, on which most research attention has focused.

Strains of *P. falciparum* with reduced sensitivity to quinine have been reported. Fortunately, increasing the dose seems to overcome this problem, although this increases the risk of side effects. Quinine resistance appears to be an independent phenotype, sometimes but not always associated with mefloquine or chloroquine resistance. Compounds that reverse chloroquine resistance also reverse quinine resistance but not mefloquine resistance (see below). Penfluridol (Peters and Robinson, in press), which reverses resistance to mefloquine, halofantrine, and artemisinin, has no influence on quinine or chloroquine resistance. Although quinine and chloroquine resistance are affected similarly in a pharmacological sense, the two traits occur independently. The molecular basis for resistance to quinine is not well understood.

Just as malaria has historically shaped the outcomes of some wars, so too have wars determined some approaches to malaria chemotherapy. For example, attempts by the Dutch to transport cinchona trees from Peru to other sites in the tropics resulted in the establishment of a cinchona plantation in Java. Eventually, this area accounted for 90 percent of the world's supply of quinine. The seizure of Java by the Japanese during World War II interrupted this supply and forced the Allied nations to begin an intensive search for synthetic quinine replacements, which eventually led to the discovery of nearly all currently available antimalarial drugs.

Chloroquine This 4-aminoquinoline was initially synthesized in Germany as part of that country's antimalarial medicinal chemistry program. The drug was thought to be too toxic, however, and development was rejected in favor of its 3-methyl analog, sontoquine. Allied interest in this series was stimulated by the capture of supplies of German sontoquine in Tunis during World War II.

Chloroquine was identified anew as a highly effective antimalarial compound by the American drug screening program during World War II. Further development resulted in its becoming a very useful antimalarial drug. It is relatively safe, inexpensive, and in the absence of resistance, highly effective. In fact, the major limitation to its usefulness is the emergence of drug-resistant strains of *P. falciparum* and, recently, *P. vivax*.

The mechanism of action of chloroquine and other quinoline-containing antimalarial drugs, including other 4-aminoquinolines, quinine, and mefloquine, is not known. Various mechanisms have been proposed, including DNA binding, formation of cytolytic complexes with ferriprotoporphyrin IX (a breakdown product of heme, stored in granules by the parasite), and variants of the lysosomotropic hypothesis, which holds that accumulation of the drug in the acidic food vacuole of the parasite somehow disrupts its function. None of these hypotheses is supported by conclusive proof, and all have been questioned on the basis of experimental results and theoretical considerations (Ginsburg and Geary, 1986; Schlesinger et al., 1988; Geary et al., 1990; Meshnick, 1990). It is not known whether these drugs share a common mechanism of action. It is particularly distressing that quinine was the first drug whose structure was determined, 170 years ago, yet very little is known about how it exerts its therapeutic effects.

Considerable effort has been spent investigating the mechanism by which malaria parasites develop resistance to chloroquine (Krogstad et al., 1988). Most research favors the hypothesis that in resistant strains, a specific protein that transports the drug out of the parasite is either amplified or altered to increase its activity (Martin et al., 1987). The process is probably similar to the glycoprotein-mediated efflux of antitumor drugs observed in multidrug-resistant tumor cells (Foote et al., 1990). Although this is an attractive theory with a considerable body of supporting evidence, there may be other explanations of the efflux process (Ginsburg and Stein, in press), and some complicating pharmacological questions need to be resolved. Furthermore, recent genetic evidence suggests that the efflux genes are not linked to resistance (Wellems et al., 1990).

Other 4-aminoquinolines, including amodiaquine, hydroxychloroquine, amopyroquine, and pyronaridine, are also occasionally used to treat malaria. Of these, amodiaquine has been used the most, but none of these agents has a significant advantage over chloroquine. Although cross-resistance to amodiaquine is not uniformly observed in chloroquine-resistant *P. falciparum*, it is common enough to prevent routine use of the drug in these cases. Because amodiaquine often causes agranulocytosis and hepatitis—extremely serious side effects—its use is no longer recommended under any circumstances.

Pyrimethamine and Pyrimethamine-Antimetabolite Combinations   Pyrimethamine is a diaminopyrimidine derivative. Like the biguanides discussed below, it is an inhibitor of the enzyme dihydrofolate reductase. Inhibition of this enzyme disrupts DNA synthesis. Pyrimethamine, which was developed at Burroughs Wellcome in the 1940s, is structurally homologous to the biguanide compound, proguanil.

Pyrimethamine has two major disadvantages: it does not work well against some strains of *P. vivax*; and when used alone, it quickly selects for resistant strains of *P. falciparum*. Currently, pyrimethamine is used only in combination with one of several PABA antimetabolites, including sulfadoxine or sulfalene (both sulfonamides) or dapsone (a sulfone).

The potential antimalarial activity of sulfonamides was demonstrated when the sulfonamide-containing azodye prontosil was found to be active against *P. falciparum* and the primate malaria parasite *P. knowlesi.* Specific antimalarial activity was discovered during the development of the sulfonamide antibiotics. Interestingly, the sulfonamides are not very effective against *P. vivax,* suggesting that folate synthesis is unnecessary for this parasite.

By themselves, the sulfa drugs act slowly against *P. falciparum* which reduces their clinical utility. Since in combination with a dihydrofolate reductase inhibitor these compounds have such enhanced activity, there is little reason to consider using them as single agents for treating malaria. The choice of dapsone, sulfalene, or sulfadoxine (from among many active compounds) is made on the basis of their half-life in humans. These compounds are relatively long acting, as is pyrimethamine, and drug synergy is most beneficial when drugs with similar pharmacokinetics are combined.

The long half-life of the sulfa component of the two-drug combination has, unfortunately, meant the occurrence of a major and serious side effect, skin reactions. In their most severe form, these can progress to a sometimes fatal condition known as Stevens-Johnson syndrome, which may be a type of idiosyncratic or allergotoxic effect. The incidence of the syndrome depends in part on the duration of treatment and is apparently more common with longer-acting drugs, such as the antimalarial agents (Miller et al., 1986).

Because of the risk of Stevens-Johnson syndrome, combinations of sulfa drugs and pyrimethamine are no longer recommended for prophylaxis of falciparum malaria. However, combinations still play a role in the treatment of *P. falciparum* infections, though their utility has been eroded by the widespread development of resistance. Only the pyrimethamine-sulfadoxine combination is marketed in the United States.

The mechanism of action of pyrimethamine and its synergism with the sulfa drugs are understood in elegant detail (Vennerstrom et al., 1991). Pyrimethamine binds tightly to dihydrofolate reductase from malaria parasites but poorly to its mammalian counterpart. Inhibition of this enzyme prevents nucleic acid synthesis. Dihydrofolate reductase from *P. falciparum* has been cloned, sequenced, and modeled on the basis of crystallographic analyses of similar reductases from other organisms. PABA is a component of folic acid; PABA antimetabolites act to decrease the synthesis (and thus intracellular concentrations) of folate. Only organisms that cannot acquire folate from the environment are adversely affected by sulfa drugs. By reducing folate concentrations, sulfa drugs enhance the inhibition of dihydrofolate reductase by pyrimethamine (Milhous et al., 1985).

Resistance to pyrimethamine is also well understood. Isolates of *P. falciparum* resistant to the drug consistently show substitution of a single amino acid at one location in dihydrofolate reductase. Proguanil resistance is associated with substitution at a different amino acid location, and strains resistant to both drugs show substitutions at both sites (Peterson et al., 1990).

A detailed understanding of the inhibitor-enzyme interaction offers an opportunity for rational drug design or discovery. It should be possible to identify compounds that bind to dihydrofolate reductase but are unaffected by the mutations associated with pyrimethamine and proguanil resistance. Drugs derived from such a program would restore the usefulness of this strategy for treating falciparum malaria.

Proguanil (Chlorguanil) and Chlorproguanil   The discovery of antimalarial activity of the biguanides predates the development of the diaminopyrimidines. These compounds were initially prepared as acyclic analogs of a series of anilino pyrimidines under investigation at Imperial Chemical Industries in the United Kingdom. Like pyrimethamine, proguanil is a causal prophylactic agent for *P. falciparum*, but it acts slowly against the blood-stage parasite. It is not particularly useful for treating vivax malaria. Unlike pyrimethamine, proguanil has a short half-life, and so prophylactic use requires daily dosing. Strains of *P. falciparum* resistant to proguanil are common, seriously limiting its use in therapy.

Chlorproguanil contains one more chlorine atom than proguanil, which increases the drug's potency and half-life (Peters, 1990b). Neither drug is currently marketed as a single oral dose in combination with a PABA antimetabolite, however, and clinical trials conducted in Thailand with proguanil in combination with sulfonamide suggest that these drugs may have utility in areas endemic for multidrug-resistant malaria (Karwacki et al., 1990). Neither proguanil nor chlorproguanil is marketed in the United States.

The mechanism of action of the biguanides is the same as that of pyrimethamine. Technically, the biguanides are "prodrugs" that must be metabolically converted by the human host to a cyclic compound, cycloguanil, that inhibits dihydrofolate reductase (Webster, 1990).

Mefloquine   The development of mefloquine was a collaborative achievement of the U.S. Army Medical Research and Development Command, the World Health Organization (WHO), and Hoffman-LaRoche, Inc. The drug was recently licensed in the United States and several other countries. A 4-quinoline methanol, mefloquine may be considered a quinine analog. It was first synthesized by the Army's medicinal chemistry program in the late 1960s.

Clinical and field trials during the past 17 years have confirmed the effectiveness of a single dose of mefloquine for rapidly clearing *P. falciparum* parasitemia and alleviating symptoms. Preliminary studies of mefloquine in pregnant women (beyond the first trimester) with falciparum malaria indicate tolerance comparable to that with quinine (World Health Organization, 1990). The triple-drug combination mefloquine-sulfadoxine-pyrimethamine is registered in at least 11 countries. WHO no longer recommends its use, however, since its effectiveness in areas of pyrimethamine-sulfadoxine resistance is unproven. Mefloquine itself is reserved for use in regions where drug resistance is a serious problem (World Health Organization, 1990).

Recently, problems have arisen with mefloquine use. The cure rate for mefloquine-sulfadoxine-pyrimethamine treatment of *P. falciparum* in Thailand fell from 96 percent in 1985 to as low as 50 percent in 1990 in some areas of the country (W. Rooney, Ministry of Health, Thailand, personal communication). Indications that the cure rate was dropping came from follow-up data of patients treated in clinics at the Cambodia-Myanmar border. Field studies are under way.

Mefloquine can produce adverse neurological and psychiatric reactions. Data from clinical trials testing the drug's therapeutic potential and surveys of travelers taking mefloquine for malaria prophylaxis suggests that its use is associated with a wide range of side effects, including ataxia, depression, stupor, and seizures. The risk of such adverse reactions is on the order of 1 percent following a treatment dose of 1 gram or more, and is 1 in 5,000 following a prophylactic dose. It is not known whether these complications can be reduced by altering the drug's formulation (Lobel et al., 1991).

The mechanism of action of mefloquine, like that of quinine, remains a matter of conjecture. Strains of *P. falciparum* resistant to mefloquine may export the drug more efficiently than sensitive strains. However, mefloquine resistance is pharmacologically distinguishable from resistance to the structurally similar drug quinine.

Halofantrine   Halofantrine, an aminoalcohol, is a member of the 9-phenanthrenemethanol class of drugs. It was first identified as a potential antimalarial agent during World War II. In the 1960s, when it became clear that chloroquine would have a limited life span, further work was done on this compound by the Walter Reed Army Institute of Research (WRAIR) (Horton, 1988). Commercial development of halofantrine began in 1984. Clinical trials have confirmed its efficacy in both *P. falciparum* and *P. vivax* infections in semi-immune patients in Malawi, the Solomon Islands, Thailand, Pakistan, France, French Guyana, Gabon, and parts of East and West Africa (Horton and Parr, 1989).

The drug is effective against chloroquine-resistant falciparum malaria, although it shares a few structural features with quinine and mefloquine, the mechanism of action is thought to differ and may be unique. Data that both support and refute cross-resistance among halofantrine, mefloquine, and quinine have been reported. The mechanism of resistance has not been conclusively proven (Cosgriff et al., 1985; Peters, 1990a).

As an antimalarial compound, halofantrine has some clear disadvantages. It is poorly soluble in water, which might explain the wide inter- and intrasubject variability in bioavailability seen in clinical and field trials. Absorption is slow but may be enhanced by intake of food (Milton et al., 1989), suggesting that a modification in dosing in relationship to food intake may improve absorption. The manufacturer has recommended not only that the drug be given in divided doses but also that the course of treatment be repeated after a week in nonimmune individuals and in children.

More research on halofantrine's efficacy, toxicity, and pharmacokinetics in patients is needed before the drug can be considered an effective antimalarial agent (Editorial, 1989). Halofantrine is not licensed for use in the United States, but it is hoped the drug may be clinically useful in areas of the world where mefloquine is not. Long-term chronic toxicity studies are under way to validate halofantrine's safety and tolerance when used as a prophylactic agent. Smith-Kline Beckman is the U.S. Army's partner in development of this drug.

Artemisinin, Artesunate, and Artemether Artemisinin was isolated from the wormwood plant, *Artemisia annua*, used for centuries in Chinese herbal medicine. It is an endoperoxide of a sesquiterpene lactone, unrelated in structure to any other known antimalarial agent. Its development was supported by the Chinese government and WHO.

Since artemisinin is poorly water soluble and rapidly metabolized, the methyl ether derivative, artemether, and a salt of a succinate ester of dihydroartemisinin, artesunate, were prepared by the Chinese. Artesunate is water soluble but is not particularly stable. Artemether, less water soluble (and apparently more toxic) than artesunate, is being developed for therapeutic administration, using an oil formulation for intramuscular administration. These drugs are produced in China and have limited but increasing geographic distribution. Side effects do not seem to be a common problem, except that artemisinin and its analogs are not recommended for use during pregnancy, since in rodent studies they have been shown to be fetotoxic. The advantage of these drugs is their ability to reduce high-level parasitemias very quickly, which is of great benefit for treatment of severely ill patients. However, complete clearance of parasites is uncommon and supplementing those agents with another antimalarial drug is recommended for curative therapy (Wernsdorfer and Trigg, 1988).

Little is known about the mechanism of action of these drugs. Resistance is known to occur in vitro. At least one phenotype appears to be linked to resistance to mefloquine and halofantrine (Peters, 1990b).

Antimalarial Antibiotics Certain antibiotics, especially the tetracyclines and clindamycin, have useful antimalarial properties (Rieckmann, 1984; Kremsner, 1990). Erythromycin, chloramphenicol, and rifampicin have activity in vitro (Geary and Jensen, 1983) but have not yet found clinical application. Antimalarial activity is not found in the beta-lactam or aminoglycoside antibiotics.

The tetracyclines and clindamycin can cure falciparum malaria in humans. They show activity against *P. vivax* as well, and there is evidence that they act on liver- and blood-stage parasites. The resolution of symptoms and clearance of parasitemia occur slowly, however, and extended courses of therapy are needed to effect a cure. The most common use of the tetracyclines is in combination with quinine for the treatment of infections resistant to chloroquine or other drugs. In addition, prophylactic use of doxycycline has received recent attention (see above). While the tetracyclines and clindamycin can be used alone to cure uncomplicated cases of falciparum malaria, they have no advantages over other antimalarial agents when multidrug resistance is not a problem. Strains of *P. falciparum* with reduced sensitivity to tetracycline have been found. To avoid the selection of parasite strains resistant to them, the use of the tetracyclines and clindamycin should be restricted to cases in which resistance is a problem.

The antimalarial mechanism of action of the tetracyclines and clindamycin is unknown. It has been proposed that they inhibit protein synthesis in parasite mitochondria (Geary and Jensen, 1983; Prapunwattana et al., 1988), but this has not yet been proven. In this respect, the recent report that *P. falciparum* expresses a rifampicin-sensitive, prokaryotic-like RNA polymerase, apparently encoded in the mitochondrial genome, is extremely interesting (Gardner et al., 1991). Further research is needed to explain the surprising antimalarial properties of these antibiotics, which are generally not toxic to eukaryotic cells. Nothing is known about parasite mechanisms of resistance to antibiotics.

Drug Discovery and Development

Although botanical preparations—most notably cinchona bark—have been used to treat malaria for thousands of years, credit for the first efforts to systematically develop synthetic antimalarial agents belongs to the Germans (Schulemann, Schonhofer, and Wingler), who synthesized pamaquine in 1926 (see discussion of primaquine above). Outside of Germany, medicinal chemistry resources became the focus of the United States Cooperative Wartime Program during World War II. This program was coordinated by various committees of the National Research Council and later the Board for the Co-ordination of Malaria Studies. This massive, national screening program allowed for a systematic exploitation of certain chemical classes of compounds (Clark, 1946). By the 1950s, after primaquine, chloroquine, pyrimethamine, and proguanil had been introduced, the arsenal of antimalarial drugs seemed to be complete and antimalarial drug discovery seemed to lapse on a global basis. Chloroquine resistance was first reported in South America in the early 1960s. Around the same time, chloroquine-resistant malaria was appearing among U.S. forces stationed in southern Vietnam (World Health Organization, 1981).

In 1964, the Army reestablished its antimalarial research program in order to develop new prophylactic and therapeutic drugs for use against resistant parasite strains. The program had a basic science component focused on the biology of the malaria parasite and research on malaria immunology, with the long-range goal of developing a vaccine. The Division of Experimental Therapeutics (formerly the Division of Medicinal Chemistry) at WRAIR was put in charge of a multidisciplinary antimalarial drug development program that combined both in-house and contract research with complementary elements in the pharmaceutical industry (Milhous and Schuster, 1990).

Walter Reed Army Institute of Research

WRAIR has the expertise and laboratory capability to carry a potential antimalarial compound from the chemist's bench, through efficacy testing, toxicity testing, and clinical trials, to registration by the U.S. Food and Drug Administration (FDA). In recent years, the institute has collaborated increasingly with the pharmaceutical industry and WHO to expedite the development process.

While basic and field research activities in malaria are conducted by the National Institutes of Health, United States Agency for International Development, and Centers for Disease Control, WRAIR is the only federal body with a discrete program for development of drugs for treatment of tropical diseases.

Various approaches have been used by WRAIR scientists to identify, design, and synthesize new antimalarial drugs, including empirical screening, screening of plant extracts from traditional medicines, synthesis of analogs to compounds known to have antimalarial (or antimicrobial or antitumor) activity, and selective targeting of specific parasite enzymes (so-called rational drug design).

Historically, rodent models of malaria have been the primary tool for identifying drug candidates. Compounds that lack toxicity and demonstrate efficacy in preliminary animal testing are selected for advanced testing in rodent or simian models. During the past 10 years, methods of in vitro drug screening using radioisotopes have been developed to complement animal testing in the drug discovery process. Well-characterized clones of falciparum malaria parasites have been derived by a specialized process of direct visualization and single cell micromanipulation. A stable and well-defined pattern of drug susceptibility makes these clones extremely useful for evaluating candidate drugs of diverse chemical classes (Milhous et al., 1989).

World Health Organization

The Special Programme for Research and Training in Tropical Diseases (TDR), a joint project of the United Nations Development Programme, the World Bank, and WHO, administers an extensive antimalarial drug development program. TDR efforts include the further development of mefloquine, particularly for use in pregnant women and children; studies of the arteether and artemether derivatives of artemisinin; development and evaluation of halofantrine, with an emphasis on improving bioavailability; research on the blood schizonticides, such as the biguanides already on the market; and the development of novel blood and tissue schizonticides, such as the 1,2,4-trioxanes and hydroxynaphthoquinones.

Researchers supported by TDR also are working to develop in vitro drug susceptibility tests and tests for detecting the presence of antimalarial drugs in blood and urine. The mechanisms of antimalarial drug resistance, the efficacy of drugs that may reverse resistance, and drug combinations that might delay the development of resistance are under investigation. Other TDR-supported scientists are attempting to synthesize antimalarial drugs for use in preclinical studies, investigate alternatives to microscopy for diagnosing malaria, identify potential drug targets in the malaria parasite's metabolic pathways, and develop cultivation methods for vivax and malariae bloodstage parasites.

Role of Drug Companies

Unfortunately, antimalarial drug discovery and development is of little interest to pharmaceutical firms. Because the vast majority of malaria cases occur in poor individuals living in less developed countries with nonconvertible currencies, even if a new and highly effective antimalarial compound were developed, a drug company likely would suffer a poor return on the money it invested in research and development.

The ease with which novel antimalarial drugs are developed depends on the structural diversity and number of compounds available for screening and the strategies used to identify them. Although WHO supports research related to malaria chemotherapy, the only centralized facility devoted to antimalarial drug screening is WRAIR. Pharmaceutical companies possess collections of compounds which, for the most part, have never been screened for antimalarial activity.

A number of pharmaceutical companies are investigating drugs with antiprotozoal activity, including activity against *Eimeria* species, *Toxoplasma gondii*, and *Cryptosporidium* species. Although these organisms are related to *Plasmodium* species, the drugs under study have not been tested for antimalarial qualities.

Other Participants

A variety of academic, national, and industrial laboratories are or have previously been involved in antimalarial drug development. Several are mentioned in the next section.

Drugs Under Development

When a candidate antimalarial drug moves from being evaluated in animals to being assessed in humans, the first step of the process—phase I testing—uses incrementally increasing doses given to healthy volunteers in an effort to determine the drug's safety and patients' tolerance for it. Once the drug's safety is assured, phase II testing is conducted to judge its efficacy in volunteers or naturally infected patients with low-level parasitemias and mild clinical illness. In phase III testing, the drug is initially given only to patients hospitalized with moderately severe disease; later, wide-scale use of the drug in a limited area, with careful monitoring to evaluate efficacy and detect low frequency side effects, takes place. Following phase III, an application may be submitted to FDA for licensure of the drug. Phase IV, post-marketing surveillance, involves careful scrutiny for low-prevalence side effects (Fernex, 1984a,b). Although there are several promising leads, few antimalarial drug candidates have reached phase I testing.

Arteether

This ethyl ether derivative of artemisinin has been selected by WHO and the U.S. Army for collaborative development as an intramuscular formulation to treat malaria. It may have some advantages over artemether, another artemisinin analog, in terms of toxicity.

WR 238605

Extensive primate studies suggest that this 8-aminoquinoline, a product of WRAIR drug development efforts, will have better efficacy, less toxicity, better oral bioavailability, and a longer half-life than primaquine. Human testing awaits the filing of an investigational new drug application with FDA. It is of considerable interest that WR 238605 has also shown activity against the opportunistic pathogen *Pneumocystis carinii* in rodents (Bartlett et al., 1991). *Pneumocystis carinii* pneumonia is a common and serious infection in AIDS patients. A partner for development of the drug has not yet been selected.

BW566c

This compound is a member of the hydroxynaphthoquinone class of compounds. The antimalarial activity of these compounds was discovered in the 1940s, when they were synthesized and tested as part of an effort to develop a synthetic replacement for quinine. Several drugs in this class, including menoctone, have gone on to human testing, but further development proved unwarranted.

BW566c was identified as an antimalarial candidate at the British drug company Burroughs Wellcome (Gutteridge, 1989). Interest intensified when, like WR 238605, it was found to possess anti-*P. carinii* activity. It is now in human trials for the treatment of *P. carinii* pneumonia. Development of BW566c as an antimalarial agent depends on the results of these studies; it is not likely to undergo further research and development if it has only antimalarial potential, since Burroughs Wellcome, like most other pharmaceutical companies, has terminated its antimalarial drug discovery program.

There is some evidence that the hydroxynaphthoquinones act by inhibiting electron transport at ubiquinone-sensitive sites in the parasite mitochondria. This inhibition is coupled to inhibition of the enzyme dihydroorotate dehydrogenase, which is necessary for pyrimidine (and thus nucleic acid) synthesis.

Antibiotics

Antimalarial activity has been found in various fluoroquinoline antibiotics and newer erythromycin derivatives, including azithromycin and roxithromycin. Most research has focused on the quinolones, which are already approved by the FDA for human use. One of these, ciprofloxacin, is now in human trials for malaria. Whether or not these drugs will have advantages over the tetracyclines and clindamycin remains to be seen.

Agents That Reverse Chloroquine Resistance

A wide variety of drugs have been found to restore the potency of chloroquine against resistant strains of *P. falciparum* in vitro. None of these compounds have yet been tested in clinical trials. These drugs may act by blocking the active efflux of chloroquine from the parasite, a process that can be measured in vitro (Krogstad et al., 1987). Similar compounds inhibit the efflux of anticancer drugs from resistant tumor cells.

A number of compounds with pharmacokinetics similar to that of chloroquine, including verapamil (and its analogs), desipramine, ketotifen, cyproheptadine, nifedipine, diltiazem, and chlorpromazine, have been tested in animals (Bitonti et al., 1988; Peters, 1990b). All but chlorpromazine have been found wanting because of toxicity, an inability to cure infection, or both (Vennerstrom et al., 1991). The combination of chloroquine and chlorpromazine can cure experimental *P. falciparum* infections in aotus monkeys (Rossan et al., 1990).

Like chloroquine, chlorpromazine has a long half-life. A great deal of clinical experience has been obtained with this drug. It has a good safety profile at the doses required to treat malaria and is inexpensive. Other phenothiazines should be evaluated for their ability to reverse chloroquine resistance.

If the efficacy of a chloroquine-chlorpromazine combination is supported by field studies, the addition of chlorpromazine or similar drugs to preparations of chloroquine could have tremendous potential for treating falciparum malaria. It should also be determined whether the chloroquine-chlorpromazine combination is useful for chloroquine-resistant *P. vivax* malaria.

Agents in Preclinical Development

Three classes of compounds are in various stages of pre-human testing. These include analogs of floxacrine, which has unsuitable toxicity; quinazoline folate antimetabolites; and 1,2,4-trioxane derivatives, which are synthetic analogs of artemisinin.

Pharmaceutics and Clinical Pharmacology

The discovery and subsequent development of novel antimalarial drugs have little value unless those compounds reach the people who can benefit from their use. The way drugs are manufactured, packaged, stored, distributed, and marketed is crucial to this end. Although these processes are dependent to some degree on the management of malaria control programs and the infrastructure of malarious countries, they are very much part of the drug development process. These issues are too broad to discuss in detail here, but it is essential to recognize that the development of antimalarial drugs is futile unless those drugs reach the populations that require them: the residents of malarious regions.

Great advances in the use of an antimalarial drug can be expected once the compound is made available. Studies in clinical pharmacology often lead to better ways of using drugs, better formulations or delivery systems, the optimization of dosing regimens in various populations, and the recognition and alleviation of side effects. A thorough understanding of clinical pharmacology is not achieved during drug development, but support for such studies, devoted to both established and new drugs, can be expected to improve the quality of care for those who suffer from or are at risk of contracting malaria.

RESEARCH AGENDA

Artemisinin

The need for new classes of antimalarial drugs is urgent because of the spread of resistance to most existing classes of compounds.

> **RESEARCH FOCUS:** Acceleration of the clinical development of artemisinin and its derivatives.

Drug Mechanisms of Action

With the exception of the dihydrofolate reductase inhibitors, the mechanisms of action of antimalarial drugs are poorly understood. Identification of these mechanisms is important because it may reveal new targets for drug discovery and provide specific screens for new compounds that operate by the same or similar mechanisms. In this way, drugs might be developed with an eye toward avoiding parasite resistance while retaining the antiparasite selectivity of the prototype.

> **RESEARCH FOCUS:** The basic pharmacological mechanisms of action of all available antimalarial drugs.

> **RESEARCH FOCUS:** A mechanism-based screening strategy that identifies compounds of interest by their ability to bind to or otherwise inhibit specific proteins (enzymes or receptors) or processes thought to be critical for parasite viability, development, or reproduction.

Quinoline Resistance

The emergence of resistance to the quinoline family of schizonticidal antimalarial drugs (chloroquine and its analogs; mefloquine, halofantrine, and quinine) has had a major impact on the prophylaxis and treatment of falciparum malaria. Although enhanced drug efflux does appear to play a role in this phenomenon, uncertainties remain about the functional mechanism of antimalarial drug resistance. Certain compounds containing protonatable amines reverse resistance both in vitro and in vivo, but there is a lack of conclusive data on how this effect is mediated.

RESEARCH FOCUS: The molecular biological basis of parasite resistance to the quinoline antimalarial drugs.

New Drug Targets

While great benefit can be obtained from further discovery efforts aimed at known parasite targets of drug action, it is equally important to identify new targets. This may require determining the functional role of the parasite mitochondria, the functional physiology and biochemistry of the food vacuole (including proton pumps, digestive enzymes, and the biochemistry of pigment formation and iron metabolism), the enzymology of lipid synthesis and membrane formation, the enzymology of glycolysis, and the molecular biology of parasite development.

RESEARCH FOCUS: Evaluation of parasite biochemistry and physiology, with the goal of cloning key parasite proteins—such as phosphofructokinase, tubulin, and the vacuolar proton pump—that might be useful drug targets. These proteins can then be compared with their human homologues.

Transformation

To get the most out of studies of mechanisms of drug action and of parasite drug resistance, a method by which genes can be introduced into *P. falciparum* is required. The ability to clone the genes responsible for resistance would be greatly enhanced if they in turn could be transferred into (or "transform") drug-sensitive strains.

RESEARCH FOCUS: Develop a transformation system for *P. falciparum*.

Plasmodium vivax Culture System

Unlike *P. falciparum*, *P. vivax* cannot be grown in the laboratory. This fact makes conducting basic studies on *P. vivax* biochemistry and pharmacology problematic and hinders other important research activities, such as analysis of chloroquine uptake and efflux in resistant strains and development of a convenient assay system for screening candidate antimalarial drugs for *P. vivax* activity.

> **RESEARCH FOCUS:** Development of an in vitro culture system for *P. vivax*.

Drug Delivery

Some antimalarial medications must be administered by injection, a method that has several drawbacks. For one, the use of contaminated hypodermic needles is a significant risk factor for contracting a number of serious diseases, including AIDS and hepatitis, in many areas of the world. The discomfort and inconvenience of injections also reduces patient compliance with drug regimens.

> **RESEARCH FOCUS:** New drug delivery approaches, especially transdermal (skin patch) methods.

Botanical Preparations

Two of the most important antimalarial drugs, quinine and artemisinin, were derived from plants, and many indigenous populations have developed botanical preparations to treat the symptoms associated with malaria. While not all of these preparations contain medically useful substances, it is not unreasonable to believe that novel compounds with potential antimalarial activity could be found through an organized screening effort.

> **RESEARCH FOCUS:** A systematic method for identifying plants of interest, screening them, and characterizing the structures or compounds responsible for their antimalarial activity.

Secondary Metabolites

The secondary metabolites of bacteria and fungi have many interesting pharmacologic properties. Microbial fermentations, which contain a rich variety of organic molecules, have not yet been exploited for their potential antimalarial properties. While performance of such assays is not difficult and can be contracted out, considerable research on the chemistry of natural products is needed to identify active components.

> **RESEARCH FOCUS:** Extension of the technology of de-

riving new medically important compounds from microorganisms to the field of antimalarial drug discovery.

REFERENCES

Arthur, J. D., P. Echeverria, G. D. Shanks, J. Karwacki, L. Bodhidatta, and J. E. Brown. 1990. A comparative study of gastrointestinal infections in United States soldiers receiving doxycycline or mefloquine for malaria prophylaxis. American Journal of Tropical Medicine and Hygiene 43:608-613.

Bartlett, M. S., S. F. Queener, R. R. Tidwell, W. K. Milhous, J. D. Berman, W. Y. Ellis, and J. W. Smith. 1991. 8-Aminoquinolines from Walter Reed Army Institute of Research for treatment and prophylaxis of *Pneumocystis* pneumonia in rat models. Antimicrobial Agents and Chemotherapy 35:277-282.

Bates, M. D., S. R. Meshnick, C. I. Sigler, P. Leland, and M. R. Hollingdale. 1990. In vitro effects of primaquine and primaquine metabolites on exoerythrocytic stages of *Plasmodium berghei*. American Journal of Tropical Medicine and Hygiene 42:532-537.

Bitonti, A. J., A. Sjoerdsma, P. P. McCann, D. E. Kyle, A. M. J. Oduola, R. N. Rossan, W. K. Milhous, and D. E. Davidson Jr. 1988. Reversal of chloroquine resistance in malaria parasite *Plasmodium falciparum* by desipramine. Science 242:1301-1303.

Bruce-Chwatt, L. J. 1987. Doxycycline prophylaxis in malaria. Lancet 2:1487.

Carson, P. E. 1984. 8-Aminoquinolines. Pp. 83-121 in Antimalarial Drugs, Vol I. Biological Background, Experimental Models, and Drug Resistance, Peters, W., and W. H. G. Richards, eds. New York: Springer-Verlag.

Clark, W. M. 1946. History of the co-operative wartime program. Pp. 2-27 in Survey of Antimalarial Drugs, F. Y. Wiselogle, ed. Ann Arbor: J. W. Edwards.

Cosgriff, T. M., C. L. Pamplin, C. J. Canfield, and G. P. Willet. 1985. Mefloquine failure in a case of falciparum malaria induced with a multidrug-resistant isolate in a nonimmune subject. American Journal of Tropical Medicine and Hygiene 34:692-693.

Editorial. 1989. Halofantrine in the treatment of malaria. Lancet 2:537-538.

Fernex, M. 1984a. Clinical trials—Phases I and II. Pp. 375-395 in Antimalarial Drugs, Vol I. Biological Background, Experimental Models, and Drug Resistance, Peters, W., and W. H. G. Richards, eds. New York: Springer-Verlag.

Fernex, M. 1984b. Clinical trials—Phases III and IV and field trials. Pp. 399-408 in Antimalarial Drugs, Vol I. Biological Background, Experimental Models, and Drug Resistance, Peters, W., and W. H. G. Richards, eds. New York: Springer-Verlag.

Foote, S. J., D. E. Kyle, R. K. Martin, A. M. J. Oduola, K. Forsyth, D. J. Kemp, and A. F. Cowman. 1990. Several alleles of the multidrug-resistance gene are closely linked to chloroquine resistance in *Plasmodium falciparum*. Nature 345:255-258.

Gardner, M. J., D. H. Williamson, and R. J. M. Wilson. 1991. A circular DNA in malaria parasites encodes an RNA polymerase like that of prokaryotes and chloroplasts. Molecular and Biochemical Parasitology 44:115-124.

Geary, T. G., and J. B. Jensen. 1983. Effects of antibiotics on *Plasmodium falciparum* in vitro. American Journal of Tropical Medicine and Hygiene 32:221-225.

Geary, T. G., A. A. Divo, J. B. Jensen, M. Zangwill, and H. Ginsburg. 1990. Kinetic modeling of the response of *Plasmodium falciparum* to chloroquine and its experimental testing in vitro. Implications for mechanism of action of and resistance to the drug. Biochemical Pharmacology 40:685-691.

Ginsburg, H., and T. G. Geary. 1986. Current concepts and new ideas on the mechanism of action of quinoline-containing antimalarials. Biochemical Pharmacology 36:1567-1576.

Ginsburg, H., and W. D. Stein. In press. Kinetic modeling of chloroquine uptake by malaria-infected erythrocytes: assessment of the factors that may determine drug resistance. Biochemical Pharmacology.

Gutteridge, W. E. 1989. Antimalarial drugs currently in development. Journal of the Royal Society of Medicine 82(Suppl 17):63-66.

Horton, R. J. 1988. Introduction of halofantrine for malaria treatment. Parasitology Today 4:238-239.

Horton, R. J., and S. N. Parr. 1989. Halofantrine: an overview of efficacy and safety. Pp. 65-80 in Halofantrine in the Treatment of Multidrug Resistant Malaria, Warhurst, D. C., and C. J. Schofield, eds. New York: Elsevier Scientific Publications.

Karwacki, J. J., D. Shanks, N. Limsommwong, and P. Singhara. 1990. Proguanil-sulphonamide for malaria prophylaxis. Transactions of the Royal Society of Tropical Medicine and Hygiene 84:55-57.

Kremsner, P. G. 1990. Clindamycin in malaria treatment. Journal of Antimicrobial Chemotherapy 25:9-14.

Krogstad, D. J., I. Y. Gluzman, D. E. Kyle, A. M. J. Oduola, S. K. Martin, W. K. Milhous, and P. H. Schlesinger. 1987. Efflux of chloroquine from *Plasmodium falciparum*: mechanism of chloroquine resistance. Science 238:1283-1285.

Krogstad, D. J., P. H. Schlesinger, and B. L. Herwaldt. 1988. Antimalarial agents: mechanisms of chloroquine resistance. Antimicrobial Agents and Chemotherapy 32:799-801.

Lobel, H. O., K. W. Bernard, S. L. Williams, A. W. Hightower, L. C. Patchen, and C. C. Campbell. 1991. Effectiveness and tolerance of long-term malaria prophylaxis with mefloquine. JAMA 265(3):361-364.

Martin, S. K., A. M. J. Oduola, and W. K. Milhous. 1987. Reversal of chloroquine resistance in *Plasmodium falciparum* by verapamil. Science 235:899-901.

Meshnick, S. R. 1990. Chloroquine as an intercalator: a hypothesis revisited. Parasitology Today 6:77-79.

Milhous, W. K., and B. G. Schuster. 1990. Malaria studies aim at drug resistance. U.S. Medicine 26:27-28.

Milhous, W. K., N. F. Weatherly, J. H. Bowdre, and R. E. Desjardins. 1985. In vitro activities of and mechanisms of resistance to antifol antimalarial drugs. Antimicrobial Agents and Chemotherapy 27:525-530.

Milhous, W. K., L. G. Gerena, D. E. Kyle, and A. M. J. Oduola. 1989. In vitro strategies for circumventing antimalarial drug resistance. Progress in Clinical and Biological Research 313:61-72.

Miller, K. D., H. O. Lobel, R. F. Satriale, J. N. Kuritsky, R. Stern, and C. C. Campbell. 1986. Severe cutaneous reactions among American travelers using pyrimethamine-sulfadoxine (Fansidar) for malaria prophylaxis. American Journal of Tropical Medicine and Hygiene 35:451-458.

Milton, K. A., G. Edwards, S. A. Ward, M. L. Orme, and A. M. Breckenridge. 1989. Pharmacokinetics of halofantrine in man: effect of food and dose size. British Journal of Clinical Pharmacology 28:71-77.

Moran, J. S., and K. W. Bernard. 1989. The spread of chloroquine-resistant malaria in Africa. Implications for travelers. JAMA 262:245-248.

Pang, L., N. Limsomwong, E. F. Boudreau, and P. Singharaj. 1987. Doxycycline prophylaxis for falciparum malaria. Lancet 1:1161-1164.

Pang, L., N. Limsomwong, and P. Singharaj. 1988. Prophylactic treatment of vivax and falciparum malaria with low-dose doxycycline. Journal of Infectious Diseases 158:1124-1127.

Payne, D. 1987. Spread of chloroquine resistance in *Plasmodium falciparum*. Parasitology Today 3:241-246.

Peters, W. 1990a. *Plasmodium*: resistance to antimalarial drugs. Annales de Parasitologie et Humaine Comparé 65(Suppl. I):103-106.

Peters, W. 1990b. The prevention of antimalarial drug resistance. Pharmacology and Therapeutics 47:499-508.

Peters, W., and B. L. Robinson. In press. The chemotherapy of rodent malaria. XLVI. Reversal of mefloquine resistance in rodent *Plasmodium*. Annals of Tropical Medicine and Parasitology.

Peterson, D. S., W. K. Milhous, and T. E. Wellems. 1990. Molecular basis of differential resistance to cycloguanil and pyrimethamine in *Plasmodium falciparum* malaria. Proceedings of the National Academy of Sciences of the United States of America 87:3018-3022.

Prapunwattana, P., W. J. O'Sullivan, and Y. Yuthavong. 1988. Depression of *Plasmodium falciparum* dihydroorotate dehydrogenase activity in in vitro culture by tetracycline. Molecular and Biochemical Parasitology 27:119-124.

Rieckmann, K. H. 1984. Antibiotics. Pp. 443-470 in Antimalarial Drugs, Vol. II. Current Antimalarials and New Drug Developments, Peters, W., and W. H. G. Richards, eds. New York: Springer-Verlag.

Rieckmann, K. H., D. R. Davis, and D. C. Hutton. 1989. *Plasmodium vivax* resistance to chloroquine? Lancet 2:1183-1184.

Rossan, R. N., W. K. Milhous, and D. E. Kyle. 1990. Cure of *Plasmodium falciparum* infections in aotus by in vivo reversal of chloroquine resistance with phenothiazines. Abstract 351, 39th Annual Meeting of the American Society of Tropical Medicine and Hygiene, New Orleans, Louisiana, November 4-8.

Schlesinger, P. H., D. J. Krogstad, and B. L. Herwalt. 1988. Antimalarial agents: mechanisms of action. Antimicrobial Agents and Chemotherapy 32:793-798.

Taylor, T. E., M. E. Molyneux, J. J. Wirima, K. A. Fletcher, and K. Morris. 1988. Blood glucose levels in Malawian children before and during the administration of intravenous quinine for severe falciparum malaria. New England Journal of Medicine 319:1040-1047.

Vennerstrom, J. L., J. W. Eaton, W. Y. Ellis, and W. K. Milhous. 1991. Antimalarial synergism and antagonism. Pp. 188-222 in Molecular Mechanisms and Chemotherapeutic Synergism, Potentiation and Antagonism, Chou, T.-C., and D. C. Rideout, eds. Orlando: Academic Press.

Webster, L. T. 1990. Drugs used in the chemotherapy of protozoal infections. Pp. 978-987 in Goodman and Billmans. The Pharmacological Basis of Therapeutics, Gilman, A. G., T. W. Rall, A. S. Nies, and P. Taylor, eds. New York: Pergamon Press.

Wellems, T. E., L. J. Panton, I. Y. Gluzman, V. E. do Rosario, R. W. Gwadz, A. Walker-Jonah, and D. J. Krogstad. 1990. Chloroquine resistance not linked to mdr-like genes in a *Plasmodium falciparum* cross. Nature 345:253-255.

Wernsdorfer, W. H., and P. I. Trigg. 1988. Recent progress of malaria research: chemotherapy. Pp. 1569-1674 in Malaria: Principles and Practice of Malariology, Wernsdorfer, W. H., and I. McGregor, eds. Edinburgh: Churchill Livingstone.

White, N. J., S. Looareesuwan, D. A. Warrell, M. J. Warrell, P. Chanthavanich, D. Bunnag, and T. Harinasuta. 1983a. Quinine loading dose in cerebral malaria. American Journal of Tropical Medicine and Hygiene 32:1-5.

White, N. J., D. A. Warrell, P. Chanthavanich, S. Looareesuwan, M. J. Warrell, S. Krishna, D. H. Williamson, and R. C. Turner. 1983b. Severe hypoglycemia and hyperinsulinemia in falciparum malaria. New England Journal of Medicine 309:61-66.

World Health Organization. 1981. Chemotherapy of Malaria, 2nd ed. Geneva: World Health Organization.

World Health Organization. 1990. Practical Chemotherapy of Malaria. World Health Organization Technical Report Series, No. 805. Geneva: World Health Organization.

9

Vaccines

WHERE WE WANT TO BE IN THE YEAR 2010

After years of research, several different malaria vaccines will be available and licensed for use in humans. For infants and children in highly endemic regions of the world, an inexpensive, safe, and stable vaccine that gives long-lasting protection from death and severe clinical illness will be integrated into existing immunization programs. For nonimmune visitors to malarious areas and for the control of epidemics, there will be a vaccine that gives complete short-term protection against malaria with few side effects. Finally, a vaccine that confers no individual protection, but prevents the development of the parasite in the mosquito, will be used in combination with the other vaccines and control measures to reduce, and in some areas even interrupt, malaria transmission.

WHERE WE ARE TODAY

Prospects for a Vaccine

Vaccination is an exceptionally attractive strategy for preventing and controlling malaria. Clinical and experimental data support the feasibility of developing effective malaria vaccines. For example, experimental vaccination with irradiated sporozoites can protect humans against malaria, suggesting that immunization with appropriate sporozoite and liver-stage antigens can prevent infection in individuals bitten by malaria-infected mosquitoes. In addition, repeated natural infections with the malaria parasite induce immune responses that can prevent disease and death in infected individuals, and the administration of serum antibodies obtained from repeatedly infected adults can control malaria infections in children who have not yet acquired protective immunity. These data suggest that immunization with appropriate blood-stage antigens can drastically reduce the consequences of malaria infection. Finally, experimental evidence shows that immunization with sexual-stage antigens can generate an immune response that prevents parasite development in the vector, offering a strategy for interrupting malaria transmission.

Prospects for the development of malaria vaccines are enhanced by the availability of suitable methods for evaluating candidate antigens. These include protocols that allow human volunteers to be safely infected with malaria, and the identification of many areas in the world where more than 75 percent of individuals can be expected to become infected with malaria during a three-month period. In contrast to vaccines for diseases of low incidence, for which tens of thousands of immunized and nonimmunized controls must be studied over several years, malaria vaccines could be evaluated in selected areas in fewer than 200 volunteers in less than a year.

Developments in molecular and cellular biology, peptide chemistry, and immunology provide the technological base for engineering subunit vaccines composed of different parts of the malaria parasite, an approach that was not possible 10 years ago. During the last 5 years, more than 15 experimental malaria vaccines have undergone preliminary testing in human volunteers. Although none of these vaccines has proven suitable for clinical implementation, progress has been made in defining the parameters of a successful vaccine and the stage has been set for further advancement.

Despite the inherent attractiveness and promise of this approach, there remain a number of obstacles to vaccine development. With the exception of the erythrocytic (blood) stages of *P. falciparum*, human malaria parasites cannot be readily cultured in vitro, limiting the ability of researchers to study other stages of this parasite and all stages of the other three human malaria parasite species.

In vitro assays, potentially useful for screening candidate vaccines for effectiveness, do not consistently predict the level of protective immunity seen in vivo. The only laboratory animals that can be infected with human malaria parasites are certain species of nonhuman primates, which are not naturally susceptible to these organisms. This makes it difficult to compare the results of many studies done in animals with what happens in human malaria infection.

The promises of modern vaccinology, while potentially revolutionary, have so far proved elusive. Few commercially available vaccines have been produced by this technology, for both scientific and economic reasons. Scientists have not yet been able to assemble defined synthetic peptides and recombinant proteins and combine them with new adjuvants and delivery systems into a practical human malaria vaccine. However, as discussed above and in the remainder of this chapter, there are good reasons to believe that this approach will ultimately succeed.

Approaches to Vaccine Development

The complex life cycle of the malaria parasite provides a number of potential targets for vaccination (Figure 9-1). Under investigation are vaccines that would be effective against the extracellular sporozoite, during the short period it spends in the bloodstream; the exoerythrocytic (or liver-stage) parasite, during the roughly seven days it develops within liver cells; the extracellular merozoite, released from liver cells or infected erythro-

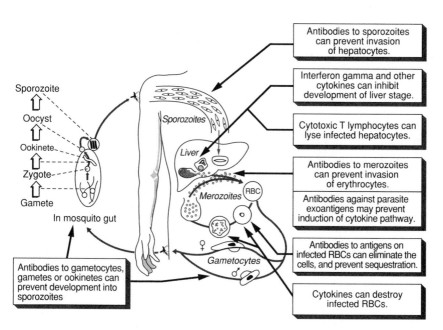

FIGURE 9-1 Host defense against malaria. (Adapted, with permission, from Rickman, L. S., and S. L. Hoffman. 1991. Malaria. Pg. 1039 in Medical Microbiology, 3rd Ed., S. Baron, ed. New York: Churchill Livingstone)

cytes and free in the circulation prior to invading other erythrocytes; the asexual parasite that develops within red blood cells; exogenous parasite material released from infected erythrocytes; and the sexual-stage parasite, which occurs both inside erythrocytes and in mosquitoes. The optimal vaccine would include antigens from the sporozoite, asexual, and sexual stages of the parasite, thus providing multiple levels of control, but vaccines effective against individual stages could also prove highly useful. In addition, a vaccine against the *Anopheles* mosquito itself, which reduced the insect's life span and prevented complete development of the parasite, could be valuable.

Regardless of the stage of parasite targeted for vaccine development, a similar strategy is envisioned. Based on knowledge of the mechanisms of protective immunity, specific parasite antigens (immunogens) are identified that induce a protective immune response, and synthetic or recombinant vaccines that accurately mimic the structure of that antigen are prepared.

In the subunit approach to vaccine development, this is done by combining the immunogen with carrier proteins, adjuvants, and live vectors or other delivery systems. This approach is being pursued throughout the world in laboratories studying infectious diseases. Clinical utility has yet to be demonstrated for the majority of these efforts, and barriers to obtaining satisfactory immunization by the subunit approach remain. Nevertheless, research on malaria subunit vaccines will continue to be at the cutting edge of this innovative and important approach to vaccine development.

Pre-Erythrocytic Vaccines

A pre-erythrocytic vaccine is designed to prevent malaria infection. If all sporozoites and liver stages of the parasite are destroyed before they can mature to cause blood-stage infection, all clinical manifestations of malaria will be prevented. Such a vaccine, even if it induced protection that lasted for only a few months, would be especially useful for tourists, diplomats, businessmen, military personnel, and other short-term visitors to malarious areas, since nonimmune individuals are highly susceptible to the rapid development of severe and fatal malaria. A pre-erythrocytic vaccine could be useful for long-term residents of malarious areas if it induced long-lasting protection, or if immunity could be boosted by natural exposure to malaria.

Mechanisms of Immunity

In the 1960s and 1970s a number of researchers showed that immunization with live sporozoites that were treated in such a way as to be noninfective (attenuated) confers protection against subsequent sporozoite-induced malaria infection in mice, monkeys, and humans (Nussenzweig et al., 1967; Clyde et al., 1973a,b, 1975; Rieckmann et al., 1974, 1979; Gwadz et al., 1979). In the human studies, mosquitoes infected with malaria sporozoites were exposed to x-rays, and the resulting radiation-attenuated sporozoites were introduced into human volunteers during the mosquitoes' blood meal.

Immunization with radiation-attenuated sporozoites induces protection unlike that found after natural infection. Naturally acquired immunity seems to be directed primarily against the erythrocytic stages of the parasite, so that infection per se is not prevented, but people are protected from severe disease and death. Individuals who have lived for 20 or more years in endemic regions still become infected, although they may have few or no symptoms (Hoffman et al., 1987). In contrast, volunteers immunized with irradiated sporozoites do not develop any detectable blood-stage infection. The differences may be due in part to the fact that even in areas of the highest malaria transmission, naturally exposed individuals are bitten by relatively few infective mosquitoes (fewer than 50 per month) (Beier et al., 1990). Thus they may not receive sufficient stimulation by sporozoite antigens to induce the protective immune responses achieved by repeated exposure to many hundreds of irradiated, infected mosquitoes over a few weeks or months (Clyde et al., 1973a,b, 1975; Rieckmann et al., 1974, 1979).

Vaccinating people with irradiated sporozoites cannot be routinely done. No culture system capable of producing large numbers of sporozoites is available or perhaps even feasible. Dissecting sporozoites from infected mosquitoes is far too labor intensive, and exposing people to mosquitoes containing irradiated sporozoites is not a tenable strategy. Given these limitations, the only hope for a pre-erythrocytic vaccine lies in the construction of a subunit vaccine, and researchers have been focusing on this objective. Identifying the mechanisms of protective immunity and the parasite antigens against which these protective immune responses are directed is a prerequisite to the development of this type of vaccine. Both antibodies and cellular immune responses contribute to this protection.

Antibody-Mediated Immunity   Mice and humans immunized with irradiated sporozoites develop antibodies directed against sporozoites. When administered to animals, some of these antisporozoite antibodies can protect against sporozoite-induced malaria infection (Potocnjak et al., 1980; Egan et al., 1987; Charoenvit et al., 1991a,b). Protective antisporozoite antibodies generally react with only a single species of malaria parasite and thus confer protection only against that species. This is similar to the species-specific immunity induced by immunization with irradiated sporozoites (Clyde et al., 1975).

The mechanisms by which antibodies confer protection are not certain. Antibodies can prevent the invasion of sporozoites into liver cells in culture (Hollingdale et al., 1984; Mazier et al., 1986), and it is likely these antibodies inhibit parasite binding to or invasion of liver cells. Antibodies appear to have other damaging effects on sporozoites, since those that successfully invade liver cells in the presence of antisporozoite antibodies often do not develop normally and fail to release merozoites that can initiate a blood-stage infection (Mazier et al., 1986). Conceivably, antibodies might also kill sporozoites directly or make them more susceptible to phagocytosis.

Cell-Mediated Immunity   Cell-mediated immunity is a broad classification that includes all immune responses that involve antigen-primed white blood cells (lymphocytes) or their products, other than antibodies. These are produced by B lymphocytes (so called because their maturation occurs in the bone marrow). The site on an antigen recognized by an antibody is known as a B-cell epitope. The cellular portion of the immune response includes T lymphocytes (so called because their maturation occurs in the thymus), natural killer cells, and monocytes. T lymphocytes have been further subdivided into helper cells (which enhance the production of antibody or stimulate other lymphocytes), suppressor cells (which suppress the production of antibody or inhibit other lymphocytes), and cytotoxic T lymphocytes (which directly kill other cells, including malaria-infected cells). The site on an antigen recognized by a T cell is known as a T-cell epitope.

Both lymphocytes and monocytes secrete proteins, called cytokines, that affect the function of other cells. Some of these cytokines regulate the function of lymphocytes. Other cytokines act to destroy cells, including those that contain infectious agents such as malaria parasites.

Cell-mediated immunity is an important part of the protection induced by immunization with irradiated sporozoites. For example, mice that are unable to produce antibodies can be successfully immunized with irradiated sporozoites (Chen et al., 1977). In addition, administration of immune lymphocytes to normal mice can protect them from sporozoite-induced malaria infection in the absence of anti-sporozoite antibodies (Egan et al., 1987). Experimental subunit sporozoite vaccines that elicit cell-mediated immunity without inducing antisporozoite antibodies also can protect mice against sporozoite-induced malaria (Sadoff et al., 1988). These studies suggest the presence of protective cell-mediated immune responses.

There are a number of mechanisms by which cell-mediated immunity could protect against sporozoite-induced malaria. Cytokines such as gamma-interferon may play a role. Gamma-interferon inhibits the development of malaria parasites in cultured liver cells (Ferreira et al., 1986; Mellouk et al., 1987). Treatment with agents that induce interferon production (Jahiel,

1968a,b), or administration of purified gamma-interferon (Maheshwari et al., 1986; Schofield et al., 1987a) will protect animals from sporozoite-induced malaria.

Cytotoxic T lymphocytes are also important. In some mouse strains, these cells appear to be the principal mechanism of protective immunity, since treatment of immunized mice with antibodies that destroy cytotoxic T lymphocytes renders them susceptible to sporozoite-induced malaria (Schofield et al., 1987b; Weiss et al., 1988). Some cytotoxic T lymphocytes recognize malaria-infected liver cells (Hoffman et al., 1989b; Weiss et al., 1990); administration of these cells can protect mice from sporozoite-induced malaria infection (Romero et al., 1989; Tsuji et al., 1990).

A general feature of T lymphocytes is that they do not recognize whole antigens directly. Instead, they recognize fragments of antigens presented as a complex with certain host proteins (the major histocompatibility complex, or MHC, proteins) on the surface of cells. Thus, cell-mediated immune responses will not be directed against extracellular sporozoites in the circulation, but will instead be directed against malaria-infected liver cells (Hoffman et al., 1989b). Because sporozoites invade liver cells within a few minutes or hours but parasite maturation within liver cells takes many days, protective cell-mediated immune responses directed against infected liver cells may be more effective than antisporozoite antibodies.

Targets of Pre-Erythrocytic Immunity

In both humans and laboratory animals, immunity induced by irradiated sporozoites is both stage specific and species specific; that is, immunization with sporozoites does not protect against infection with blood-stage parasites, and immunization with *P. falciparum* sporozoites does not protect against infection with *P. vivax* (and vice versa). This suggests that the immune response is directed against species-specific antigens on the sporozoite or the host's infected liver cells. Significantly, the protection is not strain specific; immunization with one *P. falciparum* isolate elicits protective immunity against isolates from other regions of the world (Clyde et al., 1973b).

Circumsporozoite Protein For a number of reasons, initial efforts to develop a pre-erythrocytic vaccine have focused heavily on one protein found on the surface of the sporozoite, the circumsporozoite (CS) protein. The CS protein is a target of both protective antibody and cell-mediated immune responses. The gene encoding the CS protein was one of the first malaria genes to be cloned by using molecular biology techniques, and CS genes have been cloned from a large number of human and animal malaria parasites (Chulay, 1989), which facilitates the testing of vaccines in various animal model systems.

The CS proteins of all malaria parasites studied thus far are similar in size and overall structure but vary considerably in specific composition. All have a central region consisting of tandem repeats of species-specific amino acids (Dame et al., 1984). After immunization with irradiated sporozoites, most of the antibodies that develop are directed against the repetitive region of the CS protein (Zavala et al., 1983). Antibodies directed against the CS repetitive region inhibit sporozoite invasion into cultured liver cells (Mazier et al., 1986), and administration of such antibodies can completely protect against sporozoite-induced malaria in mouse and monkey model systems (Potocnjak et al., 1980; Egan et al., 1987; Charoenvit et al., 1991a,b). In *P. falciparum*, the repetitive region contains a series of four amino acids (asparagine-alanine-asparagine-proline) that has been detected in all isolates analyzed (Zavala et al., 1985). Thus, protective immunity directed against the repetitive region of *P. falciparum* would be expected to be species specific but not isolate specific.

Antibodies against non-repetitive regions of the CS protein have also been shown to inhibit sporozoite invasion into cultured liver cells (Aley et al., 1986; D. M. Gordon, Department of Immunology, Walter Reed Army Institute of Research, personal communication, 1990).

The CS protein is also a target of cell-mediated immunity. Mice and humans immunized with irradiated sporozoites develop cytotoxic T lymphocytes directed against portions of the CS protein (Kumar et al., 1988; Romero et al., 1989; Weiss et al., 1990; Malik et al., 1991). Such cytotoxic T lymphocytes can destroy malaria-infected liver cells in culture (Weiss et al., 1990), and administration of cloned T lymphocytes specific for portions of the CS protein can protect mice against sporozoite-induced malaria (Romero et al., 1989; Del Giudice et al., 1990).

The CS protein also contains epitopes recognized by helper T lymphocytes. These T helper epitopes are present in both the repetitive and flanking non-repetitive regions of the CS protein (Good et al., 1987).

Sporozoite Surface Protein 2   A second sporozoite surface protein (SSP2) that is a target of protective immunity has recently been identified in *P. yoelii* (Charoenvit et al., 1987; Hedstrom et al., 1990). Antibodies against SSP2 partially inhibit sporozoite invasion into liver cells in culture (S. Mellouk, unpublished), and administration of a cloned T lymphocyte that recognizes SSP2 can protect mice against sporozoite-induced malaria (S. Khusmith, unpublished). Immunization of mice with either a CS protein vaccine alone or an SSP2 vaccine alone can protect a proportion of mice against sporozoite-induced malaria, while concurrent immunization with both vaccines protects all mice (Khusmith et al., 1991). This synergistic effect emphasizes one of the advantages of including multiple antigens from a single parasite stage in a multicomponent malaria vaccine.

Other Sporozoite Proteins Antibodies directed against other sporozoite antigens can inhibit sporozoite invasion into liver cells in culture, and when administered to mice can protect them from sporozoite-induced malaria (Hollingdale et al., 1990). Administration of a cloned T lymphocyte that recognizes another sporozoite antigen, that is also expressed by infected erythrocytes, can also protect mice against sporozoite-induced malaria (Tsuji et al., 1990).

Liver-Stage Antigens CS protein and other sporozoite antigens are expressed in malaria-infected liver cells. There are other antigens not found on sporozoites that are first produced by parasites developing within liver cells (Guerin-Marchand et al., 1987; Hollingdale et al., 1990). It is likely that some of these liver-stage antigens contain epitopes that are targets for protective cell-mediated immune responses.

Impediments to Pre-Erythrocytic Vaccine Development

Production of Antigen Sporozoites, like other stages of malaria parasites, cannot be produced in sufficient quantity or purity to be used to immunize humans. Malaria vaccine development has therefore relied on subunit vaccines. A subunit vaccine is generally constructed in three parts: the target of the desired protective immune response (e.g., B-cell epitopes as targets for antibodies and T-cell epitopes as targets for cytotoxic T lymphocytes); carrier peptide(s) to stimulate helper T lymphocytes; and an adjuvant or other delivery system to improve the magnitude and quality of the immune response.

The first malaria sporozoite vaccines tested in humans contained the repetitive B-cell epitope of the CS protein plus T-cell epitopes from nonmalaria proteins and were constructed by using recombinant DNA technology or synthetic peptide chemistry (Ballou et al., 1987; Herrington et al., 1987). Other approaches have utilized entirely synthetic vaccines consisting of B- and T-cell epitopes from the CS protein (Tam et al., 1990) or malaria B-cell epitopes coupled to selected proteins or peptides that have helper but not suppressor epitopes. A peptide from tetanus toxoid with these latter properties has been described (Etlinger et al., 1990). In mice primed with bacillus Calmette-Guerin (BCG), a live, avirulent strain of tuberculosis bacterium, immunization with a vaccine consisting of the B-cell epitope of the *P. falciparum* CS protein coupled to a purified tuberculosis protein produced high titers of antibodies to sporozoites without the use of any other adjuvant (Lussow et al., 1990). Given the widespread sensitization of humans to tuberculosis proteins and BCG, this vaccine, or a recombinant BCG expressing the CS protein, might be effective.

Recombinant live attenuated vaccines might also be used. For example, insertion of the CS protein gene into attenuated strains of *Salmonella* creates a vaccine that can protect mice from sporozoite-induced malaria (Sadoff et al., 1988; Aggarwal et al., 1990). Although it is relatively easy to produce vaccines for animal immunization studies, production of subunit vaccine antigens of sufficient purity for trials in human volunteers is more difficult and expensive. Research laboratories studying malaria immunity are not equipped to produce these high-quality vaccines, and collaboration with pharmaceutical or biotechnology companies is generally necessary.

Induction of the Appropriate Immune Response

ANTIBODIES   Administration of monoclonal antibodies directed against specific sporozoite B-cell epitopes can protect animals against sporozoite-induced malaria. Inducing high levels of antibody is thus one objective of immunization with sporozoite vaccines. Early subunit vaccines conferred complete protection from sporozoite-induced malaria in a small number of immunized volunteers who were experimentally exposed to the bites of infected mosquitoes, and they delayed the onset of blood-stage infection in other volunteers who had antibodies (Ballou et al., 1987; Herrington et al., 1987). Overall, however, these vaccines induced relatively low levels of antibody (Chulay, 1989). These antibody levels were lower than those to the same vaccine in mice and rabbits. They were also lower than the highest antibody levels induced by natural exposure to the bites of sporozoite-infected mosquitoes (Hoffman et al., 1987), and such levels of antibody are not protective.

One way to increase the level of antibody induced by sporozoite vaccines is to change the carrier protein and the adjuvant. Early results suggest this approach can increase the level of antibody 10-fold (Rickman et al., 1991).

The quantity of antibody is not the only determinant of protection, however. High levels of antisporozoite antibodies were achieved after immunization with the *P. falciparum* repetitive B-cell epitope coupled to a bacterial protein, but only one of eight volunteers was protected against malaria, and that individual did not have one of the highest levels of antibody (L. Fries, Associate Professor of International Health, Center for Immunization Research, Johns Hopkins School of Hygiene and Public Health, personal communication, 1990). The specificity of the antibody response is also important. For example, monkeys can be protected from sporozoite-induced *P. vivax* malaria by administration of a monoclonal antibody directed against the CS protein (Charoenvit et al., 1991b). This monoclonal antibody recognizes a four-amino-acid B-cell epitope contained within the nine amino acids of the repetitive portion of the CS protein (Charoenvit et al., 1991b).   A recombinant *P. vivax* sporozoite vaccine containing all nine amino acids of the CS repeat section that contained only the repetitive amino acids of the CS protein induced high levels of antisporozoite antibodies in monkeys and humans (Collins et al., 1989; Gordon et al., 1990), but these antibodies were not directed against the four-amino-acid B-cell epitope recognized by the protective monoclonal antibody (Charoenvit et al., 1991b).

Protection does not appear to be a function of the specific immunoglobulin G (IgG) subclass of antibodies, since monoclonal antibodies of the IgG1, IgG2b, and IgG3 subclasses, as well as Fab fragments (antibodies lacking their subclass-specific portion), have all been shown to transfer protection passively in mice (Potocnjak et al., 1980; Egan et al., 1987; Charoenvit et al., 1991a,b). Protection also does not appear to be explained by differences between the structure of the native sporozoite protein and the synthetic and recombinant peptide subunit vaccines, since monoclonal antibodies produced by immunization with short peptides can also confer protection when administered to animals.

Immunization undoubtedly produces polyclonal antibodies of varying affinities and specificities. To achieve consistent antibody-mediated protection, a vaccine may have to focus the immune response, or dramatically increase the overall production of antibody, to achieve appropriate concentrations of the "correct" antibodies.

PASSIVE IMMUNIZATION   Because passive transfer of monoclonal antibodies is so effective in protecting against sporozoite-induced malaria in animals, some researchers are working to develop human monoclonal antibodies against the repeat regions of the human malaria CS protein. These antibodies could be used to passively immunize short-term visitors to malarious areas in the same way that gamma globulin is used to prevent hepatitis A.

CELL-MEDIATED IMMUNE RESPONSE   Little is known about how to induce protective cell-mediated immune responses with subunit vaccines. Cytotoxic T lymphocytes generally are not induced by immunization with standard preparations of inactivated microbial antigens. Cytolytic T lymphocytes can be induced by immunization with recombinant live attenuated vaccines, such as those for salmonella, BCG, and vaccinia (smallpox vaccine). Work is in progress to construct recombinant live attenuated vaccines that express malaria genes and that might induce protective cell-mediated immune responses in humans.

Cytotoxic T lymphocytes can also be induced by immunization with antigens contained within liposomes (small lipid-bound vesicles that can interact with cells of the immune system), immunostimulatory complexes (particles formed by antigen complexed with the detergent saponin) (Takahashi et al., 1990), and peptides containing a cytotoxic T-lymphocyte epitope coupled to a lipid structure (Deres et al., 1989). These offer additional possible approaches to induction of protective cell-mediated immune responses.

Antigenic Diversity Most malaria antigens appear to have significant antigenic diversity. Much of this diversity may be an adaptive response of the parasite to host immunity, and it is theoretically possible that an initially effective malaria vaccine might select for parasite variants, leading to vaccine-resistant strains.

For example, there are at least two major variants of the repetitive region of the CS protein of *P. vivax*, and antibodies that recognize one variant do not react with the other (and vice versa) (Rosenberg et al., 1989; Wirtz et al., 1990). Extensive variation in the CS protein repetitive region occurs in the monkey malaria parasites *P. knowlesi* and *P. cynomolgi* (Sharma et al., 1985; Galinski et al., 1987). For vaccines intended to induce antibodies directed against the CS repetitive epitope, variability in the repetitive region would complicate vaccine formulation, since a useful vaccine must protect against all variants. For *P. falciparum*, variation in the repeat region of the CS protein has thus far been limited to minor changes in the numbers of repeating units and, occasionally, changes in a few of the individual repetitive epitopes. All *P. falciparum* isolates obtained from different parts of the world are recognized by monoclonal antibodies directed against the predominant repetitive epitope (Zavala et al., 1985).

Variability in T-cell epitopes may also be important. For example, the DNA sequence of the CS protein gene from several different isolates has been determined. It is highly conserved, and the variations that do occur are clustered within regions that code for T-cell epitopes (Good et al., 1987; Kumar et al., 1988; Lockyer and Schwarz, 1987). Variation in helper T-cell epitopes may potentially limit the ability of sporozoites to boost the antibody response to CS protein B-cell epitopes, and variations in cytotoxic T-lymphocyte epitopes may allow liver-stage parasites to evade killing by cytotoxic T lymphocytes.

Genetic Restriction of the Immune Response T lymphocytes recognize fragments of antigens that are presented as a complex with host MHC proteins on the surface of cells (see above). The antigen fragments (T-cell epitopes) are formed by the action of cellular enzymes that digest the antigen into small pieces of about 8 to 12 amino acids.

The interaction of T-cell epitopes with MHC proteins is highly specific. Changing a single amino acid in either the T-cell epitope or the region of the MHC protein that binds to the T-cell epitope can completely prevent the interaction. There is tremendous variability among individuals in the genetically determined amino acid sequence of the region of the MHC protein that binds to T-cell epitopes. This means that only the T lymphocytes of some individuals (those with suitable MHC proteins) can recognize a given T-cell epitope. Genetic restriction is most easily studied in inbred mouse strains that have MHC proteins that are identical for all individuals of that strain but different from the MHC proteins of other strains. Most T-cell epitopes on malaria antigens appear to be genetically restricted (Del Giudice et al., 1986; Good et al., 1986, 1987, 1988a,b,c; Good, 1988; Hoffman et al., 1989a). That is, only mice of a few strains can recognize these epitopes. The human cell-mediated immune response to malaria antigens also appears to be genetically restricted (Good, 1988; Good et al., 1988d; Hoffman et al., 1989c; de Groot et al., 1989).

If only a minority of individuals can mount effective immune responses against protective T-cell epitopes after immunization, a vaccine would have to include multiple T epitopes, perhaps from different target antigens, to increase the probability that at least one T-cell epitope was recognized by almost every individual within a population. Indeed, the apparently universal ability of live attenuated sporozoite vaccines to induce protective immunity may result in part from the presence of multiple T-cell epitopes on multiple different target antigens. Although knowledge in this area is limited, it is encouraging that three of four volunteers immunized with irradiated sporozoites produced cytotoxic T lymphocytes against a defined T-cell epitope in the *P. falciparum* CS protein (Malik et al., 1991). The importance of genetic restriction to malaria antigens in humans remains to be determined.

Assays Predictive of Protection   One of the major obstacles to malaria vaccine development is the lack of laboratory assays that correlate with protective immunity (Hoffman et al., 1987). The only certain way to test vaccine efficacy is to immunize volunteers and determine whether they are protected after exposure to malaria-infected mosquitoes. Development of laboratory assays that predict protective immunity would be a major advancement.

Length of Protection   Nonimmune visitors to endemic areas may need a vaccine that protects them for only several weeks or months. In contrast, long-term residents of endemic regions require a vaccine that provides protection for years.

Immunization with live attenuated sporozoites induces long-lasting protective immunity in mice, but in the few humans tested protection disappears after a few months (Clyde et al., 1973b, 1975; Rieckmann et al., 1979). The early experience with malaria subunit vaccines based on the *P. falciparum* CS protein and tested in humans indicates that antibody levels generally decline quickly. Approaches that may overcome this problem include the use of adjuvants that increase the antibody response, so that protective levels of antibody are maintained for longer periods; the addition of helper T-cell epitopes from malaria antigens to boost antibody levels after natural exposure to sporozoites; and the use of new vaccine formulations that provide prolonged release of antigen, thereby providing their own booster doses over time. It must be acknowledged that such formulations have not been developed for any vaccine and represent a considerable technological challenge.

Asexual Blood-Stage Vaccines

An erythrocytic (blood-stage) or merozoite vaccine is intended to control parasite numbers after their release from the liver, thus preventing or reducing malaria-related morbidity and mortality. Even partial immunity to the asexual blood-stage parasites could be important, since disease severity is related to the level of parasitemia. This can be visualized by considering a hypothetical "typical" *P. falciparum* infection. In a nonimmune individual (Figure 9-2A), no blood-stage parasites would be present until about day 5, and clinical illness would not appear until several days later, after one or more cycles of parasite multiplication within red blood cells. Unless the individual were treated or rapidly developed a protective immune response, the parasitemia would increase exponentially to reach life-threatening levels within about a week, and death would follow shortly thereafter.

In an individual with immunity directed against only the pre-erythrocytic stages of the parasite (Figure 9-2B), 80 percent, 90 percent, or 95 percent inhibition of parasite multiplication would delay the onset of clinical illness by two to four days, but would have no effect on the subsequent exponential increase in parasitemia and progression to life-threatening infection.

In an individual with immunity directed against only blood-stage parasites (Figure 9-2C), 80 percent inhibition of parasite multiplication would delay the onset of clinical illness by about one week and markedly prolong the time until development of life-threatening infection. Assuming a 10-fold multiplication rate in a nonimmune individual, 90 percent inhibition of parasite multiplication would result in no net increase in parasitemia, and thus theoretically could prevent clinical illness without resolving the infection. With 95 percent inhibition, there would be a progressive decrease in parasitemia and eventual resolution of infection.

Thus, many believe that the most important and realistic goal for malaria vaccine development is to identify antigens and immune responses that protect adults and children living in endemic areas from becoming severely ill or dying of the disease. This immune response seems primarily to target the erythrocytic stage of the parasite.

A. Hypothetical Course of Malaria Infection in a Non-immune Person

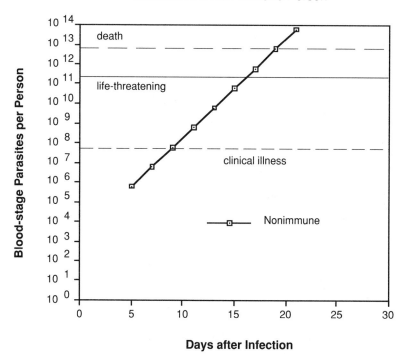

Days after Infection

FIGURE 9-2 Hypothetical course of *Plasmodium falciparum* infection in a nonimmune individual (A) and the effect of various levels of host immunity to sporozoites (B) or to blood-stage parasites (C). Note: Graphs were generated assuming (1) a mosquito injects 20 sporozoites, (2) each sporozoite yields a liver-stage parasite that gives rise to 30,000 merozoites that infect red blood cells, (3) the individual has 5 million red blood cells per microliter of blood and 6 liters total blood volume, (4) the blood-stage parasites multiply 10-fold every 48 hours, (5) clinical illness develops when parasitemia reaches about 10 per microliter of blood, (6) life-threatening illness develops when about 1 percent of the red blood cells are parasitized, and (7) death is almost inevitable when more than 20 percent of the red blood cells are parasitized. Based on unpublished calculations supplied by J. D. Chulay (Institute of Medicine Malaria Committee member) and J. D. Haynes (Walter Reed Army Institute of Research, Washington, D.C.)

Mechanisms of Immunity

Antibody Mediated Epidemiologists and clinicians working in malarious areas have long recognized there is an exposure-dependent acquisition of immunity to malaria. Because they benefit from maternal antibodies, infants are less likely than young children to become ill or die from malaria;

B. Hypothetical Effects of Incomplete
Pre-erythrocytic Immunity

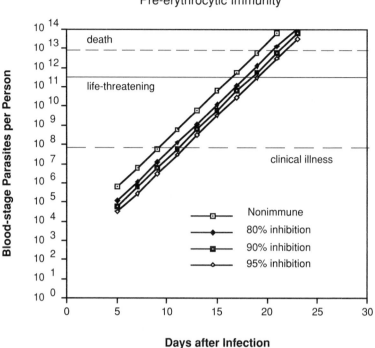

Days after Infection

FIGURE 9-2 *Continued*

in older children and adults, illness and death caused by malaria decrease with increasing exposure. This immunity is mediated primarily by antibodies against blood-stage parasites, and children with *P. falciparum* malaria who are treated with antibodies from the serum of hyperimmune adults show a dramatic reduction or even an elimination of parasitemia (Cohen et al., 1961; Bouharoun-Tayoun et al., 1990).

In infancy, these antibodies are transferred across the placenta to the fetus. In older children and adults, they are produced as a result of infection with malaria parasites. This protective immune response is not strain specific, since West African gamma globulin is effective in reducing parasitemia in children with malaria in East Africa (McGregor et al., 1963) and Thailand (Bouharoun-Tayoun et al., 1990).

The mechanisms by which antibodies confer protection from malaria are not completely understood. Antibodies could inhibit parasite invasion of red blood cells by agglutinating merozoites as they are released from schizont-infected erythrocytes, thus rendering them incapable of invasion (Miller et al., 1975;

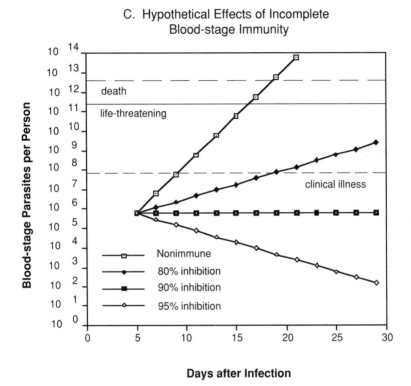

C. Hypothetical Effects of Incomplete Blood-stage Immunity

Days after Infection

FIGURE 9-2 *Continued*

Chulay et al., 1981), by blocking the binding of merozoites to erythrocytes (Thomas et al., 1984; Sim et al., 1990), or by interfering with the function of parasite proteins, such as proteases or rhoptry/microneme proteins, that mediate the invasion process (Holder and Freeman, 1984). Antimerozoite antibodies might also conceivably kill the parasites directly or make them more susceptible to phagocytosis (Khusmith and Druihle, 1983).

Antibodies that recognize parasite proteins on the surface of infected erythrocytes could contribute to the destruction of the cells. The process could be accomplished through complement-mediated lysis; by phagocytosis and antibody-dependent cellular inhibition (Bouharoun-Tayoun et al., 1990); by inhibition of the transport of nutrients essential to parasite growth (Cabantchik et al., 1983; Elford et al., 1985); or by inhibition of the attachment of infected erythrocytes to endothelial cells, thus preventing them from obstructing the microcirculation and diverting them to the spleen, where they will be removed from the circulation (David et al., 1983; Udeinya et al., 1983).

Antibodies also could react with parasite antigens, released from infected erythrocytes, that mediate the disease process (Playfair et al., 1990). This could occur through direct inhibition of parasite toxins, or by blockage of the interaction of antigens with host cells (such as macrophages), thereby preventing the release of toxic substances like tumor necrosis factor (TNF) and other cytokines. It is not clear that this response would resolve the infection or completely prevent the pathology resulting from infection.

Cell Mediated Cell-mediated immune responses appear to be important in malarial immunity, at least in animal models, but the mechanisms involved are unclear. Helper and suppressor T lymphocytes are undoubtedly important in modulating antibody levels. Because T lymphocytes recognize antigens on the surface of cells only in conjunction with MHC molecules, and mature human erythrocytes do not express MHC molecules, it is unlikely that T cells could recognize infected erythrocytes directly.

Some parasite antigens are secreted from malaria-infected erythrocytes (Howard et al., 1986) and, when taken up by macrophages or other antigen-presenting cells, may stimulate T-cell secretion of cytokines, some of which are known to be toxic to malaria parasites (Ockenhouse et al., 1984). It is possible that local concentrations of cytokines may be high enough to cause the destruction of the intra-erythrocytic malaria parasites.

Targets of Blood-Stage Immunity

The identification of targets of protective immunity has been based in part on an understanding of the mechanisms of immunity to blood-stage malaria parasites and in part on empirical observations. Several candidate proteins have been identified and are listed in Table 9-1. Some of the criteria used to select candidate vaccine antigens are discussed below.

Merozoite Invasion Interference with merozoite attachment to and invasion of erythrocytes has been a major focus of many research groups. Invasion is a multistep process involving receptor binding, "tight-junction" formation, erythrocyte-membrane invagination, vacuole formation, and closure (Hadley and Miller, 1988; Perkins, 1989). Parasite proteins involved in each of these steps are potential vaccine candidates.

There are at least two erythrocyte receptors to which *P. falciparum* merozoites bind. One of these is probably a member of a family of sialic acid-rich glycoproteins, the glycophorins (Jungery, 1985), while the other is unre-

TABLE 9-1 Candidate Antigens for Blood-Stage Malaria Vaccines

Antigen	Synonyms	Target of Inhibitory Antibodies	Protection in Primate Trial	Model Homologue	ICM	Sequence Diversity[a]
MSA-1	PMMSA, PSA, p185, p190	+	+	+	+	+
MSA-2	Gymmsa, gp56, 38-45 kDa antigen	+	n.d.	n.d.	+	+
RESA	Pf155	+	+	+	?	-
EBA		+	n.d.	n.d.	-	minor
AMA-1	Pf83	-	n.d.	+	-	minor
SERA	p113, p126 SERP, Pf140	+	+	n.d.	+	minor
RAP-1		+	+	n.d.	-	n.d.
RAP-2		-	+	n.d.	-	n.d.
Rhoph3		+	+	n.d.	-	-
PfHRP-II		-	+	n.d.	-	-
Pf55		-	+	n.d.	-	n.d.
Pf35		-	+	n.n.	-	n.d.
GBP	96-R	-	-	n.d.	+	-
ABRA	p101	-	n.d.	n.d.	+	-
Exp-1	CRA, Ag5.1	+	+	n.d.	?	minor
Aldolase		-	-	n.d.	-	n.d.
HSP70-1	p75	-	-	-	-	-

[a]Single amino acid changes may cause changes in antigenicity for B and T-cells (see Chapter 6).

Abbreviations used in this table: 96-R, 96 kDa thermostable protein; ABRA, acidic base repeat antigen; Ag5.1, antigen 5.1; AMA-1, apical merozoite antigen 1; CRA, circumsporozoite protein related antigen; Exp-1, exported protein 1; EBA, erythrocyte binding antigen; gp56, glycoprotein with an apparent molecular mass of 56 kDa; GBP, glycophorin binding protein; Gymmsa, glycosylated and major merozoite surface antigen; HSP70-1, 70-kDa heat shock protein 1; ICM = Immune clustered merozoites; kDa, kilodaltons; MSA-1, merozoite surface antigen 1; MSA-2, merozoite surface antigen 2; n.d., not determined; p75, p101, etc., proteins with an apparent molecular mass of 75 kDa, 101 kDa, etc.,; Pf83, Pf155, etc., *P. falciparum* protein with an apparent molecular mass of 83 kDa, 155 kDa, etc.; PfHRP-II, *P. falciparum* histidine rich protein II; PMMSA, precursor to the major merozoite surface antigen; PSA, polymorphic schizont antigen; RESA, ring-infected surface antigen; RAP-1, rhoptry associated protein 1; RAP-2, rhoptry associated protein 2; RhopH3, rhoptry high molecular weight complex protein 3; SERA, serine rich antigen; SERP, serine rich protein.

lated to the glycophorins (Mitchell et al., 1986). In addition, it has been proposed that the parasite itself releases proteins, called erythrocyte-binding antigens, that act as a bridge between the merozoite and the erythrocyte. At least one of these has been identified (Camus and Hadley, 1985) and characterized (Orlandi et al., 1990; Sim et al., 1990).

For *P. vivax*, the Duffy blood group antigen is the major erythrocyte receptor (Miller et al., 1976). The parasite antigens that bind to these receptors are potential vaccine candidates. Where merozoites of a single

Plasmodium species can invade by binding to one of several erythrocyte receptors, a multivalent vaccine will be required to completely inhibit merozoite invasion of red blood cells.

Rhoptries and micronemes are organelles located near the anterior end of the merozoite. Release of the contents of these organelles is essential to erythrocyte invasion, and there is evidence this process is susceptible to antibody attack (Holder and Freeman, 1984).

Antibodies from immune individuals can bind to the surface of merozoites as they are released from schizont-infected erythrocytes, forming large merozoite clusters incapable of invading erythrocytes (Chulay et al., 1981). Antibodies dissociated from these immune complexes have been used to identify the antigens involved (Chulay et al., 1987; Lyon et al., 1989). These include integral membrane proteins present on the merozoite surface as well as proteins that are only loosely associated with the merozoite surface.

Erythrocyte Surface Antigens   Antigens on the surface of infected erythrocytes are a particularly attractive target for vaccine intervention because of the long period during which they are exposed to the immune system. In *P. falciparum*, some of these antigens mediate the adherence of infected erythrocytes to endothelium, which causes mature-stage erythrocytic parasites to become sequestered in blood capillaries, where they are able to avoid destruction by the spleen (Howard et al., 1990).

Erythrocytes parasitized by mature *P. falciparum* in vitro can adhere to at least three different host endothelial cell molecules: CD-36, thrombospondin, and ICAM-1 (CD-54) (Howard and Gilladoga, 1989; Chulay and Ockenhouse, 1990). Parasitized erythrocytes can also adhere to (rosette with) normal erythrocytes, another type of cell-to-cell interaction (Udomsangpetch et al., 1989). The parasite molecules responsible for adherence have not been completely identified, but it appears that at least one is a high molecular weight (250 to 300 kilodaltons) variable antigen called *P. falciparum* erythrocyte membrane protein 1 (Leech et al., 1984; Howard et al., 1990). This protein has multiple distinct serotypes and may also undergo true antigenic variation. There is evidence that partially immune adults develop antibodies able to recognize epitopes that are conserved among all serotypes (Marsh and Howard, 1986).

Antigens Crucial to Parasite Growth   Monoclonal or polyclonal antibodies have been added to in vitro culture systems and screened to identify those that inhibit parasite growth (Perrin et al., 1981; Saul et al., 1984, 1985; Schofield et al., 1986; Lew et al., 1989). Protection of animals by passive transfer of these antibodies can confirm their value. The antigens recognized by such inhibitory antibodies are of obvious interest.

Antigens That Induce Protective Immunity in Animal Models A number of animal malarias, such as those caused by *P. chabaudi* and *P. yoelii* in mice, *P. lophurae* in ducklings, and *P. fragile* and *P. knowlesi* in rhesus monkeys, have been used to identify antigens that can induce protective immunity. The hope is that homologous molecules from human malaria parasite species will make good vaccine candidates. Experimental immunization with merozoite surface antigen 1 (MSA-1) in various animal models supports this hope (Holder and Freeman, 1981; Schmidt-Ullrich et al., 1983; Patarroyo et al., 1987; Siddiqui et al., 1987).

P. falciparum has been adapted to grow in aotus and saimiri monkeys, and partially purified parasite antigens that confer protection have been identified (Patarroyo et al., 1987). A number of blood-stage proteins were purified and tested individually for protective efficacy in aotus monkeys. The sequence of proteins that induced a degree of protection was determined, and synthetic peptides were made and used to immunize aotus monkeys. A combination of peptides from three proteins induced a protective immune response that resulted in survival from an otherwise lethal infection, often with little or no parasitemia.

Pathogenic Immune Factors Efforts to produce vaccines that prevent the most severe symptoms and signs of malaria disease represent an exciting new approach to malaria vaccine development. The impetus for research in this area comes from the observation that older children and repeatedly infected adults in endemic areas may harbor significant parasite concentrations without showing symptoms of disease. This tolerance is lost fairly quickly after exposure to malaria ceases. There is also similarity between the symptoms of malaria and the symptoms produced in nonmalarious individuals by treatment with TNF, interferons, and some of the interleukins. There is also a correlation between the severity of symptoms in severe malaria and the level of circulating TNF (see Chapter 4).

Soluble exoantigens of bloodstage *P. yoelii*, *P. berghei*, and *P. falciparum*, probably released at the time of schizont rupture, induce the secretion of TNF from mouse peritoneal macrophages and human peripheral blood lymphocytes in vitro (Bate et al., 1988; Taverne et al., 1990). These exoantigens, which appear to be phospholipids, also induce TNF production in vivo and can kill mice made sensitive to it (Bate et al., 1989). When exoantigens are used as immunogens, they induce a T-cell-independent IgM antibody response (Bate et al., 1990) that protects mice from dying from what would ordinarily be a lethal malaria infection (Playfair et al., 1990). This antibody response also blocks the ability of exoantigens to induce TNF production in vitro. Exoantigens appear to be conserved across animal species, since antisera against rodent malaria exoantigens recognize human exoantigens, and vice versa.

Preclinical and Clinical Trials

To date, the only reported human trials of asexual-stage malaria vaccines have been performed by Dr. Patarroyo and his colleagues in Colombia (Patarroyo et al., 1988). The vaccines were synthetic peptides based on studies in aotus monkeys (Patarroyo et al., 1987). All immunized subjects became clinically ill, but the infection in three of five volunteers receiving one of the vaccines was controlled without treatment, while all nonimmunized control subjects required treatment. This trial called for treatment only for individuals with more than 0.5 percent of their erythrocytes infected with parasites. No efficacy would have been demonstrated in this trial if a more conservative threshold for starting treatment had been used (see below). The mechanism of immunity, and the role of immune responses against the different antigens included in the vaccine, have not been established. Results of more recent clinical trials with this vaccine are not available for analysis.

Impediments to Asexual Blood-Stage Vaccine Development

Many of the same obstacles to the development of pre-erythrocytic vaccines are relevant to asexual blood-stage vaccines. Several additional impediments are worth mentioning.

Animal Models Animal models for vaccine challenge with *P. falciparum* and *P. vivax* are not optimal. Parasites often require extensive adaptation before they will grow in aotus monkeys, and splenectomy is required to get reproducible infections in saimiri monkeys. Further, there are only a few parasite isolates adapted to monkeys, making testing of antigenically diverse vaccine antigens difficult. Variation in the course of infection in control-group monkeys has made interpreting results difficult for vaccines that produce only partial protection. Despite its shortcomings, the aotus monkey model system remains the best available for simulating human *P. falciparum* infection.

Clinical Trials The outcome of a sporozoite vaccine trial is relatively simple to measure, since any appearance of parasites in the bloodstream signals failure. In contrast, an asexual-stage vaccine that controls parasite multiplication and protects against morbidity and mortality would be considered useful, even if it allowed moderate levels of parasitemia. Because the clinical effects of parasitemia vary with the immune status of the individual, determining when such a vaccine is effective is problematic. Trials performed in nonimmune volunteers, for example, may have to be terminated when only 0.05 percent of erythrocytes are infected. Parasitemia may increase 10- or 20-fold during the next cycle of asexual development, and parasitemias of about 1 percent may be associated with severe disease and some risk of death, despite appropriate treatment. Vaccines that control infection only after higher levels of parasitemia are reached would not be recognized in such a trial, even though such vaccines might be beneficial in partially immune individuals who were tolerant to modest levels of parasitemia. Candidate vaccine antigens may therefore need to be tested twice before efficacy is known: once in nonimmune volunteers and a second time in individuals living in an endemic area. This adds a further layer of logistical complexity to the vaccine evaluation process.

Antigen Complexity Malaria infection stimulates immune responses to a vast array of asexual blood-stage antigens. It is difficult to predict a priori whether a particular antigen will stimulate a protective immune response. Many of these antigens show considerable sequence variability, and some appear to undergo antigenic variation. In addition, many are too large to be expressed efficiently in recombinant vector systems, and because of their size they are difficult to analyze with use of synthetic peptides. A detailed look at one blood-stage antigen will illustrate many of the problems that are faced.

Merozoite Surface Antigen 1: A Case Study in Vaccine Development

MSA-1 is a glycoprotein (Holder, 1988) anchored by myristic acid to the surface of the schizont (Haldar et al., 1985). When the schizont ruptures, the antigen is processed into a number of discrete products residing on the surface of the merozoite, most of which disappear at the time the merozoite invades red blood cells. Only the carboxy-terminus of MSA-1 carries over into the ring-form trophozoite stage of the parasite (see Figure 9-1). MSA-1 from different *P. falciparum* isolates varies in size from 180 to 220 kilodaltons, and homologues are present in all *Plasmodia* species studied. The protein is encoded by a single exon on parasite chromosome 9 (Holder et al., 1985; Mackay et al., 1985; Tanabe et al., 1987; Peterson et al., 1988a).

Monoclonal antibody-binding studies have demonstrated that MSA-1 from different strains contains both conserved and variable regions (McBride et al., 1985). Gene-sequencing studies have confirmed this, and results from several groups have allowed the gene coding region to be subdivided into conserved, semivariable, and variable blocks (Tanabe et al., 1987; Peterson et al., 1988a,b). The variable blocks are generally one of two types (alleles), raising the possibility that a limited number of antigens could be used to protect against all variants of MSA-1. In addition to the two alleles, there are isolate-specific mutations that might allow the parasite to evade allele-specific immunity.

There is considerable evidence that MSA-1 is the target of a protective immune response. Two groups have reported that human monoclonal antibodies against *P. falciparum* MSA-1 inhibit growth of the parasite in vitro (Brown, 1986; Schmidt-Ullrich et al., 1986). Passive transfer experiments using anti-MSA-1 monoclonal antibodies have demonstrated protection against *P. yoelii* and *P. chabaudi* infection in mice (Boyle et al., 1982; Majarian et al., 1984; Burns et al., 1989). These monoclonal antibodies recognize epitopes in the carboxy-terminal half of MSA-1, the portion of the antigen that carries over into the trophozoite stage of the parasite (Burns et al., 1989; Lew et al., 1989).

Active immunization studies with purified MSA-1 have shown protection against *P. yoelii* in mice (Holder and Freeman, 1981), *P. knowlesi* in saimiri monkeys (Schmidt-Ullrich et al., 1983), and *P. falciparum* in saimiri and aotus monkeys (Hall et al., 1984; Cheung et al., 1985; Siddiqui et al., 1987). Immunization with synthetic peptide fragments of MSA-1 has demonstrated some efficacy in saimiri and aotus monkeys (Cheung et al., 1986; Patarroyo et al., 1987). Finally, MSA-1 has been used as part of a combination-peptide antigen in the human trial reported by Patarroyo et al. (1988). Of some concern, however, is the report that mice immunized with MSA-1 and challenged with a different *P. chabaudi* strain were unprotected (Brown et al., 1985). The full meaning of such results can be determined only after the structure of MSA-1 in different parasite strains is known.

Since immunization with MSA-1 provides at least partial protection against malaria, it is likely that immunogens derived from MSA-1 will be included in a successful multivalent malaria vaccine. Efforts to express MSA-1 by recombinant DNA techniques have so far failed, due in part to the difficulty in obtaining the correct conformational structure of the protein. Recent research using baculovirus vectors may have solved this problem (Murphy et al., 1990), and it is likely that recombinant MSA-1 fragments will soon be tested in humans.

Transmission-Blocking Vaccines

A vaccine that induces an immune response to the sexual stages of the malaria parasite will not necessarily protect against infection with sporozoite or blood-stage parasites. It may, however, have a dramatic effect on reducing malaria transmission by slowing or halting human-to-mosquito (and thus mosquito-to-human) spread of infectious parasites. A transmission-blocking vaccine can be considered "altruistic," as it benefits primarily the uninfected or nonimmune individuals in a community, providing little or no benefit to those actually immunized. (Carter et al., 1988; Kaslow, 1990; Targett et al., 1990).

Mechanisms of Immunity

Antibodies Sera from animals immunized with gametocyte-rich blood develop antibodies that, when mixed with gametocytes before ingestion by mosquitoes, will inhibit parasite development and maturation to oocysts within the mosquito (Carter and Chen, 1976; Gwadz, 1976). Monoclonal antibodies directed against gamete and zygote antigens will also inhibit parasite development in mosquitoes via several mechanisms. Some monoclonal antibodies require serum complement and act before fertilization to lyse gametes (Quakyi et al., 1987). Other monoclonal antibodies are complement independent and act either before fertilization, inhibiting zygote formation (Rener et al., 1983; Vermeulen et al., 1985), or work after fertilization (Vermeulen et al., 1985), inhibiting zygote penetration through the peritrophic membrane (Sieber et al., 1991). It is theoretically possible that antibodies could also inhibit zygote-ookinete transformation, inhibit ookinete motility, or inhibit ookinete penetration at later stages of parasite development.

Cell-Mediated Immunity Administration of immune T lymphocytes can reduce the density of gametocytes in the blood of recipient animals and reduce the ability of mosquitoes to transmit parasites by 95 percent (Harte et al., 1985). Helper and suppressor T lymphocytes are presumably also important for modulating antibody production. There is no evidence that ingestion of immune T cells can inhibit parasite development in the mosquito.

Targets of Transmission-Blocking Immunity

The sexual stage of the parasite life cycle provides several potential targets for immunological attack. As with the asexual stages, parasite antigens on the surface of erythrocytes infected with sexual stages could be targeted. Most of the research on transmission-blocking vaccines has focused on the extracellular sexual stages (gametes, zygotes, and ookinetes) found in the mosquito, in part because it is easy to measure antibodies against them, by feeding mosquitoes on infected blood mixed with antibodies and looking for inhibition of parasite development within the mosquito.

A number of proteins on the surface of sexual stages of malaria parasites have been identified by using monoclonal antibodies that inhibit parasite development in mosquitoes (Carter et al., 1988). These antigens are generally named by the initials of the parasite species (e.g., Pf for *P. falciparum*), the letter "s" (for sexual), and the approximate molecular weight in kilodaltons of the protein (Kaslow et al., 1988). Pfs230, Pfs48/45, and Pfs40/10 are expressed predominantly by gametes. Pfs25 is expressed predominantly by zygotes (Kaslow et al., 1988). Analogous targets of transmission-blocking antibodies have been identified for *P. vivax* (Peiris et al., 1988) and various animal malaria parasites.

Impediments to Transmission-Blocking Vaccine Development

Production of Antigen It has been difficult to clone the genes encoding the antigens that are targets of transmission-blocking immunity. Monoclonal antibodies against these antigens appear to recognize conformational epitopes that are not faithfully reproduced by the bacteria in which recombinant DNA libraries are prepared. The use of polyclonal antisera has resulted in cloning other, nontarget antigen genes. It is difficult to culture amounts of sexual stage parasites sufficient to determine the amino acid sequence, which would allow an alternative approach to antibody-based identification. This has slowed the research pace, but various groups appear to have cloned the genes for most or all of the *P. falciparum* sexual-stage target antigens. Even when the genes are cloned, however, the fact that protective monoclonal antibodies recognize conformational epitopes suggests that expression of recombinant proteins or synthetic peptides that mimic that conformation may be difficult.

Genetic Restriction of the Immune Response Target antigens of transmission blocking antibodies appear to fall into two categories. For Pfs230, Pfs48/45, and Pfs40/10, there is significant genetic restriction of T-cell responses in inbred mice (Good et al., 1988b), and only a minority of people living in malaria-endemic areas develop antibodies against these antigens after repeated malaria infections (Graves et al., 1988; Carter et al., 1989; Quakyi et al., 1989). In addition, antigenic variants of Pfs48/45 have been detected (Graves et al., 1985). If genetic restriction proves to be responsible for the limited human immune response to these antigens, this could have an impact on the development of subunit vaccines.

In contrast, Pfs25 is immunogenic and induces transmission-blocking antibodies in all congenic mouse strains tested (Good et al., 1988b; Kaslow et al., 1991), and antibodies are never found in humans living in endemic regions. Pfs25 also was found to lack significant antigenic diversity (Kaslow et al., 1989).

These data suggest that the first group of antigens has been under selective pressure by the host immune system. The absence of genetic restriction in mice and the lack of antibodies to Pfs25 in people living in endemic areas suggest that Pfs25 may be expressed in abundant amounts only when the parasite is in the mosquito midgut, not while circulating in the host's blood, and thus has not been under immune pressure. In either case, the poor or absent human immune response suggests that we may not be able to rely on natural boosting after primary immunization with a transmission-blocking vaccine. The use of novel adjuvants, carrier proteins, and slow-release vaccine formulations may overcome this problem.

Enhancement of Infectivity At least with *P. vivax* and the monkey malaria parasite *P. cynomolgi*, many naturally infected individuals develop antibodies that inhibit parasite development in mosquitoes (Mendis et al., 1987). Early in the course of infection and very late after infection, when the levels of transmission-blocking antibodies are low, parasite development and transmission may be enhanced (Peiris et al., 1988). Enhancement is also observed with low concentrations of some inhibitory monoclonal antibodies, although not with antibodies to Pfs25 and its homologous antigens in other malaria parasites. Although this may superficially suggest that transmission-blocking vaccines may actually enhance transmission as vaccine-induced antibody levels decline, it seems unlikely that vaccination would exacerbate the enhancement that occurs naturally (and may be an important factor sustaining malaria transmission in some areas).

Cost and Acceptability of an Altruistic Vaccine Because transmission-blocking vaccines will not protect individuals, they would not be used alone in nonimmune visitors to malaria-endemic areas. Consequently, there is even less commercial incentive to develop these vaccines than pre-erythrocytic or blood-stage vaccines. Vaccines that protect populations but not individuals might also have to be safer and have fewer side effects than vaccines that provided protection to the vaccinated individual. It is likely that transmission-blocking vaccines will be used primarily in conjunction with pre-erythrocytic and blood-stage vaccines, in which case they may have the added benefit of reducing the transmission of vaccine-resistant parasite strains.

Antimosquito Vaccines

Of the many methods proposed and tested for controlling mosquito populations, one of the most unusual is the use of antimosquito vaccines. In this approach, humans would be vaccinated with mosquito proteins critical for insect viability. The resulting human antimosquito antibodies are ingested in the mosquito's blood meal. The goal is to reduce parasite transmission by reducing the vitality or vector capability of the mosquito. An antimosquito vaccine that reduced the adult mosquito's life span, so that parasite development would be interrupted, might have a significant effect on transmission.

Early studies reported that mortality of *Anopheles stephensi* was increased when these mosquitoes fed on rabbits that had been immunized with mosquito midgut extracts (Alger and Cabrera, 1972). Another mosquito, *Aedes aegypti*, when fed on rabbits immunized with whole *Ae. aegypti* extracts, suffered reduced reproductive capability (Sutherland and Ewen, 1974). Further work with *Ae. aegypti* fed on mice or rabbits immunized with selected mosquito body-part extracts demonstrated reduced viability of first generation offspring (Ramasamy et al., 1988) and increased mortality associated with the level and specificity of antibodies ingested (Hatfield, 1988a). Antibodies retained their immunological properties for two to three days and bound to the mosquito midgut epithelium (Hatfield, 1988b). Ramasamy and Ramasamy (1989) and Ramasamy et al. (1990) reported significant reductions in susceptibility to Ross River virus and Murray Valley encephalomyelitis virus in *Ae. aegypti* previously fed on rabbit blood-virus mixtures containing high levels of antibody against mosquito midgut extracts.

Recent work utilizing *An. farauti* (a vector of human malaria) and *P. berghei* (a rodent malaria parasite) showed that antibodies from mice immunized against mosquito midgut antigens appeared to prevent parasite ookinetes from penetrating the midgut of engorged mosquitoes (Ramasamy and Ramasamy, 1990). Interestingly, these same antibodies also reduced mosquito mortality rates, an undesirable outcome.

Although studies of antimosquito vaccines have used anthropophilic mosquitoes in unnatural animal host systems, they nevertheless hold promise for a new approach to reducing parasite transmission. This work is, however, in its early stages, and the opposing results obtained by Ramasamy and Ramasamy (1990) suggest that the immunological interactions among mosquitoes, host antibodies, and parasites are more complex than previously thought.

RESEARCH AGENDA

Identification of Mechanisms and Targets of Protective Immunity

Protective immunity can be induced in humans or experimental animals by repeated natural infection, by passive transfer of immune serum or cells, by immunization with radiation-attenuated parasites, or by immunization with subunit vaccines prepared by using purified parasite fractions, synthetic peptides or recombinant proteins. Identifying the mechanisms of such protective immunity will facilitate the development of subunit vaccines. Research on animal model systems will continue to be critical to the growth of basic knowledge in this area.

> **RESEARCH FOCUS:** Continued use of animal model systems to identify and characterize mechanisms of protective antimalarial immunity.

RESEARCH FOCUS: Expanded studies in humans, including further immunization trials with radiation-attenuated sporozoites, to characterize the mechanisms of protective immunity.

Identification of antigens that are targets of protective immunity is incomplete. Successful approaches have included identification of antigens that are the target of protective immune responses; empiric screening of antigens, using monoclonal antibodies or recombinant DNA expression libraries; and identification of parasite molecules that perform an essential function and that are potentially accessible to immune attack. Further expansion of our knowledge of such target antigens is essential.

RESEARCH FOCUS: Continued identification of parasite antigens that are targets of protective immune responses.

Little is known about how malaria sporozoites invade liver cells. Our understanding of the process of merozoite invasion into erythrocytes is incomplete. The role of parasite proteases and other enzymes in parasite development is poorly characterized. The factors controlling transition from one parasite stage to the next are unknown. The parasite molecules involved in sequestration are poorly characterized. Tumor necrosis factor and other cytokines have been implicated in the pathogenesis of malaria disease, but little is known about the parasite molecules that induce such cytokines. Increased understanding of these and related aspects of parasite biology could provide important avenues for vaccine development.

RESEARCH FOCUS: Expanded studies of parasite biology.

Vaccine Formulation

The ideal malaria vaccine would be composed of multiple antigens from two or more stages of the parasite. The most useful of such proteins, the relevant epitopes in these molecules, the best way to combine them, and the appropriate adjuvants, dosage regimens, and routes of administration remain to be determined. It is unclear whether an effective immune response can be elicited against variant forms of the parasite by immunizing with conserved regions of these proteins.

RESEARCH FOCUS: Improved vaccine construction and delivery techniques, including the use of more potent adjuvants, time release preparations, live vectors, and better carrier proteins.

RESEARCH FOCUS: Better methods of assessing vaccine efficacy, with consideration given to conducting well-designed human vaccine trials at an early stage of antigen assessment.

In Vitro Assays

There is an immediate need for validated, reproducible, quantitative in vitro assays that correlate with and are predictive of protective immunity in humans. Such assays not only would permit candidate vaccines to be screened prior to human challenge studies, but also would facilitate field evaluations of vaccine effectiveness.

RESEARCH FOCUS: Development of in vitro tests predictive of protective immunity.

Culture Systems

Currently, only the asexual and sexual blood stages of *P. falciparum* can be easily cultured in vitro, and only in erythrocytes. The understanding of the basic biology and biochemistry of other species and stages of the malaria parasite could be dramatically improved with appropriate culture systems. *P. vivax*, for example, causes roughly half the world's malaria, but because it cannot be grown continuously in culture, relatively little research has gone into developing a vaccine against this parasite species. If sporozoites or blood-stage parasites could be cultured in the absence of contaminating cells, serious consideration could be given to developing whole-organism vaccines.

RESEARCH FOCUS: Methods for culturing *P. falciparum* sporozoites, improving culture techniques for *P. falciparum* liver-stage parasites, culturing the erythrocytic stages of *P. falciparum* in nonerythrocyte systems, and culturing *P. vivax*.

REFERENCES

Aggarwal, A., S. Kumar, R. Jaffe, D. Hone, M. Gross, and J. Sadoff. 1990. Oral *Salmonella*: malaria circumsporozoite recombinants induce specific CD8+ cytotoxic T cells. Journal of Experimental Medicine 172:1083-1090.

Aley, S. B., M. D. Bates, J. P. Tam, and M. R. Hollingdale. 1986. Synthetic peptides from the circumsporozoite proteins of *Plasmodium falciparum* and *Plasmodium knowlesi* recognize the human hepatoma cell line HepG2-A16 in vitro. Journal of Experimental Medicine 164:1915-1922.

Alger, N. E., and E. J. Cabrera. 1972. An increase in death rate of *Anopheles stephensi* fed on rabbits immunized with mosquito antigen. Journal of Economic Entomology 65:165-168.

Ballou, W. R., S. L. Hoffman, J. A. Sherwood, M. R. Hollingdale, F. A. Neva, W. T. Hockmeyer, D. M. Gordon, I. Schneider, R. A. Wirtz, J. F. Young, G. F. Wasserman, P. Reeve, C. L. Diggs, and J. D. Chulay. 1987. Safety and efficacy of a recombinant DNA *Plasmodium falciparum* sporozoite vaccine. Lancet 1:1277-1281.

Bate, C. A. W., J. Taverne, and J. H. L. Playfair. 1988. Malarial parasites induce tumour necrosis factor production by macrophages. Immunology 64:227-231.

Bate, C. A. W., J. Taverne, and J. H. L. Playfair. 1989. Soluble malarial antigens are toxic and induce the production of tumour necrosis factor in vivo. Immunology 66:600-605.

Bate, C. A. W., J. Taverne, A. Dave, and J. H. L. Playfair. 1990. Malaria exoantigens induce T-independent antibody that blocks their ability to induce TNF. Immunology 70:315-320.

Beier, J. C., P. V. Perkins, F. Onyango, T. P. Gargan, C. N. Oster, R. E. Whitmire, D. K. Koech, and C. R. Roberts. 1990. Characterization of malaria transmission by *Anopheles* (Diptera: Culicidae) in western Kenya in preparation for malaria vaccine trials. Journal of Medical Entomology 27:570-577.

Bouharoun-Tayoun, H., P. Attanath, A. Sabchareon, T. Chongsuphajaisiddhi, and P. Druihle. 1990. Antibodies that protect humans against *Plasmodium falciparum* blood stages do not on their own inhibit parasite growth and invasion in vitro, but act in cooperation with monocytes. Journal of Experimental Medicine 172:1633-1641.

Boyle, D. B., C. I. Newbold, C. C. Smith, and K. N. Brown. 1982. Monoclonal antibodies that protect in vivo against *Plasmodium chabaudi* recognize a 250,000-dalton parasite polypeptide. Infection and Immunity 38:94-102.

Brown, G. V. 1986. Prospects for a vaccine against malaria. Medical Journal of Australia 144:703-704.

Brown, K. N., W. Jarra, C. I. Newbold, and M. Schryer. 1985. Variability in parasite protein antigen structure and protective immunity to malaria. Annales de l'Institut Pasteur, Immunologie 136C:11-23.

Burns, J. M. Jr., W. R. Majarian, J. F. Young, T. M. Daly, and C. A. Long. 1989. A protective monoclonal antibody recognizes an epitope in the carboxyl-terminal cysteine-rich domain in the precursor of the major merozoite surface antigen of the rodent malarial parasite, *Plasmodium yoelii*. Journal of Immunology 143:2670-2676.

Cabantchik, Z. I., S. Kutner, M. Krugliak, and H. Ginsburg. 1983. Anion transport inhibitors as suppressors of *Plasmodium falciparum* growth in in vitro cultures. Molecular Pharmacology 23:92-99.

Camus, D., and T. J. Hadley. 1985. A *Plasmodium falciparum* antigen that binds to host erythrocytes and merozoites. Science 230:553-556.

Carter, R., and D. H. Chen. 1976. Malaria transmission blocked by immunisation with gametes of the malaria parasite. Nature 263:57-60.

Carter, R., N. Kumar, I. Quakyi, M. Good, K. Mendis, P. Graves, and L. Miller. 1988. Immunity to sexual stages of malaria parasites. Progress in Allergy 41:193-214.

Carter, R., P. M. Graves, I. A. Quakyi, and M. F. Good. 1989. Restricted or absent immune responses in human populations to *Plasmodium falciparum* gamete antigens that are targets of malaria transmission-blocking antibodies. Journal of Experimental Medicine 169:135-147.

Charoenvit, Y., M. F. Leef, L. F. Yuan, M. Sedegah, and R. L. Beaudoin. 1987. Characterization of *Plasmodium yoelii* monoclonal antibodies directed against stage-specific sporozoite antigens. Infection and Immunity 55:604-608.

Charoenvit, Y., W. E. Collins, T. R. Jones, P. Millet, L. Yuan, G. H. Campbell, R. L. Beaudoin, J. R. Broderson, and S. L. Hoffman. 1991a. Inability of malaria vaccine to induce antibodies to a protective epitope within its sequence. Science 251:668-671.

Charoenvit, Y., S. Mellouk, C. Cole, R. Bechara, M. F. Leef, M. Sedegah, L. F. Yuan, F. A. Robey, R. L. Beaudoin, and S. L. Hoffman. 1991b. Monoclonal, but not polyclonal, antibodies, protect against *Plasmodium yoelii* sporozoites. Journal of Immunology 146:1020-1025.

Chen, D. H., R. E. Tigelaar, and F. I. Weinbaum. 1977. Immunity to sporozoite-induced malaria infection in mice. I. The effect of immunization of T and B cell-deficient mice. Journal of Immunology 118:1322-1327.

Cheung, A., A. R. Shaw, J. Leban, and L. H. Perrin. 1985. Cloning and expression in *Escherichia coli* of a surface antigen of *Plasmodium falciparum* merozoites. EMBO Journal 4:1007-1012.

Cheung, A., J. Leban, A. R. Shaw, B. Merkli, J. Stocker, C. Chizzolini, C. Sander, and L. H. Perrin. 1986. Immunization with synthetic peptides of a *Plasmodium falciparum* surface antigen induces antimerozoite antibodies. Proceedings of the National Academy of Sciences of the United States of America 83: 8328-8332.

Chulay, J. D. 1989. Development of sporozoite vaccines for malaria. Transactions of the Royal Society of Tropical Medicine and Hygiene 83(Suppl.):61-66.

Chulay, J. D., and C. F. Ockenhouse. 1990. Host receptors for malaria-infected erythrocytes. American Journal of Tropical Medicine and Hygiene 43(Suppl):6-14.

Chulay, J. D., M. Aikawa, C. Diggs, and J. D. Haynes. 1981. Inhibitory effects of immune monkey serum on synchronized *Plasmodium falciparum* cultures. American Journal of Tropical Medicine and Hygiene 30:12-19.

Chulay, J. D., J. A. Lyon, J. D. Haynes, A. I. Meierovics, C. T. Atkinson, and M. Aikawa. 1987. Monoclonal antibody characterization of *Plasmodium falciparum* antigens in immune complexes formed when schizonts rupture in the presence of immune serum. Journal of Immunology 139:2768-2774.

Clyde, D. F., V. C. McCarthy, R. M. Miller, and R. B. Hornick. 1973a. Specificity of protection of man immunized against sporozoite-induced falciparum malaria. American Journal of the Medical Sciences 266:398-403.

Clyde, D. F., H. Most, V. C. McCarthy, and J. P. Vanderberg. 1973b. Immunization of man against sporozoite-induced falciparum malaria. American Journal of the Medical Sciences 266:169-177.

Clyde, D. F., V. C. McCarthy, R. M. Miller, and W. E. Woodward. 1975. Immunization of man against falciparum and vivax malaria by use of attenuated sporozoites. American Journal of Tropical Medicine and Hygiene 24:397-401.

Cohen, S., I. A. McGregor, and S. P. Carrington. 1961. Gamma globulin and acquired immunity to human malaria. Nature 192:733-737.

Collins, W. E., R. S. Nussenzweig, W. R. Ballou, T. K. I. I. Ruebush, E. H. Nardin, J. D. Chulay, W. R. Majarian, J. F. Young, G. F. Wasserman, I. Bathurst, H. L. Gibson, P. J. Barr, S. L. Hoffman, S. S. Wasserman, J. R. Broderson, J. C. Skinner, P. M. Procell, V. K. Filipski, and C. L. Wilson. 1989. Immunization of *Saimiri sciureus boliviensis* with recombinant vaccines based on the circumsporozoite protein of *Plasmodium vivax*. American Journal of Tropical Medicine and Hygiene 40:455-464.

Dame, J. B., J. L. Williams, T. F. McCutchan, J. L. Weber, R. A. Wirtz, W. T. Hockmeyer, W. L. Maloy, J. D. Haynes, I. Schneider, D. Roberts, G. S. Sanders, E. P. Reddy, C. L. Diggs, and L. H. Miller. 1984. Structure of the gene encoding the immunodominant surface antigen on the sporozoite of the human malaria parasite *Plasmodium falciparum*. Science 225:593-599.

David, P. H., M. Hommel, L. H. Miller, I. J. Udeinya, and L. D. Oligino. 1983. Parasite sequestration in *Plasmodium falciparum* malaria: spleen and antibody modulation of cytoadherence of infected erythrocytes. Proceedings of the National Academy of Sciences of the United States of America 80:5075-5079.

de Groot, A. S., A. H. Johnson, W. L. Maloy, I. A. Quakyi, E. M. Riley, A. Menon, S. M. Banks, J. A. Berzofsky, and M. F. Good. 1989. Human T cell recognition of polymorphic epitopes from malaria circumsporozoite protein. Journal of Immunology 142:4000-4005.

Del Giudice, G., J. A. Cooper, J. Merino, A. S. Verdini, A. Pessi, A. R. Togna, H. D. Engers, G. Corradin, and P.-H. Lambert. 1986. The antibody response in mice to carrier-free synthetic polymers of *Plasmodium falciparum* circumsporozoite repetitive epitope is I-Ab-restricted: possible implications for malaria vaccines. Journal of Immunology 137:2952-2955.

Del Giudice, G., D. Grillot, L. Renia, I. Mullere, G. Corradin, J. A. Louis, D. Mazier, and P.-H. Lambert. 1990. Peptide-primed CD4+ cells and malaria sporozoites. Immunology Letters 25:59-64.

Deres, K., H. Schild, K.-H. Wiesmuller, G. Jung, and H.-G. Rammensee. 1989. In vivo priming of virus-specific cytotoxic T lymphocytes with synthetic lipopeptide vaccine. Nature 342:561-564.

Egan, J. E., J. L. Weber, W. R. Ballou, M. R. Hollingdale, W. R. Majarian, D. M. Gordon, W. L. Maloy, S. L. Hoffman, R. A. Wirtz, I. Schneider, G. R. Woollett, J. F. Young, and W. T. Hockmeyer. 1987. Efficacy of murine malaria sporozoite vaccines: implications for human vaccine development. Science 236:453-456.

Elford, B. C., J. D. Haynes, J. D. Chulay, and R. J. M. Wilson. 1985. Selective stage-specific changes in the permeability to small hydrophilic solutes of human erythrocytes infected with *Plasmodium falciparum*. Molecular and Biochemical Parasitology 16:43-60.

Etlinger, H. M., D. Gillessen, H.-W. Lahm, H. Matile, H.-J. Schonfeld, and A. Trzeciak. 1990. Use of prior vaccinations for the development of new vaccines. Science 249:423-425.

Ferreira, A., L. Schofield, V. Enea, H. Shellekens, P. Van der Meide, W. E. Collins, R. S. Nussenzweig, and V. Nussenzweig. 1986. Inhibition of development of exoerythrocytic forms of malaria parasites by gamma-interferon. Science 232:881-884.

Galinski, M. R., D. E. Arnot, A. H. Cochrane, J. W. Barnwell, R. S. Nussenzweig, and V. Enea. 1987. The circumsporozoite gene of the *Plasmodium cynomolgi* complex. Cell 48:311-319.

Good, M. F. 1988. T cells, T sites, and malaria immunity—further optimism for vaccine development. Journal of Immunology 140:1715-1716.

Good, M. F., J. A. Berzofsky, W. L. Maloy, Y. Hayashi, N. Fujii, W. T. Hockmeyer, and L. H. Miller. 1986. Genetic control of the immune response in mice to a *Plasmodium falciparum* sporozoite vaccine. Widespread nonresponsiveness to single malaria T epitope in highly repetitive vaccine. Journal of Experimental Medicine 164:655-660.

Good, M. F., W. L. Maloy, M. N. Lunde, H. Margalit, J. L. Cornette, G. L. Smith, B. Moss, L. H. Miller, and J. A. Berzofsky. 1987. Construction of synthetic immunogen: use of new T-helper epitope on malaria circumsporozoite protein. Science 235:1059-1062.

Good, M. F., J. A. Berzofsky, and L. H. Miller. 1988a. The T cell response to the malaria circumsporozoite protein: an immunological approach to vaccine development. Pp. 663-688 in Annual Review of Immunology, Paul, W. E., C. G. Fathman, R. Germain, and H. Metzger, eds. Palo Alto: Annual Reviews, Inc.

Good, M. F., L. H. Miller, S. Kumar, I. A. Quakyi, D. Keister, J. H. Adams, B. Moss, J. A. Berzofsky, and R. Carter. 1988b. Limited immunological recognition of critical malaria vaccine candidate antigens. Science 242:574-577.

Good, M. F., D. Pombo, W. L. Maloy, V. F. de la Cruz, L. H. Miller, and J. A. Berzofsky. 1988c. Parasite polymorphism present within minimal T cell epitopes of *Plasmodium falciparum* circumsporozoite protein. Journal of Immunology 140:1645-1650.

Good, M. F., D. Pombo, I. A. Quakyi, E. M. Riley, R. A. Houghten, A. Menon, D. W. Alling, J. A. Berzofsky, and L. H. Miller. 1988d. Human T-cell recognition of the circumsporozoite protein of *Plasmodium falciparum*: immunodominant T-cell domains map to the polymorphic regions of the molecule. Proceedings of the National Academy of Sciences of the United States of America 85:1199-1203.

Gordon, D. M., T. M. Cosgriff, I. Schneider, G. F. Wasserman, W. R. Majarian, M. R. Hollingdale, and J. D. Chulay. 1990. Safety and immunogenicity of a *Plasmodium vivax* sporozoite vaccine. American Journal of Tropical Medicine and Hygiene 42:527-531.

Graves, P. M., R. Carter, T. R. Burkot, J. Rener, D. C. Kaushal, and J. L. Williams. 1985. Effects of transmission-blocking monoclonal antibodies on different isolates of *Plasmodium falciparum*. Infection and Immunity 48:611-616.

Graves, P. M., R. Carter, T. R. Burkot, I. A. Quakyi, and N. Kumar. 1988. Antibodies to *Plasmodium falciparum* gamete surface antigens in Papua New Guinea sera. Parasite Immunology 10:209-218.

Guerin-Marchand, C., P. Druilhe, B. Galey, A. Londono, J. Patarpotikul, R. L. Beaudoin, C. Dubeaux, A. Tartar, O. Mercereau-Puijalon, and G. Langsley. 1987. A liver-stage-specific antigen of *Plasmodium falciparum* characterized by gene cloning. Nature 329:164-167.

Gwadz, R. W. 1976. Malaria: successful immunization against the sexual stages of *Plasmodium gallinaceum*. Science 193:1150-1151.

Gwadz, R. W., A. H. Cochrane, V. Nussenzweig, and R. S. Nussenzweig. 1979. Preliminary studies on vaccination of rhesus monkeys with irradiated sporozoites of *Plasmodium knowlesi* and characterisation of surface antigens of these parasites. Bulletin of the World Health Organization 57(Suppl 1):165-173.

Hadley, T. J., and L. H. Miller. 1988. Invasion of erythrocytes by malaria parasites: erythrocyte ligands and parasite receptors. Progress in Allergy 41:49-71.

Haldar, K., M. A. J. Ferguson, and G. A. M. Cross. 1985. Acylation of a *Plasmodium falciparum* merozoite surface antigen via sn-1,2-diacyl glycerol. Journal of Biological Chemistry 260:4969-4974.

Hall, R., J. E. Hyde, M. Goman, D. L. Simmons, I. A. Hope, M. Mackay, J. Scaife, B. Merkli, R. Richle, and J. Stocker. 1984. Major surface antigen gene of a human malaria parasite cloned and expressed in bacteria. Nature 311:379-382.

Harte, P. G., N. C. Rogers, and G. A. T. Targett. 1985. Role of T cells in preventing transmission of rodent malaria. Immunology 56:1-7.

Hatfield, P. R. 1988a. Anti-mosquito antibodies and their effects on feeding, fecundity and mortality of *Aedes aegypti*. Medical and Veterinary Entomology 2:331-338.

Hatfield, P. R. 1988b. Detection and localization of antibody ingested with a mosquito bloodmeal. Medical and Veterinary Entomology 2:339-345.

Hedstrom, R. C., J. R. Campbell, M. L. Leef, Y. Charoenvit, M. Carter, M. Sedegah, R. L. Beaudoin, and S. L. Hoffman. 1990. A malaria sporozoite surface antigen distinct from the circumsporozoite protein. Bulletin of the World Health Organization 68(Suppl):152-157.

Herrington, D. A., D. F. Clyde, G. Losonsky, M. Cortesia, J. R. Murphy, J. Davis, S. Baqar, A. M. Felix, E. P. Heimer, D. Gillessen, E. Nardine, R. S. Nussenzweig, V. Nussenzweig, M. R. Hollingdale, and M. M. Levine. 1987. Safety and immunogenicity in man of a synthetic peptide malaria vaccine against *Plasmodium falciparum* sporozoites. Nature 328:257-259.

Hoffman, S. L., C. N. Oster, C. V. Plowe, G. R. Woollett, J. C. Beier, J. D. Chulay, R. A. Wirtz, M. R. Hollingdale, and M. Mugambi. 1987. Naturally acquired antibodies to sporozoites do not prevent malaria: vaccine development implications. Science 237:639-642.

Hoffman, S. L., J. A. Berzofsky, D. Isenbarger, E. Zeltser, W. R. Majarian, M. Gross, and W. R. Ballou. 1989a. Immune response gene regulation of immunity to *Plasmodium berghei* sporozoites and circumsporozoite protein vaccines: overcoming genetic restriction with whole organism and subunit vaccines. Journal of Immunology 142:3581-3584.

Hoffman, S. L., D. Isenbarger, G. W. Long, M. Sedegah, A. Szarfman, L. Waters, M. R. Hollingdale, P. H. van der Meide, D. S. Finbloom, and W. R. Ballou. 1989b. Sporozoite vaccine induces genetically restricted T cell elimination of malaria from hepatocytes. Science 244:1078-1081.

Hoffman, S. L., C. N. Oster, C. Mason, J. C. Beier, J. A. Sherwood, W. R. Ballou, M. Mugambi, and J. D. Chulay. 1989c. Human lymphocyte proliferative response to a sporozoite T cell epitope correlates with resistance to falciparum malaria. Journal of Immunology 142:1299-1303.

Holder, A. A. 1988. The precursor to major merozoite surface antigens: structure and role in immunity. Progress in Allergy 41:72-97.

Holder, A. A., and R. R. Freeman. 1981. Immunization against blood-stage rodent malaria using purified parasite antigens. Nature 294:361-364.

Holder, A. A., and R. R. Freeman. 1984. Protective antigens of rodent and human bloodstage malaria. Philosophical Transactions of the Royal Society of London, Series B: Biological Sciences 307:171-177.

Holder, A. A., M. J. Lockyer, K. G. Odink, J. S. Sandhu, V. Riveros-Moreno, S. C. Nicholls, Y. Hillman, L. S. Davey, M. L. Tizard, R. T. Schwarz, and R. R. Freeman. 1985. Primary structure of the precursor to the three major surface antigens of *Plasmodium falciparum* merozoites. Nature 317:270-273.

Hollingdale, M. R., E. H. Nardin, S. Tharavanij, A. L. Schwartz, and R. S. Nussenzweig. 1984. Inhibition of entry of *Plasmodium falciparum* and *P. vivax* sporozoites into cultured cells; an in vitro assay of protective antibodies. Journal of Immunology 132:909-913.

Hollingdale, M. R., M. Aikawa, C. T. Atkinson, W. R. Ballou, G. Chen, J. Li, J. F. G. M. Meis, B. Sina, C. Wright, and J. Zhu. 1990. Non-CS pre-erythrocytic protective antigens. Immunology Letters 25:71-76.

Howard, R. J., and A. D. Gilladoga. 1989. Molecular studies related to the pathogenesis of cerebral malaria. Blood 74:2603-2618.

Howard, R. J., S. Uni, M. Aikawa, S. B. Aley, J. H. Leech, A. M. Lew, T. E. Wellems, J. Rener, and D. W. Taylor. 1986. Secretion of a malarial histidine-rich protein (PfHRP II) from *Plasmodium falciparum*-infected erythrocytes. Journal of Cell Biology 103:1269-1277.

Howard, R. J., S. M. Handunnetti, T. Hasler, A. Gilladoga, J. C. de Aguiar, B. L. Pasloske, K. Morehead, G. R. Albrecht, and M. R. van Schravendijk. 1990. Surface molecules on *Plasmodium falciparum*-infected erythrocytes involved in adherence. American Journal of Tropical Medicine and Hygiene 43(Suppl.):15-29.

Jahiel, R. I., R. S. Nussenzweig, J. Vanderberg, and J. Vilcek. 1968a. Antimalarial effect of interferon inducers at different stages of development of *Plasmodium berghei* in the mouse. Nature 220:710-711.

Jahiel, R. I., J. Vilcek, R. Nussenzweig, and J. Vanderberg. 1968b. Interferon inducers protect mice against *Plasmodium berghei* malaria. Science 161:802-804.

Jungery, M. 1985. Studies on the biochemical basis of the interaction of the merozoites of *Plasmodium falciparum* and the human red cell. Transactions of the Royal Society of Tropical Medicine and Hygiene 79:591-597.

Kaslow, D. C. 1990. Immunogenicity of *Plasmodium falciparum* sexual stage antigens: implications for the design of a transmission blocking vaccine. Immunology Letters 25:83-86.

Kaslow, D. C., I. A. Quakyi, C. Syin, M. G. Raum, D. B. Keister, J. E. Coligan, T. F. McCutchan, and L. H. Miller. 1988. A vaccine candidate from the sexual stage of human malaria that contains EGF-like domains. Nature 333:74-76.

Kaslow, D. C., I. A. Quakyi, and D. B. Keister. 1989. Minimal variation in a vaccine candidate from the sexual stage of *Plasmodium falciparum*. Molecular and Biochemical Parasitology 32:101-103.

Kaslow, D. C., S. N. Isaacs, I. A. Quakyi, R. W. Gwadz, B. Moss, and D. B.

Keister. 1991. Induction of *Plasmodium falciparum* transmission-blocking antibodies by recombinant vaccinia virus. Science 252:1310-1313.

Khusmith, S., and P. Druihle. 1983. Antibody-dependent ingestion of *P. falciparum* merozoites by human blood monocytes. Parasite Immunology 5:357-368.

Khusmith, S., Y. Charoenvit, S. Kumar, M. Sedegah, R. L. Beaudoin, and S. L. Hoffman. 1991. Protection against malaria by vaccination with sporozoite surface protein 2 plus CS protein. Science 252:715-718.

Kumar, S., L. H. Miller, I. A. Quakyi, D. B. Keister, R. A. Houghten, W. L. Maloy, B. Moss, J. A. Berzofsky, and M. F. Good. 1988. Cytotoxic T cells specific for the circumsporozoite protein of *Plasmodium falciparum*. Nature 334:258-260.

Leech, J. H., J. W. Barnwell, L. H. Miller, and R. J. Howard. 1984. Identification of a strain-specific malarial antigen exposed on the surface of *Plasmodium falciparum*-infected erythrocytes. Journal of Experimental Medicine 159:1567-1575.

Lew, A. M., C. J. Langford, R. F. Anders, D. J. Kemp, A. Saul, C. Fardoulys, M. Geysen, and M. Sheppard. 1989. A protective monoclonal antibody recognizes a linear epitope in the precursor to the major merozoite antigens of *Plasmodium chabaudi adami*. Proceedings of the National Academy of Sciences of the United States of America 86:3768-3772.

Lockyer, M. J., and R. T. Schwarz. 1987. Strain variation in the circumsporozoite protein gene of *Plasmodium falciparum*. Molecular and Biochemical Parasitology 22:101-108.

Lussow, A. R., G. Del Giudice, L. Renia, D. Mazier, J. P. Verhave, A. S. Verdini, A. Pessi, J. A. Louis, and P. H. Lambert. 1990. Use of a tuberculin purified protein derivative—Asn-Ala-Asn-Pro conjugate—in bacillus Calmette-Guerin primed mice overcomes H-2 restriction of the antibody response and avoids the need for adjuvants. Proceedings of the National Academy of Sciences of the United States of America 87:2960-2964.

Lyon, J. A., A. W. Thomas, T. Hall, and J. D. Chulay. 1989. Specificities of antibodies that inhibit merozoite dispersal from malaria-infected erythrocytes. Molecular and Biochemical Parasitology 36:77-86.

Mackay, M., M. Goman, N. Bone, J. E. Hyde, J. Scaife, U. Certa, H. Stunnenberg, and H. Bujard. 1985. Polymorphism of the precursor for the major surface antigens of *Plasmodium falciparum* merozoites: studies at the genetic level. EMBO Journal 4:3823-3829.

Maheshwari, R. K., C. W. Czarniecki, G. P. Dutta, S. K. Puri, B. N. Dhawan, and R. M. Friedman. 1986. Recombinant human gamma interferon inhibits simian malaria. Infection and Immunity 53:628-630.

Majarian, W. R., T. M. Daly, W. P. Weidanz, and C. A. Long. 1984. Passive immunization against murine malaria with an IgG3 monoclonal antibody. Journal of Immunology 132:3131-3137.

Malik, A., J. E. Egan, R. Houghten, and S. L. Hoffman. 1991. Human cytotoxic T lymphocytes against the *Plasmodium falciparum* circumsporozoite protein. Proceedings of the National Academy of Sciences of the United States of America 88:3300-3304.

Marsh, K., and R. J. Howard. 1986. Antigens induced on erythrocytes by *P. falciparum*: expression of diverse and conserved determinants. Science 231:150.

Mazier, D., S. Mellouk, R. L. Beaudoin, B. Texier, P. Druilhe, W. Hockmeyer, J.

Trosper, C. Paul, Y. Charoenvit, J. Young, F. Miltgen, L. Chedid, J. P. Chigot, B. Galley, O. Brandicourt, and M. Gentilini. 1986. Effect of antibodies to recombinant and synthetic peptides on *P. falciparum* sporozoites in vitro. Science 231:156-159.

McBride, J. S., C. I. Newbold, and R. Anand. 1985. Polymorphism of a high molecular weight schizont antigen of the human malaria parasite *Plasmodium falciparum*. Journal of Experimental Medicine 161:160-180.

McGregor, I. A., S. P. Carrington, and S. Cohen. 1963. Treatment of East African *P. falciparum* malaria with West African human gammaglobulin. Transactions of the Royal Society of Tropical Medicine and Hygiene 57:170-175.

Mellouk, S., R. K. Maheshwari, A. Rhodes-Feuillette, R. L. Beaudoin, N. Berbiguier, H. Matile, F. Miltgen, I. Landau, S. Pied, J. P. Chigot, R. M. Friedman, and D. Mazier. 1987. Inhibitory activity of interferons and interleukin 1 on the development of *Plasmodium falciparum* in human hepatocyte cultures. Journal of Immunology 139:4192-4195.

Mendis, K. N., Y. D. Munesinghe, Y. N. Y. deSilva, I. Keragalla, and R. Carter. 1987. Malaria transmission-blocking immunity induced by natural infections of *Plasmodium vivax* in humans. Infection and Immunity 55:369-372.

Miller, L. H., M. Aikawa, and J. A. Dvorak. 1975. Malaria (*Plasmodium knowlesi*) merozoites: immunity and the surface coat. Journal of Immunology 114:1237-1242.

Miller, L. H., S. J. Mason, D. F. Clyde, and M. H. McGinniss. 1976. The resistance factor to *Plasmodium vivax* in blacks. The Duffy-blood-group genotype, FyFy. New England Journal of Medicine 295:302-304.

Mitchell, G. H., T. J. Hadley, M. H. McGinniss, F. W. Klotz, and L. H. Miller. 1986. Invasion of erythrocytes by *Plasmodium falciparum* malaria parasites: evidence for receptor heterogeneity and two receptors. Blood 67:1519-1521.

Murphy, V. F., W. C. Rowan, M. J. Page, and A. A. Holder. 1990. Expression of hybrid malaria antigens in insect cells and their engineering for correct folding and secretion. Parasitology 100(Pt. 2):177-183.

Nussenzweig, R. S., J. Vanderberg, H. Most, and C. Orton. 1967. Protective immunity induced by the injection of X-irradiated sporozoites of *Plasmodium berghei*. Nature 216:160-162.

Ockenhouse, C. F., S. Schulman, and H. L. Shear. 1984. Induction of crisis forms in the human malaria parasite *Plasmodium falciparum* by gamma-interferon-activated, monocyte-derived macrophages. Journal of Immunology 133:1601-1608.

Orlandi, P. A., B. K. L. Sim, J. D. Chulay, and J. D. Haynes. 1990. Characterization of the 175-kilodalton erythrocyte binding antigen of *Plasmodium falciparum*. Molecular and Biochemical Parasitology 40:285-294.

Patarroyo, M. E., P. Romero, M. L. Torres, P. Clavijo, A. Moreno, A. Martinez, R. Rodriguez, F. Guzman, and E. Cabezas. 1987. Induction of protective immunity against experimental infection with malaria using synthetic peptides. Nature 328:629-632.

Patarroyo, M. E., R. Amador, P. Clavijo, A. Moreno, F. Guzman, P. Romero, R. Tascon, A. Franco, L. A. Murillo, G. Ponton, and G. Trujillo. 1988. A synthetic vaccine protects humans against challenge with asexual blood stages of *Plasmodium falciparum* malaria. Nature 332:158-161.

Peiris, J. S. M., S. Premawansa, M. B. R. Ranawaka, P. V. Udagama, Y. D. Munasinghe, M. V. Nanayakkara, C. P. Gamage, R. Carter, P. H. David, and K. N. Mendis. 1988. Monoclonal and polyclonal antibodies both block and enhance transmission of *Plasmodium vivax* malaria. American Journal of Tropical Medicine and Hygiene 39:26-32.

Perkins, M. E. 1989. Erythrocyte invasion by the malarial merozoite: recent advances. Experimental Parasitology 69:94-99.

Perrin, L. H., E. Ramirez, P. H. Lambert, and P. A. Miescher. 1981. Inhibition of *P. falciparum* growth in human erythrocytes by monoclonal antibodies. Nature 289:301-303.

Peterson, M. G., R. L. Coppel, P. McIntyre, C. J. Langford, G. Woodrow, G. V. Brown, R. F. Anders, and D. J. Kemp. 1988a. Variation in the precursor to the major merozoite surface antigens of *Plasmodium falciparum*. Molecular and Biochemical Parasitology 27:291-302.

Peterson, M. G., R. L. Coppel, M. B. Moloney, and D. J. Kemp. 1988b. Third form of the precursor to the major merozoite surface antigens of *Plasmodium falciparum*. Molecular and Cellular Biology 8:2664-2667.

Playfair, J. H. L., J. Taverne, C. A. W. Bate, and J. B. de Souza. 1990. The malaria vaccine: antiparasite or anti-disease? Immunology Today 11:25-27.

Potocnjak, P., N. Yoshida, R. S. Nussenzweig, and V. Nussenzweig. 1980. Monovalent fragments (Fab) of monoclonal antibodies to a sporozoite surface antigen (Pb44) protect mice against malarial infection. Journal of Experimental Medicine 151:1504-1513.

Quakyi, I. A., R. Carter, J. Rener, N. Kumar, M. F. Good, and L. H. Miller. 1987. The 230-kDa gamete surface protein of *Plasmodium falciparum* is also a target of transmission-blocking antibodies. Journal of Immunology 139:4213-4217.

Quakyi, I. A., L. N. Otoo, D. Pombo, L. Y. Sugars, A. Menon, A. S. DeGroot, A. Johnson, D. Alling, L. H. Miller, and M. F. Good. 1989. Differential nonresponsiveness in humans of candidate *Plasmodium falciparum* vaccine antigens. American Journal of Tropical Medicine and Hygiene 41:125-134.

Ramasamy, M. S., and R. Ramasamy. 1989. Effect of host anti-mosquito antibodies on mosquito physiology and mosquito-pathogen interactions. Pp. 142-148 in Host Regulated Developmental Mechanisms in Vector Arthropods, Borovsky, D., and A. Spielman, eds. University of Florida-IFAS: Vero Beach.

Ramasamy, M. S., and R. Ramasamy. 1990. Effect of anti-mosquito antibodies on the infectivity of the rodent malaria parasite *Plasmodium berghei* to *Anopheles farauti*. Medical and Veterinary Entomology 4:161-166.

Ramasamy, M. S., R. Ramasamy, B. H. Kay, and C. Kidson. 1988. Anti-mosquito antibodies decrease reproductive capacity of *Aedes aegypti*. Medical and Veterinary Entomology 2:87-93.

Ramasamy, M. S., M. Sands, B. H. Kay, I. D. Fanning, G. W. Lawrence, and R. Ramasamy. 1990. Anti-mosquito antibodies reduce the susceptibility of *Aedes aegypti* to arbovirus infection. Medical and Veterinary Entomology 4:49-55.

Rener, J., P. M. Graves, R. Carter, J. L. Williams, and T. R. Burkot. 1983. Target antigens of transmission blocking immunity on gametes of *Plasmodium falciparum*. Journal of Experimental Medicine 158:976-981.

Rickman, L. S., D. M. Gordon, R. Wistar, Jr., U. Krzych, M. Gross, M. R. Hollingdale,

J. E. Egan, J. D. Chulay, and S. L. Hoffman. 1991. Use of adjuvant containing mycobacterial cell-wall skeleton, monophosphoryl lipid A, and squalene in malaria circumsporozoite protein vaccine. Lancet 337:998-1001.

Rieckmann, K. H., P. E. Carson, R. L. Beaudoin, J. S. Cassells, and K. W. Sell. 1974. Sporozoite induced immunity in man against an Ethiopian strain of *Plasmodium falciparum*. Transactions of the Royal Society of Tropical Medicine and Hygiene 68:258-259.

Rieckmann, K. H., R. L. Beaudoin, J. S. Cassells, and K. W. Sell. 1979. Use of attenuated sporozoites in the immunization of human volunteers against falciparum malaria. Bulletin of the World Health Organization 57(Suppl 1):261-265.

Romero, P., J. L. Maryanski, G. Corradin, R. S. Nussenzweig, V. Nussenzweig, and F. Zavala. 1989. Cloned cytotoxic T cells recognize an epitope in the circumsporozoite protein and protect against malaria. Nature 341:323-326.

Rosenberg, R., R. A. Wirtz, D. E. Lanar, J. Sattabongkot, T. Hall, A. P. Waters, and C. Prasittisuk. 1989. Circumsporozoite protein heterogeneity in the human malaria parasite *Plasmodium vivax*. Science 245:973-976.

Sadoff, J. C., W. R. Ballou, L. S. Baron, W. R. Majarian, R. N. Brey, W. T. Hockmeyer, J. F. Young, S. J. Cryz, J. Ou, G. H. Lowell, and J. D. Chulay. 1988. Oral *Salmonella typhimurium* vaccine expressing circumsporozoite protein protects against malaria. Science 240:336-338.

Saul, A., P. Myler, L. Schofield, and C. Kidson. 1984. A high molecular weight antigen in *Plasmodium falciparum* recognized by inhibitory monoclonal antibodies. Parasite Immunology 6:39-50.

Saul, A., J. Cooper, L. Ingram, R. F. Anders, and G. V. Brown. 1985. Invasion of erythrocytes in vitro by *Plasmodium falciparum* can be inhibited by monoclonal antibody directed against an S antigen. Parasite Immunology 7:587-593.

Schmidt-Ullrich, R., J. Lightholder, and M. T. Monroe. 1983. Protective *Plasmodium knowlesi* Mr 74,000 antigen in membranes of schizont-infected rhesus erythrocytes. Journal of Experimental Medicine 158:146-158.

Schmidt-Ullrich, R., J. Brown, H. Whittle, and P.-S. Lin. 1986. Human-human hybridomas secreting monoclonal antibodies to the Mr 195,000 *Plasmodium falciparum* blood stage antigen. Journal of Experimental Medicine 163:179-188.

Schofield, L., G. R. Bushell, J. A. Cooper, A. J. Saul, J. A. Upcroft, and C. Kidson. 1986. A rhoptry antigen of *Plasmodium falciparum* contains conserved and variable epitopes recognized by inhibitory monoclonal antibodies. Molecular and Biochemical Parasitology 18:183-195.

Schofield, L., A. Ferreira, R. Altszuler, V. Nussenzweig, and R. S. Nussenzweig. 1987a. Interferon-gamma inhibits the intrahepatocytic development of malaria parasites in vitro. Journal of Immunology 139:2020-2025.

Schofield, L., J. Villaquiran, A. Ferreira, H. Schellekens, R. Nussenzweig, and V. Nussenzweig. 1987b. Gamma interferon, CD8+ T cells and antibodies required for immunity to malaria sporozoites. Nature 330:664-666.

Sharma, S., P. Svec, G. H. Mitchell, and G. N. Godson. 1985. Diversity of circumsporozoite antigen genes from two strains of the malarial parasite *Plasmodium knowlesi*. Science 229:779-782.

Siddiqui, W. A., L. Q. Tam, K. J. Kramer, G. S. N. Hui, S. E. Case, K. M. Yamaga,

S. P. Chang, E. B. T. Chan, and S.-C. Kan. 1987. Merozoite surface coat precursor protein completely protects *Aotus* monkeys against *Plasmodium falciparum* malaria. Proceedings of the National Academy of Sciences of the United States of America 84:3014-3018.

Sieber, K.-P., M. Huber, D. Kaslow, S. M. Banks, M. Torii, M. Aikawa, and L. H. Miller. 1991. The peritrophic membrane as a barrier: its penetration by *Plasmodium gallinaceum* and the effect of a monoclonal antibody to ookinetes. Experimental Parasitology 72:145-156.

Sim, B. K. L., P. A. Orlandi, J. D. Haynes, F. W. Klotz, J. M. Carter, D. Camus, M. E. Zegans, and J. D. Chulay. 1990. Primary structure of the 175K *Plasmodium falciparum* erythrocyte binding antigen and identification of a peptide which elicits antibodies that inhibit malaria merozoite invasion. Journal of Cell Biology 111:1877-1884.

Sutherland, G. B., and A. B. Ewen. 1974. Fecundity decrease in mosquitoes ingesting blood from specifically sensitized mammals. Journal of Insect Physiology 20:655-660.

Takahashi, H., T. Takeshita, B. Morein, S. Putney, R. N. Germain, and J. A. Berzofsky. 1990. Induction of CD8+ cytotoxic T cells by immunization with purified HIV-1 envelope protein in ISCOMs. Nature 344:873-875.

Tam, J. P., P. Clavijo, Y. A. Lu, V. Nussenzweig, R. Nussenzweig, and F. Zavala. 1990. Incorporation of T and B epitopes of the circumsporozoite protein in a chemically defined synthetic vaccine against malaria. Journal of Experimental Medicine 171:299-306.

Tanabe, K., M. Mackay, M. Goman, and J. G. Scaife. 1987. Allelic dimorphism in a surface antigen gene of the malaria parasite *Plasmodium falciparum*. Journal of Molecular Biology 195:273-287.

Targett, G. A. T., P. G. Harte, S. Eida, N. C. Rogers, and C. S. L. Ong. 1990. *Plasmodium falciparum* sexual stage antigens: immunogenicity and cell-mediated responses. Immunology Letters 25:77-82.

Taverne, J., C. A. Bate, D. Kwiatkowski, P. H. Jakobsen, and J. H. Playfair. 1990. Two soluble antigens of *Plasmodium falciparum* induce tumor necrosis factor release from macrophages. Infection and Immunity 58:2923-2928.

Thomas, A. W., J. A. Deans, G. H. Mitchell, T. Alderson, and S. Cohen. 1984. The Fab fragments of monoclonal IgG to a merozoite surface antigen inhibit *Plasmodium knowlesi* invasion of erythrocytes. Molecular and Biochemical Parasitology 13:187-199.

Tsuji, M., P. Romero, R. S. Nussenzweig, and F. Zavala. 1990. CD4+ cytolytic T cell clone confers protection against murine malaria. Journal of Experimental Medicine 172:1353-1357.

Udeinya, I. J., L. H. Miller, I. A. McGregor, and J. B. Jensen. 1983. *Plasmodium falciparum* strain-specific antibody blocks binding of infected erythrocytes to amelanotic melanoma cells. Nature 303:429-431.

Udomsangpetch, R., M. Aikawa, K. Berzins, M. Wahlgren, and P. Perlmann. 1989. Cytoadherence of knobless *Plasmodium falciparum*-infected erythrocytes and its inhibition by a human monoclonal antibody. Nature 338:763-765.

Vermeulen, A. N., T. Ponnudurai, P. J. A. Beckers, J.-P. Verhave, M. A. Smits, and

J. H. E. T. Meuwissen. 1985. Sequential expression of antigens on sexual stages of *Plasmodium falciparum* accessible to transmission-blocking antibodies in the mosquito. Journal of Experimental Medicine 162:1460-1476.

Weiss, W. R., M. Sedegah, R. L. Beaudoin, L. H. Miller, and M. F. Good. 1988. CD8+ T cells (cytotoxic/suppressors) are required for protection in mice immunized with malaria sporozoites. Proceedings of the National Academy of Sciences of the United States of America 85:573-576.

Weiss, W. R., S. Mellouk, R. A. Houghten, M. Sedegah, S. Kumar, M. F. Good, J. A. Berzofsky, L. H. Miller, and S. L. Hoffman. 1990. Cytotoxic T cells recognize a peptide from the circumsporozoite protein on malaria-infected hepatocytes. Journal of Experimental Medicine 171:763-773.

Wirtz, R. A., R. Rosenberg, J. Sattabongkot, and H. K. Webster. 1990. Prevalence of antibody to heterologous circumsporozoite protein of *Plasmodium vivax* in Thailand. Lancet 336:593-595.

Zavala, F., A. H. Cochrane, E. H. Nardin, R. S. Nussenzweig, and V. Nussenzweig. 1983. Circumsporozoite proteins of malaria parasites contain a single immunodominant region with two or more identical epitopes. Journal of Experimental Medicine 157:1947-1957.

Zavala, F., A. Masuda, P. M. Graves, V. Nussenzweig, and R. S. Nussenzweig. 1985. Ubiquity of the repetitive epitope of the CS protein in different isolates of human malaria parasites. Journal of Immunology 135:2790-2793.

10

Epidemiologic Approaches to Malaria Control

WHERE WE WANT TO BE IN THE YEAR 2010

Epidemiologists will have made great strides in elucidating the complex determinants of malaria, including the risk factors for severe and complicated disease and the role of acquired immunity. It will be clear how chemoprophylaxis and drug therapy reduce morbidity and mortality, and how malaria more severely affects pregnant women and young children. New techniques to measure the impact of various anti-malaria interventions, including strategies to control mosquito populations, will have been developed and will be used in different regions of the world. Advances in understanding local epidemiology will lead to better targeted and more effective malaria control programs. Malaria-related illness and death will decrease as a result. Drug and vaccine testing will be enhanced by epidemiologically based insights into the variations in parasite and human biology that determine the acquisition of immunity and the development of clinical disease.

WHERE WE ARE TODAY

Epidemiologically, malaria is extremely complex. The nature, duration, and severity of malaria infection depend not only on the species of malaria

211

parasite but also on the level of malaria-specific acquired immunity in the individual. Malaria is a focal disease whose distribution is influenced by literally dozens of factors related both to human, mosquito, and parasite populations and to the environment.

Because epidemiology is a cross-disciplinary science, many of the building blocks of malaria epidemiology are discussed in greater detail elsewhere in this report (see Chapters 4, 7, 8, and 12). No attempt will be made here to provide a comprehensive review of the status of malaria epidemiology. Rather, this chapter focuses on several key issues in this evolving science and introduces a new epidemiologically-based approach to understanding malaria.

Infection and Disease

For many years, epidemiologic studies have focused on the prevalence of malaria infection in populations, relating levels of infection to a variety of parasitologic, climatologic, and entomologic parameters. Beginning in the late 1950s and continuing through the late 1960s, when considerable effort was directed toward the global eradication of malaria, the goal was to halt malaria transmission altogether. Therefore, it was particularly important to detect and eliminate all malaria infections. The incidence of clinical disease and an understanding of risk factors for disease were considered to be of minor significance, since it was believed that malaria would soon disappear. Indeed, little research was conducted on the clinical progression of, or risk factors for, the disease itself.

This distinction between infection and disease is particularly important with respect to malaria. The vast majority of older children and adults living in some endemic areas may be infected with the parasite, but only a small proportion will suffer occasional mild or moderate illness. Knowing that someone is infected with the malaria parasite, then, is of little practical value; being able to determine which infected individuals will become ill and why would be quite useful, however.

Despite the formal abandonment by the World Health Organization (WHO) in 1969 of plans to eradicate malaria in favor of strategies to control the disease, epidemiologic studies and surveillance persisted in tracking malaria infections. Even today, many malaria control programs continue to measure the magnitude of the malaria problem and the relative success of their control efforts by using the annual parasite incidence, a calculation of the number of parasite-infected individuals as a proportion of the total population at risk for becoming infected. Millions of blood films are examined under the microscope each year in malaria-endemic countries, of which less than five percent may be found to contain parasites. The resources expended on such questionably useful surveys are enormous, and given the risk of transmitting the human immunodeficiency virus, hepatitis B virus, and other blood-borne pathogens through nonsterile finger-prick methods, such routine mass screening cannot be recommended.

In countries where malaria is highly endemic, the epidemiology is focal, the burden of disease varies greatly, and surveys that evaluate the prevalence of malaria infection can be particularly deceptive. For example, areas of both Papua New Guinea and the Gambia are highly endemic for malaria and have similar prevalences of malaria infection, yet the levels of malaria-related mortality in the two countries appear to be quite different. On the north coast of Papua New Guinea, few deaths can be traced to malaria, even among very young children (Moir et al., 1989), while in the Gambia, a quarter of all deaths in children one to four years of age are believed to be malaria related (Greenwood et al., 1987). Some of the differences may be explained by the fact that the population around Madang, Papua New Guinea, is relatively advantaged and has better access to antimalarial drugs.

Not all people in malarious areas are at the same risk of becoming sick or dying from the disease. Indeed, the risk of severe and potentially fatal infection with *Plasmodium falciparum* falls principally on nonimmunes, such as young children, immigrants from malaria-free areas, and pregnant women, in whom immunosuppression during pregnancy appears to be associated with a higher frequency of malaria infection and adverse pregnancy outcomes (Breman and Campbell, 1988). Despite this general pattern, and for reasons not well understood, not all individuals within these groups are at equal risk of becoming seriously ill or dying. Much of the most recent work in malaria epidemiology has thus concentrated on the identification of the variables that place certain groups at greater risk of illness and death. Central to this work has been a better understanding of the acquisition of immunity.

Acquired immunity appears to be relatively short-lived and depends on repeated exposure to the parasite over time. It is directly related to the level of malaria endemicity in a given area, transmission patterns, frequency of human-vector contact, and the length of time a person resides in an endemic area. The species of parasite present, the level of endemicity, and the biologic, behavioral, and socioeconomic characteristics of the human population determine the prevalence of infection and the distribution of disease.

An increasingly important issue in understanding the epidemiology of malaria disease is the availability and use of antimalarial drugs. With the spread of drug-resistant parasites, the effects of drugs on immune status and on drug resistance itself are issues of paramount concern.

By looking at malaria as a disease, epidemiologists are better equipped to assess the short- and long-term impacts of various control strategies, including antimosquito measures (e.g., insecticide-treated bednets) and antimalarial drugs (given as chemoprophylaxis, as therapy, or for both purposes), in reducing malaria-related morbidity and mortality. The shift from studying malaria as an infection to focusing on its importance as a disease is recent, and the questions being asked are a substantial departure from traditional routes of inquiry. The answers are far from apparent.

Morbidity and Mortality

In terms of its contribution to morbidity and mortality, malaria is among the world's most serious health problems. According to WHO, there are over 100 million clinical cases of malaria in the world each year (World Health Organization, 1990), and an estimated 1 to 2 million deaths. Because of the difficulty of obtaining reliable data, most of the malaria-related mortality estimates are based on extrapolations from areas and studies in which mortality has been effectively documented. One of the most widely quoted figures is that of 1 million children dying of malaria in Africa each year (Bruce-Chwatt, 1969).

When one is determining levels of morbidity, for example, a clinical diagnosis of malaria in the absence of microscopic confirmation—a frequent occurrence in many parts of the world—can have an error rate of up to 50 percent. On the other hand, the prevalence of malaria parasites in peripheral blood, particularly in children living in endemic areas, can be close to 100 percent, yet most of these children have asymptomatic infections, complicating confirmation of the diagnosis by a blood film. In addition to these inherent difficulties, there is generally uneven surveillance and incomplete and irregular reporting of malaria cases at all levels of the health system in most countries where the disease is endemic.

Estimates of malaria mortality are notoriously imprecise and particularly difficult to derive. Even in the most rigorously conducted studies, ascertaining the number of malaria deaths is not without pitfalls. This is in part because most people in the world die at home, not in the hospital. Therefore, studies that rely on hospital-based records consistently underestimate mortality attributable to a given disease. In a recent study conducted in the Gambia, for example, 23 of 25 children who died of malaria died at home; only 2 died in a dispensary, and none died in the hospital (Greenwood et al., 1987).

A number of methodologies have been developed to better determine the causes and rates of mortality in communities that lack formalized records of births and deaths. Verbal autopsy, in which the family of the deceased is interviewed about the circumstances of the death, can be useful for identifying those diseases with characteristic clinical features. Another demographic methodology, the preceding child technique, involves asking a mother about the fate of her previous child. Analysis of prospectively recorded deaths by village health workers over an extended period of time can also be helpful in determining both overall mortality and disease-specific mortality. These and other methodologies, while useful, are imperfect and often imprecise. In certain settings, however, they should be further explored in estimating the impact of malaria in childhood mortality.

Approaches to Malaria Control

Tactical Variants and Stratification

Several approaches to thinking about malaria control have been devised over the past 20 years. Two of the best known are based on tactical variants (World Health Organization, 1979) and stratification.

The resurgence of malaria in many parts of the world beginning in the mid-1960s and continuing through the mid-1970s caused a general reassessment of existing control strategies. In the most significant of these efforts, WHO proposed a way of viewing malaria control that was based on what was thought to be achievable given the epidemiologic, sociologic, managerial, logistic, and financial resources of individual malarious countries. This tactical-variant approach was adopted by the Thirty-first World Health Assembly in 1978, and the concept was further developed at the meeting of the Seventeenth WHO Expert Committee on Malaria (World Health Organization, 1979)

The four variants are (1) reduction and prevention of mortality due to malaria through drug treatment; (2) reduction and prevention of mortality and morbidity, with special attention to reduction of morbidity in high-risk groups, through prompt treatment, the distribution of prophylactic drugs to special at-risk groups, and application of vector control and personal protection measures, where appropriate; (3) in addition to the features of (1) and (2) above, a reduction in malaria prevalence through the systematic application of a malaria control program; and (4) country-wide malaria control, with the ultimate objective of eradication. These tactical variants were designed to illustrate possible malaria control objectives. They were not intended to help characterize or define the malaria problem in a country.

The concept of stratification, developed by WHO in the mid-1980s, characterizes epidemiologic zones of malaria in terms of their main determinants, including climate, the location of sources of water and of mountains, vector biology, anthropology, and social and economic factors. Using stratification, a country or continent could be broken down by geographic area and/or by population characteristics, and a number of epidemiologic, biologic, social, and economic factors could be identified that would govern the choice and intensity of antimalarial interventions. The scale of application of stratification varied considerably, from the characterization of large homogeneous areas to that of very small epidemiologic units, such as a locality. With a few exceptions, however, stratification has not been widely adopted or implemented, in part because a large amount of detailed baseline information was required.

The Epidemiologic Approach to Malaria Control

The Eighteenth Expert Committee (World Health Organization, 1986) further promoted the concept of an epidemiologic approach to malaria control. The approach emphasized the local variability in the distribution of malaria problems, calling for the design of appropriate and suitable control strategies, training of staff, and monitoring and evaluation in different ecological areas within a given country. The enormous changes that have overtaken most malaria programs in the past 10 or 15 years, in their transition from eradication to control and then, in some cases, control through primary health care, often against the background of decentralization and integration of health services, were just too much for many program managers to cope with. The problem was compounded by difficulties in interpreting guidelines about what methods of control should be used, and many managers virtually suspended their programs pending a firmer identification of what was actually to be done in the field.

Development of the Paradigms

In an attempt to make the epidemiologic approach to malaria control more user friendly and of greater practical utility to those charged with implementing and overseeing control programs, members of WHO's Division of Control of Tropical Diseases and representatives of the Institute of Medicine's Committee on Malaria Prevention and Control convened a two-day meeting in Montreux, Switzerland, in September 1990. The purpose of the meeting was to simplify the complex epidemiology of malaria by classifying the disease into a limited number of major types or paradigms, a model first discussed in 1989 (Najera, 1989). It was thought that this approach would enable program managers and nonspecialists to better understand the variability of malaria and if developed more fully, provide a method of matching the most appropriate control tools to specific situations.

Some critics of this approach considered it to be an oversimplification. Others felt that it was nothing new, a restatement of the obvious, another name for stratification, or the first step in creating another in a long line of malaria control dicta. The paradigm concept continues to generate a good deal of controversy.

While the malaria paradigms may be oversimplifications, the simplicity may allow the approach to work where others have failed. Previous epidemiologic approaches to malaria control, including stratification, have been faulted for being overly complex. Even if one accepts the underlying principles, it is difficult to know how to begin to plan malaria control interventions based on these approaches. In terms of substance, the paradigms are simply a new way of examining and understanding the sound epidemiologic principles already extensively explored. They are not dicta, but a way of thinking about and systematically organizing malaria control activities.

The paradigm approach is in an early stage of development. Even so, it may help program managers and others better define the malaria problem and prioritize control interventions. The approach will require refinement and field validation before we can adequately assess its usefulness in rationalizing malaria control.

The paradigm approach begins with the observation that most malaria problems in the world can be categorized as one or more major types: malaria of the African savannah; forest malaria; malaria associated with irrigated agriculture; highland fringe malaria; desert fringe and oasis malaria; urban malaria; plains malaria associated with traditional agriculture; and seashore malaria. Although certain situations may not fit easily into any of these categories, such cases are of limited importance on a global scale. There may also be unique hybrids of two or more of the paradigm types which will require special consideration.

Use of these easily conceptualized types, rather than more abstract epidemiologic principles, enables even nonspecialists to gain an understanding of the malaria problem. Application of the paradigm approach requires a logical progression through a series of steps in which attributes of a particular malaria problem, from the most general through the more specific, are considered (see Appendix A). The goal is to classify the situation only as narrowly as necessary, not as narrowly as possible, before choosing control tools and planning interventions.

The following is a brief description of the paradigm approach. A more complete discussion of the method and its use should soon be available from the Malaria Unit of the Control of Tropical Diseases at the World Health Organization.

Description of the Paradigms

Malaria of the African Savannah Eighty percent of the world's malaria and 90 percent of mortality due to the disease occur in Africa south of the Sahara, mostly in the savannah regions. The principal vectors, *Anopheles gambiae, An. funestus,* and *An. arabiensis* are efficient transmitters of the malaria parasite and are found in abundance. Malaria transmission is seasonal and correlates with relatively predictable patterns of rainfall, although transmission may continue at lower levels during the dry season. Because of the extremely high inoculation rates, virtually all of those living in these areas become infected early in life. For children, treatment (until recently, chloroquine was very effective) may prevent death long enough for acquired immunity to establish itself, which can provide protection from malaria-related death or illness later in life. Young children who do not acquire this protective immunity, and whose infections are not treated adequately or promptly, are at particular risk of dying from the disease. These areas, which can be further subdivided into wet and dry savannah, are characterized by high-intensity transmission by efficient vectors in abundance, resulting in immunity in those who survive initial infections and an eventual ability to tolerate parasitemia without symptomatic or serious illness.

Forest Malaria Forest malaria, the result of human incursions into forests or jungles, occurs in several regions of the world, including the Amazon basin of South America, Southeast Asia (primarily Bangladesh, Myanmar, Thailand, and the Indochinese peninsula), Borneo, equatorial Africa, and certain of the Pacific Islands. The indigenous inhabitants of these forest and jungle areas, including Indians of the Amazon, the pygmies of central Africa, and the aborigines of the Malaysian jungle, traditionally have been relatively unaffected by malaria. Recently, however, economic pressures have brought large numbers of poor nonindigenous laborers into these regions for agriculture, timbering, gem and gold mining, and road construction. The results have been serious malaria-related morbidity and considerable mortality among the newcomers and the reintroduction or increase of malaria in indigenous populations.

Typically, the mosquitoes responsible for transmitting malaria parasites in forest areas are difficult or impossible to control by traditional means. For example, *An. dirus*, the primary malaria vector in Southeast Asian jungles, can develop in almost any shaded collection of water (even in animal hoofprints and the bracts of commensal plants); this mosquito feeds in the early evening, and rests outdoors after taking a blood meal. Such characteristics make the application of traditional larval control measures and other tactics aimed at reducing the adult mosquito population, such as use of residual insecticides, relatively fruitless.

Malaria Associated with Irrigated Agriculture Irrigation for agricultural purposes may both provide breeding sites for vector mosquitoes and allow concentrated parasite reservoirs in the form of large labor forces to become established, helping maintain a high level of malaria transmission. Examples of places where this type of malaria occurs include the cotton plantations of the Gezira in the Sudan and irrigated rice cultivation areas in Sri Lanka.

Sugarcane cultivation in dry areas that require irrigation has also resulted in an increase in malaria transmission where it had not been a serious problem in the past.

Highland Fringe Malaria   Although malaria has been transmitted at altitudes of up to 2,800 meters, the disease does not generally occur above about 1,500 meters (Bruce-Chwatt, 1985). Because of fluctuations in climate, and perhaps even global warming, vector anophelines may begin to flourish at higher and higher altitudes. The altitudes subject to this type of malaria problem may vary greatly according to the local geography. Populations, in particular settled populations, living at higher, normally malaria-free altitudes may have little acquired immunity to malaria and so may suffer devastating epidemics. Such a situation recently occurred in the highland plateaus of Madagascar, where malaria had previously been eradicated or nearly so. Because of unusual climatic conditions, or perhaps as a result of a documented gradual increase in the mean temperature, the malaria vector *An. funestus* recolonized the high plateau, causing many hundreds of thousands of cases of the disease and significant mortality in the nonimmune population. Similar, less devastating epidemics have been seen in Papua New Guinea, in Ethiopia, and on the mountain slopes of Kenya. Even without an expansion in the range of vector anophelines, however, economic conditions may force nonimmune highland populations to search for work in lower highland fringe areas, where they may be exposed to intense malaria transmission.

Desert Fringe and Oasis Malaria   This paradigm shares many characteristics with highland fringe malaria, including the occurrence of periodic and serious epidemic outbreaks of disease in nonimmune populations. Since there is normally no transmission in these arid grassland areas, the populations living in or at the edge of deserts generally do not have protective immunity against malaria. When climatic conditions change—when, for example, unusually heavy rains occur that allow vector mosquitoes to develop—nonimmune populations may be at risk of infection and of severe and often fatal malaria. Such conditions have prevailed in recent years in areas of the Sahel, along the southern edge of the Sahara, and on the fringes of the Kalahari desert, where increasingly serious epidemics have occurred in northern Namibia over the past four years. Ethiopia regularly experiences such epidemics. Both settled populations and nomadic groups may be at risk near oases that support malaria transmission, such as in the western desert of Egypt.

Urban Malaria   Urban malaria can be of two basic types. Malaria can be transmitted by vectors well adapted to city conditions (e.g., *An. stephensi*, the archetypal urban vector of South Asia). This type of mosquito, which develops in domestic water sources such as wells, cisterns, and household water containers, is responsible for malaria transmission in Delhi, Karachi, Madras, and other urban centers of the Indian subcontinent.

Urban malaria may also occur when sprawling urban settlements encroach on the rural habitats of malaria vectors not usually found in city environments. This occurs in semiurban African villages where the African savannah paradigm predominates. It is important to differentiate these two situations, however, as malaria control strategies will be different even if the vector is the same. Similarly, the densely populated ramshackle settlements associated with gold mines in the Amazon basin support a type of urban malaria, which is actually the result of people moving into areas of forest malaria transmission. In areas of urban malaria, larval control may be a realistic option for reducing malaria transmission, particularly if communities become actively involved. Residual spraying of houses may also be feasible in such settings.

Plains Malaria Associated with Traditional Agriculture   Malaria transmission in plains villages involved in subsistence agriculture is usually of low to moderate intensity and fluctuates with the seasons. Such areas are prone to epidemics, particularly in association with early and prolonged rainy seasons. The predominant parasite is often *P. vivax*. While devastating epidemics are seldom seen, and childhood mortality is not a significant feature as it is with African savannah malaria, this type of malaria can cause chronic debility and suboptimal agricultural productivity. Malaria of this type is widely seen in South Asia and Central America.

Seashore Malaria   Many seashore areas of the tropics pose a malaria threat to residents and visitors alike. Such areas are becoming more and more important economically to poor countries as tourists search out unspoiled "tropical paradises" suitable as vacation sites and large numbers of workers come to support the industry. Port areas also offer the potential for malaria transmission and may be the source of infected mosquitoes transported by ships to other regions or of malaria imported by infected seamen to other countries.

Seashore malaria may be transmitted by mosquitoes that breed in brackish water such as the South China Sea. In Africa, the seashore resorts of Kenya provide another example of this type of malaria. Because there is often the potential for successful malaria control efforts, and because of the income generated by tourism, expensive interventions may be more acceptable and sustainable in these areas.

Most of the world's malaria problem can be characterized according to the paradigms described above. Certain other types represent combinations of these paradigms. Malaria on islands, for example, falls generally under one or more of the eight paradigms; many of the islands of the South Pacific have coastal and highland fringe malaria. Riverine malaria is usually an intensification of either plains malaria or African savannah malaria, associated with greater potential for vector breeding. The malaria associated with development projects is often forest malaria or irrigated agriculture malaria influenced by the specific characteristic of the development project. These characteristics will determine the feasibility of certain types of interventions to some extent irrespective of the vector mosquito or ecological setting of transmission.

Principal Determinants

Once the types of malaria present in a country have been identified and ranked in importance, the paradigm's principal determinants must be systematically considered. These determinants will point to specific control strategies that should be considered within any given paradigm. Eight principal determinants have been identified to date: level of endemicity; parasite species; mosquito vectors; characteristics of the human population; social, behavioral, and economic considerations; health infrastructure; availability and effectiveness of antimalarial drugs; and the influence of development projects. In many situations, existing sources provide the general knowledge and specific data necessary to assess the importance of these determinants in setting control strategies. In other cases, simple operational research projects will be needed to collect basic information.

Level of Endemicity   Endemicity is characterized by different patterns of malaria transmission. Levels of transmission may be high, moderate, or low, and transmission may be seasonal, perennial, or characterized by periodic epidemics. Data about transmission patterns can often be extracted from existing health facilities or records of malaria control programs. Sometimes, however, original data will need to be collected. An understanding of transmission patterns is essential to the planning of vector control operations. For example, cycles of insecticide spraying should be adjusted to anticipate increasing densities of mosquito vectors. In addition, knowledge of existing patterns of malaria transmission may provide early warning of epidemics, perhaps allowing their impact to be diminished by control efforts.

Parasite Species   *Plasmodium falciparum* is the parasite species responsible for the most serious forms of malarial illness and for essentially all fatal cases of the disease. *Plasmodium vivax*, the most widely distributed of the malaria parasites, is seen frequently in temperate regions and, because of its contribution to malaria relapse, is able to persist in areas of wide climatic fluctuation. *Plasmodium malariae* and *P. ovale* are less widely distributed. In areas where *P. falciparum* is prevalent, efforts to limit mortality must be considered first. In areas where *P. vivax* predominates, debilitating disease rather than mortality is the primary concern. Where more than one species is present, control efforts should be focused on *P. falciparum*, even when it is not the predominant parasite, because of its potentially fatal consequences.

Mosquito Vectors   There are nearly 400 *Anopheles* species, of which about 60 are proven vectors of human malaria. The existence or creation of situations favorable for particular anopheline vectors is determined largely by the eight basic types of malaria paradigms. As difficult as it is to manage clinical malaria or to prevent infection through prophylaxis given the interventions currently available, controlling populations of anopheline vectors in the long term has proven to be a nearly insurmountable challenge, at least in some of the major paradigms (e.g., African savannah and forest).

To define the risks of infection, to identify methods of reducing human-vector contact, and, where feasible, to reduce vector density, it is essential to understand the population dynamics of the predominant vector(s) in areas where antimalarial activities are being contemplated or implemented. In practice, vector identification is often based on traditional impressions and outdated data rather than on a clear understanding of the current situation.

There are a number of vector-related variables that should be considered before control interventions are selected. Such variables include the mosquito species in the area, their relative importance as vectors of malaria; their distribution, abundance, and competence; their vector feeding and resting habits; and the characteristics of larval development sites.

To determine the potential effectiveness of any antivector measures undertaken, the following factors must be considered: vector susceptibility to insecticides; the cost, safety, and acceptability of effective insecticides; the utility, acceptability, availability, and local cost of bednets; the feasibility of using bednets impregnated with insecticides on a community-wide basis; and the availability, acceptability, and cost of mosquito repellents and fumigant coils (see Chapter 7).

Characteristics of the Human Population   The most important determinant of the impact of malaria on a population is the prevailing level of immunity. For example, in the African savannah, where transmission is intense, immunity in those who survive childhood may provide protection from death and even severe clinical illness. Malaria control activities in such regions will necessarily focus on preventing death in young children and nonimmune people coming into the area. In parts of mainland Southeast Asia, however, where forest malaria prevails, exposure to malaria parasites may occur first in young adult males during work-related activities. Antimalarial efforts in these areas will focus on protecting forest workers, and military patrols, and perhaps accompanying family members. The simple observation that in Africa malaria is mainly a childhood disease, whereas in much of Asia and South America it is a disease of young adults, is often overlooked during the planning of control strategies.

Population movement also plays a role in determining the impact of malaria. For example, residents of settled villages (often settled because they are malaria free) are often at lower risk of contracting malaria than are people living in constantly shifting villages, such as members of the hill tribes of Southeast Asia, which practice slash-and-burn agriculture. If the movement of people is organized and predictable, as it is when African nomads routinely visit oases that support malaria transmission, interventions can be put in place during the times when the population is at greatest risk of disease. The role of population density and settlement patterns must also be taken into account. Amazonian Indians, who traditionally live in widely separated villages of low population density, are at much less risk of contracting malaria than are large groups of gold miners, who constantly are shifting to new exploration sites in the same geographic area. The population movement determinant should be considered in decisions on control strategies both to identify populations at greatest risk and to assess the feasibility of a given intervention.

Social, Behavioral, and Economic Considerations Several social, behavioral, and economic factors should bear on decisions as to the most appropriate and cost-effective malaria interventions. These factors, some of which are discussed below, may help determine differential exposure to malaria parasites or the likelihood that effective treatment will be administered early enough to prevent severe disease.

ACCESS TO HEALTH CARE is probably the most important socioeconomic determinant of malarial illness. People in malarious areas who live at great distances from health services, whether governmental, nongovernmental (mission, etc.), or commercial markets and pharmacists, are likely to suffer more from the disease than those who have such services close at hand. Access may be limited by more than distance, however. Close-by health centers that have unreliable drug supplies, have poorly trained and unsupervised staff, or charge fees unaffordable to affected populations are no better than nonexistent or too-distant services. Appreciation of such factors will influence the choice of malaria control interventions.

TYPE OF HOUSING may influence both the risk of infection and the potential for vector control. Houses that have integral walls and screened windows and doors will greatly limit the risk of indoor infection, particularly when used in conjunction with other measures, such as application of residual sprays. By contrast, houses constructed with semi-open bamboo or stick walls will admit insects of all sorts and are much less suitable for spraying with residual insecticides.

WATER STORAGE PATTERNS may influence malaria transmission through the provision of breeding sites, particularly in urban settings. For example, water tanks on the roofs of houses, common in many urban centers in India, may become larval development sites for *An. stephensi* and enhance the chances that malaria transmission will be maintained.

HEALTH SEEKING BEHAVIORS of populations affected by malaria will affect the outcome of clinical infections. For example, people accustomed to seeking initial treatment from traditional healers may suffer greater mortality from malaria than do those who go first to well-supplied health centers stocked with effective drugs. This is particularly true for young children, in whom the disease may rapidly become life-threatening.

SLEEPING HABITS, i.e., whether people sleep indoors or outdoors, at what time they retire in relation to the peak feeding times of vector mosquitoes, and whether or not they are accustomed to using bednets, will influence the risk of malaria infection and the choice of various antimosquito measures.

CUSTOMS AND TABOOS may affect both the risk of acquiring malaria and the outcome of infections. For example, taboos against pregnant women using drugs may influence the success of prophylactic or treatment regimens aimed at women pregnant for the first time, who are at high risk for severe and complicated malaria.

INCOME AND WEALTH clearly affect the severity of the malaria problem. If the population has the financial resources to build housing inhospitable to mosquitoes, is knowledgeable about the use of personal protection measures such as mosquito repellents, understands the importance of seeking effective treatment at the first sign of illness, and can pay for health services and drugs, the rates of severe morbidity may be low and malaria mortality nonexistent, despite being in an area of intense malaria transmission.

LOCAL UNDERSTANDING of malaria will affect decisions about whether and when to seek treatment and behaviors influencing exposure to infected mosquitoes. Populations exposed to malaria may know that the disease is transmitted by a mosquito, may feel that it is a consequence of "spirit anger," or may simply accept it as an unavoidable part of life. Whatever view is held, it will influence the degree of acceptance of measures designed to limit transmission or to increase the use of health services.

Health Infrastructure   The organization of health services in a malarious area must be known in order to determine the feasibility of potential antimalarial measures. The national health budget—both the amount available for malaria control and the relative importance assigned to health—must be known for appropriate planning to proceed and for affordable interventions to be selected. The status of health services must be critically evaluated in terms of distribution, efficiency, and effectiveness. The characteristics and orientation, whether vertical or horizontal, of the national malaria control program, as well as its strengths and weaknesses, must be understood. The effects of malaria control measures already undertaken should be known, and the adequacy of funding, availability of drugs and insecticides, level of competence among program planners, and quality of the field staff must be assessed.

In many areas, nongovernmental services can be more important than those provided by government facilities. Hospitals and district health clinics, organized and supported by religious missions, may have a greater impact on the health of the local populations than do programs administered by impoverished governments. In certain societies, traditional healers may play a major role in treating malaria patients and referring them to organized medical facilities.

Private health care, whether provided by clinics and hospitals, moonlighting governmental health staff, traditional healers, private pharmacists, medical "quacks," or drug sections of markets, are often more important for the delivery of health care at the local level than are organized governmental services. The impact of these alternatives must be understood and exploited during the planning and implementation of malaria control activities.

Availability and Effectiveness of Antimalarial Drugs   The efficacy of antimalarial drugs depends in part on cost, availability, acceptability to the local population, and patterns of parasite resistance. Highly effective drugs may be so expensive that neither patients nor control programs can afford them. A course of mefloquine, for example, may cost 25 times as much as a course of chloroquine. Programs that have been designed to use chloroquine may not be able to adapt to the use of a new, more expensive drug. Patients unable to buy a full course of medication may purchase only one or two tablets, making the treatment ineffective. If the practice is widespread enough, it may contribute to the selection of parasite populations resistant to the drug. If, because of cost, corruption, or disorganization, a program is unable to make effective drugs available to the population it serves, mortality, particularly among children in Africa, is bound to be high.

Drug resistance is becoming a major limiting factor in the use of afford-able antimalarial drugs. Chloroquine resistance in *P. falciparum* malaria in Africa has been followed by resistance to the sulfadoxine-pyrimethamine combination and even, in some areas, to mefloquine. It is important to note, however, that resistance is often confined to small geographic areas.

In terms of controlling malaria, the likelihood that patients will comply with a recommended course of treatment—the drug regimen's feasibility—is nearly as important as the drug's antiparasite efficacy. Drug regimens requiring complex administration schedules (such as quinine-tetracycline) are unlikely to be adequately followed by outpatients, resulting in partial treatment, recrudescence, and possibly the selection of drug-resistant para-site populations.

Finally, the goal of drug therapy needs to be defined. Those in charge of control efforts need to know whether it is necessary to completely elimi-nate malaria infection or simply to treat an episode of acute disease. In areas where infection is sporadic and work related, where patients have little or no acquired immunity, and where health services are far from the site where infection was acquired, it is essential to provide a reliably cura-tive regimen. In situations where immunity is the most important protec-tion against serious malaria-related morbidity or death, and where reinfection within a short period of time is certain, the aim of drug treatment may be to allow the patient to survive the current acute episode, without necessar-ily eradicating the parasitemia.

Development Projects   The local impact of development needs to be con-sidered when antimalarial interventions are planned. Development projects may be officially sanctioned by government or undertaken by private en-terprise (e.g., road building, dam construction, forestry, or agricultural projects) or they may be unofficial, uncontrolled activities, such as large-scale gem or gold mining or illegal land development. All such activities affect the epidemiologic factors relating to malaria, including population immunity, mobility, access to health services, and availability of drugs, and often represent major differences from the surrounding national or even local malaria situations. Development projects also provide a controlled setting for an effective malaria control effort specific to the labor force and their families. These settings should be exploited wherever possible and pri-vate enterprise should be enlisted to assume a major responsibility.

Malaria Control Tools

The control strategies adopted for any given paradigm and its principal determinants will be constrained by the control tools available and, of course, by their cost, effectiveness, and feasibility of implementation. The information available in the determinants of a given paradigm should allow decisions to be made regarding affordability, efficacy, and feasibility.

Antimalarial Drugs and Malaria Treatment Facilities   Drugs may be used to prevent, treat, and (theoretically) stop the transmission of malaria. Prevention through drug prophylaxis is difficult in endemic populations, since the provision and administration of safe, effective drugs is often not sustainable over the longer term. However, under certain circumstances, such as in the military and organized labor camps, it is possible to provide effective prophylaxis for an extended period of time to large numbers of people exposed to malaria. Drug prophylaxis is also used by tourists visiting malarious areas.

Antimalarial treatment drugs are used for oral treatment of uncomplicated illness on an outpatient basis, for parenteral treatment of patients unable to take oral medication, or for treatment of those requiring prolonged and supervised administration. Treatment is also required to eliminate persisting liver-stage parasites, which cause malaria relapse in the case of *P. vivax* malaria.

At present, there is only one drug (primaquine) that can be used to reduce malaria transmission by adult gametocytes. However, because of the difficulty in getting adequate drug coverage in populations, and because of the drug's short half-life in the blood, this intervention has limited utility.

In the case of epidemic outbreaks of malaria, mass administration of treatment doses of chloroquine and primaquine may be justified as an emergency measure to limit mortality and morbidity. In general, however, the temptation to use mass drug administration to combat malaria should be resisted, since supervision of such a program is difficult and resistant parasite strains may be selected. Other effective antimalarial drugs are less suitable for this purpose because of expense, toxicity, or both.

The use of microscopy to confirm the presence of malaria parasites, and to indicate the most appropriate drugs, thereby limiting the use of sometimes expensive and toxic medications to those individuals actually requiring them, should also be considered a malaria control tool.

Treatment facilities can limit the impact of malaria. The establishment and support of treatment posts throughout areas of malaria transmission, and of inpatient health care facilities capable of providing parenteral drugs and managing severe malaria and its complications, are important contributors to malaria control particularly in areas where antivector measures are not feasible.

Antivector Measures   Personal protection measures (e.g., mosquito nets, coils, repellents, and screens) can be used to limit or prevent human-mosquito contact. Insecticide-treated mosquito nets in particular are being promoted worldwide as a relatively inexpensive, nontoxic, and culturally acceptable method of reducing human-mosquito contact. Sleeping each night under an insecticide-treated bednet is likely to reduce the individual's overall risk of infection and is a useful form of personal protection. However, the impact of community-wide use of bednets on malaria transmission, morbidity, and mortality remains to be determined. Most of the studies conducted to date, which attempted to measure, among other things, the impact of insecticide-treated bednets on overall malaria transmission, infection, and illness, reported some reduction in a key measure (Rozendaal, 1989). Unfortunately, there are difficulties in interpreting and extrapolating some of the data. For example, most studies conducted in Africa south of the Sahara had a very small sample size, making it impossible to determine the overall impact of the use of bednets on transmission, morbidity, and mortality. In some of the largest trials conducted in China (Li et al., 1989), a dramatic decline in the incidence of malaria was reported over several years; however, it is difficult to ascribe this decline to the use of insecticide-treated bednets, given the tremendous variation in the epidemiology of malaria in the study areas.

Only one study to date has attempted to measure the impact of insecticide-treated bednets on child mortality (Alonso et al., 1991). This study, conducted in the Gambia, recorded substantial reductions in overall mortality and malaria-specific mortality in children one to four years of age of 63 percent and 70 percent, respectively. However, extrapolation of the results of this study to other areas is complicated by variations in infant and child mortality rates among regions, vector competence and behavior, and the acceptance and use of bednets.

There is little doubt that insecticide-treated bednets are a superior form of individual protection, but as a population-based malaria control strategy, they remain experimental. Large population-based trials of insecticide-treated bednets now in progress are expected to yield valuable information on the impact of community-wide use of bednets on malaria-related mortality and morbidity.

Environmental management includes such measures as draining larval development sites or clearing vegetation from such sites; reforestation in some areas and band deforestation in others; and flushing of streams where local vectors breed. Deliberately positioning domestic animals, such as horses, cattle, or buffalo, between vector sources and human dwellings (zooprophylaxis) has contributed to the reduction of transmission in some areas, including China and the Soviet Union.

Larviciding may be an effective antivector method where larval development sites are accessible. Chemical agents, biological agents, or larvivorous fish have been used successfully in certain situations.

Residual insecticides are useful against susceptible mosquitoes that rest on sprayed surfaces. These insecticides have been the mainstay of malaria control operations in many parts of the world for decades. This approach, which continues to be effective in some areas, can also be comparatively expensive, toxic to spray personnel, and damaging to the environment when misused. It should be evaluated carefully before it is implemented. Fogging with aerosol insecticides can be extremely effective in controlling epidemics in areas of high human population density, such as refugee camps, but only when done with the correct timing, frequency, and concentration.

Surveillance Techniques Malaria surveillance techniques are essential to establish priorities for control programs, target resources, and monitor program impact on morbidity and mortality. For example, monitoring of malaria morbidity, the incidence and frequency of severe disease and mortality, case-fatality rates, and the prevalence of parasitemia can delineate high-risk groups and guide control activities. Similarly, surveillance systems that detect early stages of epidemic malaria transmission can prevent the devastating effects of serious outbreaks. Monitoring of vector density, insecticide susceptibility, and vector behavior can greatly increase the cost-effectiveness of vector control efforts.

It is also essential to monitor the rate at which antimalarial drug regimens fail. Measurements of the susceptibility of *P. falciparum* to antimalarial drugs, using in vivo techniques to guide therapy policies and in vitro techniques to define trends over time can be undertaken. When made a routine part of antimalarial activities, such monitoring can greatly increase the effectiveness of control efforts.

Information, Education, and Communication The dissemination of information on how to avoid malaria infections and the importance of prompt treatment is an important tool for malaria control. Such information can be aimed at both the general public and health care personnel. Most decisions about malaria prevention and treatment are made by infected individuals and/or their families. School curricula, radio, newspapers, television, songs, theater, and films are among the media that can be used to convey information to families about malaria prevention and treatment.

In many parts of the world, the local market is the primary source of antimalarial drugs. These medications are much more likely to have a therapeutic effect if patients and their families are supplied with information about correct dosage, duration of treatment, and possible toxicity.

Educational campaigns that target health care providers should include information on diagnosis, correct dosage regimens, changes in the epidemiology of malaria, the characteristics of high risk-groups, the status of drug resistance, and drug toxicity.

Application of the Paradigm Approach

Logical progression through the steps (identifying the major types of malaria occurring in a country or area, considering the impact of major determinants, and matching available tools to the requirements defined should provide a shortcut to an analysis of the malaria situation and promote a better understanding of the components of the problem. The paradigm approach can serve to orient those who plan malaria control programs, reminding them that a single control strategy applied on a country-wide basis is not likely to affect the problem throughout the country. Furthermore, the paradigm approach can help planners structure evaluations of antimalarial activities by ensuring that a consistent set of basic information is included in every consultant's report. The paradigms may improve communication between malaria specialists and nonspecialists, and they have already been used successfully to teach nonspecialists about the complexity of the malaria problem. It is important to reiterate, however, that the paradigm approach is in an early stage of development, and considerable field testing is required to assess its utility and suggest modifications and refinements.

Program Planning and Evaluation[1]

Insufficient attention to good management practices has probably contributed more to the failure of malaria control programs than have technical problems. Efficient management, planning, budgeting, logistics, and monitoring are often missing from malaria control programs, with the result that antimalaria measures seldom reach their full potential. The availability of new technologies will mean little in endemic areas unless there is a responsive delivery system that can successfully introduce new drugs, vaccines, or mosquito control methods into regions of the world where they are most needed.

For too long, there has been unproductive debate among health planners about whether control programs should be run in a centralized, hierarchical fashion (vertical organization) or integrated into primary health care (horizontal organization). In reality, neither approach is inherently superior to the other, and the two are not mutually exclusive. Some malaria control activities, such as policy formulation, the design of intervention strategies, training, the reporting of epidemiologic data, operational (problem-solving) research, and program evaluation, are best conducted in a

---

[1] The information and views presented in this section are drawn heavily from Liese et al., 1991.

centralized fashion. Other activities, such as the establishment and support of treatment facilities, implementation of vector control operations, health education, and intersectoral cooperation, are more suited to a decentralized approach.

Policy Formulation

Responsibility for communication between the malaria control program and other divisions of the government for formulation of policy must rest with the central administration of the malaria program, i.e., the ministry of health, as well as other concerned ministries such as those for interior, planning, social action, and agriculture. The central administration must be able both to react to changes in political and epidemiologic situations and to define strategies for disease control.

Intervention Strategy

The central administration of each malaria control program should be responsible for developing strategies and selecting interventions to be used in malaria control. It is of primary importance that selection of the interventions be based on an understanding of the local epidemiology of the malaria problem and of the advantages and limitations of the control technologies. A single method applied across a large area in which there are a variety of environmental and epidemiologic conditions will probably fail.

Malaria control is usually constrained by the limited experience of decision makers and their tendency to apply certain interventions without careful analysis, often because they lack the training and experience to evaluate the effectiveness of current control methods. Consequently, malaria control programs frequently rely on the residual application of insecticides to reduce malaria transmission because the technique is available rather than because it is epidemiologically or biologically appropriate.

Technical and human resources are not always considered when the decision to use specific control methods is made. The absence of trained personnel, for example, constrains the ability of control programs to plan effectively and, if necessary, expand. This problem is compounded by the fact that when new resources are sought or developed the efforts tend to proceed along very traditional lines because the decision makers are not prepared to think innovatively or risk new ideas.

Training

Training has often meant sending senior program staff to the United States or Europe for master's degrees (usually in disciplines unrelated to the design or management of control programs) or for study tours or conducting low-level courses for implementing staff. The management skills of decision makers within malaria control programs have been largely ignored. Management training at this level should focus on a number of areas, including goal setting and program planning; communication and supervisory skills; personnel management techniques; budgeting, allocating, and monitoring the use of resources; and personnel training and development.

The development of skills at the central level will include training in epidemiology, entomology, vector control operations, and the planning and evaluation of field research. Skill in these disciplines can often be developed through short courses (of the type offered by the Centers for Disease Control) and on-the-job training in countries that have similar malaria problems. In addition, malaria control program staff from two countries with similar problems, e.g., forest malaria in Thailand and Brazil, can often learn more from each other (if the communication is structured around focused discussions and visits, not simply through observation tours) than by attending year-long academic programs abroad.

Training at the periphery of the health care system, if based on the results of local operational research, can be more effective than academic coursework. These training activities will include seminars, meetings, and panel discussions involving personnel from different institutions and levels of the health network. Training of this sort requires that supervisors and their subordinates communicate and cooperate.

Training, including technical training, not only must address a review of all curricula of health personnel involved in even the smallest way with malaria control but also should initiate innovative approaches in planning, designing, and implementing courses and seminars. The development, field testing, and production of training support systems such as modules, treatment charts, and other job aids should, wherever possible, be developed. Instruction of trainers of health workers and the follow-up and evaluation of all of these activities are important components of the training programs.

Reporting

The ability to collect and report data on disease incidence, prevalence and severity, mortality, parasite sensitivity to antimalarial drugs, and vector behavior and susceptibility to insecticides is an essential part of any malaria control program. The practice of mass blood slide screening, originally instituted as part of efforts during the 1950s and 1960 to eradicate malaria, is no longer advised. Further, where time-limited eradication is no longer a feasible goal, preparation for identification of the last remaining cases should not be the goal of surveillance and reporting. Instead, the malaria control program core staff must be able to design surveys to obtain the specific epidemiologic information required for operations management.

Problem Solving (Operational Research)

Operational research involves identifying a technical problem that is impeding the progress of a control program, framing an answerable question based on this problem, and designing a study that will answer the question. The questions addressed may be very straightforward: Is one drug regimen so much better than another that a change in treatment policy is justified? Does the resting behavior of the most important malaria vector warrant a program of spraying residual insecticides? Is a community likely to accept and use permethrin-impregnated bednets? A malaria control program able to make constructive changes based on the findings of operational research is more likely to be successful.

Logistical Support and Transportation

Logistical support and transportation are critical to the success of malaria control programs. Unfortunately, in many countries, poor or nonexistent logistical support and organization and the lack of transportation are major limiting factors in malaria control programs. Such problems consume inordinate time and are often beyond the immediate control of the malaria control program manager.

Evaluation

The evaluation of progress toward the stated objectives must be an integral part of every control program, and areas of success, failure, and gaps in knowledge should be identified on an ongoing basis. Any control program that receives outside support will as a matter of course periodically conduct evaluations to satisfy sponsors that progress is being made.

Central Core of Expertise

All of the activities identified above require the presence of a central, coordinated body of expertise. The precise membership of such a group will depend on the local malaria situation and the operational requirements of the control program. The group must be managed by someone whose responsibilities are matched by his or her capabilities and authority. Even in control programs in malaria-endemic countries that are fully integrated into the general health care system, there must be a technical focus for malaria. Public health generalists do not have the level of technical expertise needed to plan and guide an effective malaria control program.

Decentralized Activities

Ideally, when a policy for malaria control is established, the authority for implementing necessary control activities will be decentralized. To be responsive to any number of possible changes in the malaria situation, decision making within a control program should take place at the lowest possible level, in accordance with the capabilities of the field staff. Operational decisions should be made peripherally, and decision makers should be held accountable for their decisions.

RESEARCH AGENDA

Infection, Immunity, and Disease

The difference between malaria infection and disease is critical, since infection with the parasite does not necessarily result in disease. In the vast majority of malaria endemic countries, data on the prevalence of infection tell us very little about the incidence of clinical disease and death. Lack of immunity predisposes people to severe and complicated malaria, but very little is known about the specific factors that place certain people at greater risk than others. Further, surprisingly little is known about the acquisition of immunity among different population and age groups.

> **RESEARCH FOCUS:** Determination of epidemiologic risk factors for severe and complicated malaria.

> **RESEARCH FOCUS:** Population-based studies of parasite and human variability as they relate to the development of immunity and the evolution of clinical disease.

Pregnancy and Birth Outcome

Women pregnant for the first time who are in the last trimester of pregnancy are considered to be at particular risk for complications due to malaria. Maternal complications have also been linked to a number of poor birth outcomes, including intrauterine growth retardation and low birth weight. Despite their importance, the effects of malaria on maternal and fetal health and survival have received little recent attention.

> **RESEARCH FOCUS:** Measurement of the impact of malaria on pregnancy and on maternal and infant health.

Chemoprophylaxis and Therapy

There is conflicting evidence on the role of chemoprophylaxis and therapy in reducing overall morbidity and mortality and malaria-related morbidity and mortality, and it may well be that the efficacy of measures will vary according to the intensity of malaria transmission.

> **RESEARCH FOCUS:** Assessment of the role of therapy and chemoprophylaxis in reducing overall and malaria-related morbidity and mortality in areas of varied intensity of malaria transmission.

Drug Resistance

The development of drug-resistant strains of *P. falciparum*, particularly to strains resistant to chloroquine (the preferred antimalarial drug), is widespread and increasing in all regions of the world. Within a country or region, however, drug resistance appears to be focal. The determinants of drug resistance in different regions are largely unknown.

> **RESEARCH FOCUS:** The epidemiology of drug resistance.

Paradigms

The paradigm approach to understanding malaria is very much in its infancy. In the coming years, it will be important to test and evaluate the strategies that evolve from the paradigm approach.

> **RESEARCH FOCUS:** Field test the paradigm approach to determine its utility in helping program managers assess the malaria situation in their areas and develop viable control strategies.

Bednets

Insecticide-treated bednets are increasingly being promoted around the world as a means of reducing contact with the vectors of malaria. Use of impregnated bednets will reduce an individual's risk of infection, but the impact of community-wide use of impregnated bednets on overall malaria transmission, morbidity, and mortality is unclear.

> **RESEARCH FOCUS:** Evaluation of the impact of community-wide use of insecticide-treated bednets on ma-

laria transmission, morbidity, and mortality in areas of varying malaria endemicity.

REFERENCES

Alonso, P. L., S. W. Lindsay, J. R. M. Armstrong, M. Conteh, A. G. Hill, P. H. David, G. Fegan, A. de Francisco, A. J. Hall, F. C. Shenton, K. Cham, and B.M. Greenwood. 1991. The effect of insecticide-treated bed nets on mortality of Gambian children. Lancet 337:1499-1502.

Breman, J. G., and C. C. Campbell. 1988. Combating severe malaria in African children. Bulletin of the World Health Organization 66:611-620.

Bruce-Chwatt, L. J. 1969. Malaria eradication at the crossroads. Bulletin of the New York Academy of Medicine 45:999-1012.

Bruce-Chwatt, L. J. 1985. Essential Malariology, 2nd ed. London: Heinemann.

Greenwood, B. M., A. K. Bradley, A. M. Greenwood. 1987. Morbidity and mortality from malaria among children in a rural area of the Gambia West Africa. Transactions of the Royal Society of Tropical Medicine and Hygiene 81:478-486.

Li, Z., M. Zhang, Y. Wu, B. Zhong, G. Lin, and H. Huang. 1989. Trial of deltamethrin impregnated bed nets for the control of malaria transmitted by *Anopheles sinensis* and *Anopheles anthropophagus*. American Journal of Tropical Medicine and Hygiene 40:356-359.

Liese, B. H., P. S. Sachdeva, and D. G. Cochrane. 1991. Organizing and Managing Tropical Disease Control Programs—Lessons of Success (Draft). Vol. I and II. Washington, D. C.: World Bank.

Moir, J. S., P. A. Garner, P. F. Heywood, and M. P. Alpers. 1989. Mortality in a rural area of Madang Province, Papua New Guinea. Annals of Tropical Medicine and Parasitology 83:305-319.

Najera, J. A. 1989. Global malaria situation. Geneva: World Health Organization, unpublished.

Rozendaal, J. A. 1989. Impregnated mosquito nets and curtains for self-protection and vector control. Tropical Diseases Bulletin 86(No. 7):R1-R41.

World Health Organization. 1979. Seventeenth report of the Expert Committee on Malaria. WHO Technical Report Series No. 640. Geneva: World Health Organization.

World Health Organization. 1986. Eighteenth report of the Expert Committee on Malaria. WHO Technical Report Series No. 735. Geneva: World Health Organization.

World Health Organization. 1990. World malaria situation, 1988. Rapport Trimestriel de Sanitares Mondiales 43:68-79.

11

Economics of Malaria Control

WHERE WE WANT TO BE IN THE YEAR 2010

There will be a great change in the way economic reasoning and analysis are applied to malaria. Health priorities no longer will be set according to the absolute burden of disease, but will be based on what can actually be done about a given disease problem. Average cost-effectiveness, once an ubiquitous and poorly applied tool of analysis, will have been discarded. Improved collection and better use of data will allow for more rigorous analyses of the marginal effectiveness and costs of programs. Policymakers will recognize that malaria is a number of different diseases and that control interventions must be situation specific. Further, they will have a better understanding of how various policy instruments, applied at different levels of intensity, affect disease outcomes.

WHERE WE ARE TODAY

Applications of Economics to Malaria

Research on the economics of malaria has traditionally fallen into two categories: studies that document the economic burden (costs) of the disease, and those that examine the cost-effectiveness of interventions aimed at preventing or controlling the disease.

The Economic Costs of Malaria

The primary cost of malaria is its contribution to mortality and morbidity. Because precise data on morbidity and mortality are often lacking, it is not surprising that estimates of the disease's economic impact are vague and imprecise. A number of factors make calculating economic impact very difficult. For one, the disease affects each geographic region, and the individual communities within them, differently. The economic impact of malaria-related death also varies according to the age of those who die. In Africa and other highly endemic regions, where most deaths are among infants and young children, the impact on productivity is lower than in areas of low to moderate endemicity, where the burden of disease falls primarily on adults, who are the main breadwinners or primary caretakers (Over et al., 1990).

Most economic impact studies attempt to measure the effects of episodes of malarial illness on lowered worker productivity, a literature reviewed by Barlow and Grobar (1986). Researchers have estimated that each case of malaria causes between 5 and 20 days of disability (Van Dine, 1916; Russell and Menon, 1942; Malik, 1966; Conly, 1975). A common convention in the literature has been to use seven days of work lost per bout of malaria whenever this parameter is needed to assess a program and cannot be independently estimated (Sinton, 1935, 1936; Quo, 1959; San Pedro, 1967-1968; Niazi, 1969).

A number of studies have attempted to measure malaria's impact on worker output. One study found that malaria prevalence did have an effect on rice production (Audibert, 1986) and another that found farm families with malaria cleared 60 percent less land than did families free of the disease (Bhombore et al., 1952).

Other researchers have shown that in agricultural settings malaria can influence the choice of crops. Conly (1975) observed that farmers replaced higher-value crops, whose growing season coincided with the peak malaria season, with lower-value crops with different growing seasons. A similar analysis revealed that new settlers in agricultural areas may decide, a priori, to plant crops that are less sensitive to interruptions in cultivation (e.g., root crops) to avoid the potential impact of malaria (Rosenfield et al., 1984). De Castro (1985) showed that families with at least one sick member tended to shift the workload to healthy family members, thereby reducing (and also spreading) the net economic costs of the disease.

Despite the work of these and other researchers, the precise effect of malaria on productivity is still an open question. Using direct measurements of physical ability, for example, at least one study demonstrated that malaria had no effect at all on productivity (Brohult et al., 1981).

Another approach focuses on the potential economic benefits of new agricultural or industrial development made possible by malaria control efforts (Wernsdorfer and Wernsdorfer, 1988). For example, successful malaria control efforts may allow workers to enter previously malarious mining areas, thereby increasing an individual's or company's earnings. If successful control efforts were not undertaken, the costs of malaria in this scenario would be the potential (but unearned) profits that would have accrued from the new mining activity (Griffith et al., 1971). In a similar vein, Sinton (1935, 1936) documents a number of cases in India where malaria prevented expansion into new areas, with substantial losses in forgone earnings.

In a recent study of the impact of malaria in four African countries (Burkina Faso, Chad, Rwanda, and the Congo) a distinction was made between "direct costs" (the out-of-pocket expense of treatment, including transportation and allied expenses) and "indirect costs" (earnings forgone by adults while sick or while caring for sick children, and discounted future earnings lost due to child mortality) (Shepard et al., 1990). In these countries, between three and seven days of production were lost per case of malaria. Extrapolating to the whole of Africa, an average of 2.1 days of output per person were lost, or $1.70 per capita per year.

All of these analytical approaches have shortcomings. For instance, the focus on days lost from work or output forgone is too narrow. A more appropriate measure of "cost" might be the "compensating variation," or the amount of money necessary to return a sick individual to the same level of utility, happiness, satisfaction, and sense of well-being enjoyed prior to the onset of disease. Such a measure would capture the subjective and psychological impact of the illness and would be more inclusive than simply looking at the effect of malaria on worker productivity. Regardless of its appeal, there are no good methods for obtaining this number.

It is possible, however, to infer a lower bound for compensating variation by calculating the total costs of malaria treatment borne by families and individuals. These costs include not only payment for treatment but also the time and money spent on transportation, family care for patients, and preventive measures at the household and community levels. All of these calculations are affected by other variables, of which the most important may be access to appropriate care, and are subject to significant underestimation. (For example, there may be costs incurred by the individual before formal treatment is sought, and some individuals may decide that the costs of seeking treatment and forgoing income outweigh the uncertain costs of letting the disease run its course.)

To illustrate how this approach can be applied, a study in Thailand

(Kaewsonthi, 1989) estimated, among other things, patient costs associated with seeking local treatment for malaria prior to receiving care at a government-supported health center. These "external" expenses amounted to an average of $20 per positive case, nine times the average Thai minimum daily wage. For Thailand as a whole, external costs equaled about 45 percent of what the government itself spent to treat these patients. This is probably a considerable underestimation of actual patient costs, since productive time lost before and after seeking treatment—which may depend in part on the speed of the service provided and varies within and among countries—was not taken into account.

It is clear from this review of the literature that the analytical approaches used to study the costs of malaria are incomplete and difficult to compare with one another. The result, as noted by Andreano and Helminiak (1988), is that "we remain woefully ignorant of the social and economic effect of malaria in those countries of the world where it is prevalent."

Costs and Effects of Malaria Control

While there has been progress in estimating the economic burden of malaria, estimates of the relative costs and impacts of interventions used to control the disease are less satisfactory. The predominant analytical method has used cost-effectiveness to help policymakers choose among policy alternatives. The primary measure, the cost-effectiveness ratio, represents the costs of a given intervention divided by a given outcome, with the outcome usually expressed in terms of the number of cases prevented (lives or life-years saved, the latter sometimes corrected for quality and with future years discounted).

Average cost-effectiveness ratios are widely used, but they can be quite misleading and should be viewed with great caution (Doubilet et al., 1986). Barlow and Grobar (1986) and Mills (1987) have summarized the results of a number of studies that calculated the costs per year of life saved (Table 11-1) and cost-benefit ratios (Table 11-2) for malaria control efforts in various countries over the past two decades. Table 11-1 also includes calculations of the cost per discounted quality adjusted life-years (QALY) saved by the program under analysis (Jamison and Mosley, 1990).[1]

These data are most striking because of their variability; it is hard to make any generalizations about them. The costs per case prevented ranged from $2.10 to $260 (in 1987 dollars), and cost-benefit ratios ranged from 2.4 to 150. The higher cost-benefit figures make malaria control seem of

---

[1] QALYs attempt to adjust for sickness or premature death. Healthy years or days are given higher weights than unhealthy days or years. Often, as with basic accounting principles, the value of future years is discounted to the present.

TABLE 11-1 Cost Effectiveness of Malaria Control

			Cost (1987$)		
Author(s)	Country	Method	per Case Prevented	per Death Averted	per Discounted QALY Saved
Barlow (1968)	Sri Lanka	Insecticide		78	2.80
Cohn (1973)	India	Insecticide	2.10		7.00
Gandahusada et al. (1984)	Indonesia	Insecticide	83-102		275-618
Hedman et al. (1979)	Liberia	Vector control and chemo-therapy	14		143
Kaewsonthi and Harding (1984)	Thailand	Vector control and chemo-therapy	27-74		90-760
Mills (1987)	Nepal	Vector control and chemo-therapy	1.30-172		2.80-255
Molineaux and Gramiccia (1980)	Nigeria	Vector control and chemo-therapy	259		1,500-2,650
Ortiz (1968)	Paraguay	Insecticides	60		71
Walsh and Warren (1979)	LDCs	Vector control		990	34

SOURCES: Barlow and Grobar (1986); Mills (1987); authors' calculations.

TABLE 11-2 Cost-Benefit Ratios in Malaria Control

Author(s)	Country	Method	Cost-Benefit Ratio
Barlow (1968)	Sri Lanka	Insecticide	146
Griffith et al. (1971)	Thailand	Chemoprophylaxis	6.5
Khan (1966)	Pakistan	Eradication program	4.9
Livadas and Athanassatos (1963)	Greece	Eradication program	17.3
Niazi (1969)	Iraq	Eradication program	6.0
Ortiz (1968)	Paraguay	Insecticides	3.6
San Pedro (1967-1968)	Philippines	Eradication program	2.4
Democratic Republic of Sudan (1975)	Sudan	Control program	4.6

SOURCE: Barlow and Grobar (1986).

utmost economic importance, while the lower figures make malaria control appear no more urgent than a number of other government programs.

Unfortunately, there are no simple methodological explanations for this variability that could guide future cost-benefit calculations. Differences in data quality, the assumptions used in the analyses, the definition of relevant costs, the length of the study period, the discount rate applied, and the coverage and purpose of the original intervention all contribute to, but do not account for, the variation. For example, the Garki Project study (Molineaux and Gramiccia, 1980), which generated an estimate of $260 saved for every case of malaria prevented per year, included as part of overall project costs the expenditures on research and monitoring that accompanied the intervention. Some studies added in administrative costs to their computations, while others included only the cost of materials. While some calculations were based on small pilot projects (Gandahusada et al., 1984), others were based on large national efforts (Barlow, 1968). Finally, case fatality rates were assumed for those countries with data only on cases averted per year. Costs per QALY are sensitive to these assumptions.[2]

Even if standardized research methods were used, the cost-benefit and cost-effectiveness ratios from these studies would vary greatly. That is because this variation has more to do with the inherent variability of malaria than with differences in research design. There are four underlying reasons for the wide variations seen in these cost-effectiveness ratios: levels of endemicity, temporal variability, organization structure, and returns to scale.

Levels of Endemicity   Differences in the ecologic, epidemiologic, and social characteristics of each study region help determine the effectiveness of control programs per dollar spent (see Chapter 10). While the most crucial of these is the degree of endemicity, other factors, such as the behavior of the mosquito population, the presence of nonimmune individuals, and the degree of parasite resistance to chloroquine, also contribute.

Temporal Variability   Depending on the degree of endemicity, there can be substantial variations in malaria prevalence within the same region at different times during the year or between years. Since costs per death or illness averted are likely to vary inversely with the prevalence rate, the usefulness of cost calculations based on a single year is questionable. Consequently, policy options should be evaluated on the basis of their "ex-

---

[2] Following Lancaster (1990), case fatality rates were assumed to be 1 percent for India, 0.25 percent for Liberia and Nigeria, 3 percent for Paraguay, and a range of 0.2 to 1 percent for the rest of Asia, based on the figure for India and data from Malaysia.

pected" value, taking into account the distribution of prevalences at different times. This is particularly important if costs include a fixed component, such as the administrative costs for control organizations, that does not depend on the disease prevalence in any one year.

Organizational Structure Control programs may be highly structured and single-purpose (vertical), or they may be integrated with other components of the health care system and somewhat unstructured (horizontal). Assessing control policies in integrated settings requires that the costs of providing general health care to be separated from costs specific to malaria control. As a rule, the higher the volume of cases, the more similar the costs of integrated and free-standing programs are likely to be (Mills, 1987). In areas with few cases, however, integrated programs can cost considerably less, since health personnel can more efficiently serve patients with different health needs, as demand requires.

Returns to Scale The intensity of the intervention has a substantial effect on both costs and effectiveness. The concept of returns to scale is useful for determining what level of intervention is appropriate, given its expected effect on some desirable outcome. Although certain costs are relatively fixed (facilities, staff salaries), others increase as the workload increases. In addition, many malaria control programs that rely on single interventions experience diminishing returns. The expense of vector control activities, for example, will increase as the program moves into peripheral areas where there are fewer people and, possibly, fewer mosquitoes per unit area covered. Similarly, the costs of case management will rise when there is a shift from passive to active case detection. Analyses that estimate costs only at a single level of intensity will be of limited value if extrapolations are made to higher levels of intensity. Barlow and Grobar (1986) suggest that because cost estimates for parasitic disease control programs are uncertain, a combination of policies (a "portfolio" of instruments) should be used. However, even if program personnel were armed with perfect knowledge of the costs and effects of various strategies, a diversified approach would still be desirable given the reality of diminishing returns to any single instrument (see Example 3 below).

Operational Research

Much of the best recent research on the economics of malaria control has been designed to answer specific questions about service delivery in specific geographic areas. Using this type of operational research it is relatively easy to gauge costs, since changes in scale are not an issue. Incremental benefits can also be assessed in relation to local epidemiology and institutional and administrative conditions. Such exercises can greatly improve resource allocation and program decisions by local-level managers.

In two studies (Kaewsonthi, 1989; Mills, 1987), comparisons among techniques of vector control, and between vector control and therapy, were illuminated by carefully calculating the costs at the local level. The authors also were able to propose a set of practical recommendations based on their analyses. Mills, for example, was able to suggest reducing active malaria case detection and increasing investment in malaria clinics (or other treatment-based facilities) in Nepal. According to that study, either alternative was more cost-effective than spraying pesticide to kill mosquitoes.

Although few studies have done so, operational research can be used to assess "decreasing effectiveness"—the point at which the cost-effectiveness ratio of a given intervention drops enough to merit a reevaluation of its worth. Using such a method, Ettling et al. (1990) documented the increasing costs of expanding clinic coverage in a district in Thailand, making clear the trade-off between numbers of cases treated and the cost per case. Researchers at the Centers for Disease Control (Sudre et al., 1990) examined the relative costs of alternative drug therapies under differing degrees of chloroquine resistance. The salient variables in this decision-making process, including patient compliance with drug regimens, were also identified.

A review of the regulation and control of pharmaceuticals in Africa south of the Sahara (Foster, 1990) highlights the savings and improved health resulting from the effective use of drugs, and the costs of misdiagnosis, prescribing errors, and compliance failure. Another study took a more theoretical approach: the relative merits of over-the-counter and prescription drug sales were examined, and the possible loss of accurate drug use of the former was compared with its potential for increasing access and affordability (Hammer, in press). Other ongoing work has highlighted the problems of malaria-related infant and child mortality in endemic regions of Africa. One conclusion emerging from that work is that prenatal prophylaxis, undertaken early in pregnancy and especially for first pregnancies, can reduce low birth weight and infant mortality. From a policy perspective, this raises the issue of how women who have not felt sick from malaria for years and who do not normally seek prenatal care can be convinced to take preventive measures. All of these studies suggest that improved education of prescribers or patients about drug therapies can have beneficial effects.

Economics and Policymaking

In any analysis of any government program, such as malaria control, it is important to realize that different decision makers have fundamentally different perspectives. The top levels of government, for example, must weigh the value of resources put into the health sector as opposed to other sectors, such as education or agriculture. Within the health sector, policymakers must choose between malaria and other diseases. Administrators of malaria control or primary health care programs, for their part, must allocate resources among a variety of interventions, such as spraying or case management. Local project managers may have to select among different vector control interventions or drug protocols.

Studies of the economic costs of malaria control generally do not provide the information that would be most useful to policymakers. In lieu of firm quantitative estimates of the costs of various malaria control interventions, qualitative judgments (with variable degrees of documentation) are often made. This approach may be adequate in many cases, but local decision makers would be greatly aided if more precise estimates were available. Further, to be truly effective, decisions affecting policy must take into account what is truly within the control of the policymaker. The relationships among the various instruments available to the policymaker, the objectives of the program, and program costs also must be determined.

Determining Policy Options

Determining what policy options (instruments) are available for disease control is more complicated than it seems. Epidemiologic research typically identifies risk factors associated with a specific disease; however, the degree to which these risk factors can be affected by policy is not always clear.

Instruments In the case of malaria, while it may be possible to identify the effect of vectorial capacity on the incidence of disease, neither vectorial capacity nor any of its components are directly controllable by policymakers (see Chapter 7), nor do policymakers control the number or proportion of houses sprayed with pesticide or, by extension, the death rate of mosquitoes. The relevant instrument actually is the hiring and training of sprayers; whether they actually spray houses, or do so successfully, is another matter. Similarly, for drug therapy, although the technical effectiveness of a specific protocol may be well documented, the degree to which that protocol affects disease prevalence depends on how many people seek treatment and how well they comply with the drug regimens. In both of these instances, the intervening variable is a function of some kind of managerial or monitoring capability, the presence or absence of which determines how effectively the policy instrument affects the program in question.

In fact, many aspects of malaria case management depend on the structure of the health care system. The government's role and ability to influence outcomes thus are quite context specific. Malaria policy in situations in which health care is provided within the family or by private-sector traditional healers, physicians, nurses, or pharmacists will be different than in cases in which the bulk of services are provided by public primary health facilities or malaria clinics. The instruments applied in the former might be taxes, subsidies, or information campaigns geared to encouraging the use of certain drugs; in the latter, the instrument might be drug protocols that more directly control the types and dosages of drugs used. For example, in the case of drug therapy, the relevant policy options are more likely to include information, education, and communication (IEC) services, or active case detection methods, rather than simply the choice of drug.

Outcomes When the results, or outcome, of an intervention can be valued in some unit of account such as money, cost-benefit analysis becomes possible and investments in health can be compared with those for other government-supported activities such as road building. Short of this, intermediate outcomes can be selected and compared across projects. In health, the number of lives saved is one such measure.

Once an outcome, such as lives saved, is chosen, the impact of each dollar spent or program pursued on the outcome needs to be determined. For a number of reasons, this type of information is hard to come by. While a policy option may be directed toward a specific objective, its effects may be felt in other areas: vector control aimed at halting malaria transmission may affect the transmission of other diseases or may degrade the environment; changes in water management practices can affect agriculture; more accurate diagnostic techniques may improve the treatment of other diseases. These external effects, positive or negative, cannot be ignored in calculations of cost-effectiveness, but they are difficult to track and measure.

A policy's effectiveness (and its marginal benefit) also varies according to the extent to which it is implemented; this leads, in turn, to either higher or lower costs (the marginal cost) per life saved. If a new clinic is built, the per-capita costs of the initial investment will decline if the number of users increases over time. In contrast, the effectiveness of an information campaign may decline and per-capita costs therefore increase as more and more is spent to reach those living in remote areas.

Epidemiology and Economics

The relationship between economics and malaria epidemiology in the policy arena has largely been expressed in the rather static calculation of "burden of disease." The goal of an economics-based approach, however, is to describe how people make choices and prescribe how governments should make them. The fact that malaria affects hundreds of million of people does not, in and of itself, make the disease a priority for policymakers. What matters to the economist (and to policymakers and those directly in charge of control programs) is whether something can be done about the disease. Policy choices should be made on the basis of the effects that those policies will have on outcomes, not on the size of the problem.

An important exception to this concept is found in basic research, where the benefits of investing in a project are speculative. In cases like this, policymakers might opt to invest heavily, despite an uncertain return, in the hope that the payoff will be large. For any disease, the burden of the disease at least defines the upper bound of a control project's value.

The examples that follow illustrate four fundamental economic concepts: first, the absolute magnitude of the burden of a disease is not a proper criterion for setting priorities in health; second, changes in costs that occur at different levels of intensity of activity affect the optimal allocations of resources; third, this pattern of costs requires a mix of malaria control strategies; and fourth, average cost-effectiveness is not a proper criterion for setting policy priorities. A fifth example illustrates the use of the epidemiologic paradigms, discussed in Chapter 10, for economic decision making.

Example 1: The Burden of Disease and Priority Setting

There are two diseases. Disease A kills 1,000 people per year, and disease B kills 30 people per year. It so happens that it costs $100 per person to prevent people from dying of disease A and $50 per person to prevent death from disease B. The Ministry of Health has $10,000 for disease control. How should it spend the money?

If priorities are set by ranking diseases by "importance," as measured by mortality rates, disease A wins easily since it kills more than 30 times as many people as disease B. If all resources were devoted to disease A, the Ministry could save 100 lives ($10,000/100). However, if resources were devoted to each of the diseases in proportion to their mortality rates, disease A would receive $9,700, disease B would get the rest, and a total of 103 lives would be saved: six disease-B patients (using the $300) and 97 disease-A patients. The ministry could do even better, though, were it to give the $1,500 needed to eradicate the less important disease, disease B, and use the remaining $8,500 to treat patients who have disease A. In this case, 115 patients would be saved: 30 with disease B and 85 with disease A.

In this example, priorities set by looking only at the burden of disease are exactly backwards. It is the disease with the lower total burden that should have the first priority, not the one that is more prevalent. Interventions should be ranked in order of the marginal effect of each additional unit of input, whether in dollars, hours, or number of patients seen. Interventions are carried out in this order until the budget is exhausted (as in this case) or until the marginal effect is no longer greater than the marginal cost of other uses of these funds. For instance, if it were determined that each life saved was worth $60 (either because that is how much saving lives from all other causes would cost or, more contentiously, because someone decided that was what lives are worth), then only disease B would warrant intervention.

Example 2: Decreasing Returns

In this instance, the cost of controlling disease B remains at $50 per life saved, but costs associated with disease A are now different: 100 people can be saved at a cost of $25 apiece, but the remaining 900 would cost $100, as in example 1. This situation might arise if there were different techniques for dealing with the disease and the cheaper technique was subject to some capacity limits. Alternatively, there may be only one technique that becomes less effective as its use increases. For example, drug therapy may be inexpensive for patients treated in a clinic setting but quite expensive if health workers have to go into the field to detect and treat cases. With this cost structure and the same $10,000 budget, what should the Ministry of Health do?

If disease A is a priority because of the burden-of-disease argument, 175 lives are saved: 100 at a cost of $2,500 and 75 at a cost of $7,500. More lives could be saved, however, if the criterion used in example 1 were applied. First, $2,500 spent on disease A would save 100 lives. Next, attention would turn to disease B, where 30 lives could be saved for $1,500. The remaining $6,000 could then be spent on the more expensive technique for controlling disease A, saving 60 lives, for a total of 190 lives saved. If the marginal benefits are compared with the marginal cost of $60, as in example 1, the first 100 people suffering from disease A and the 30 people suffering from B would be saved. The rest of the money would be used elsewhere in the health sector (or in another part of the economy).

Figure 11-1 shows the relationship between money spent and lives saved in examples 1 and 2. Path OABC represents the strategy of using the $25 technique (from O to A) for disease A, followed by spending on disease B (A to B), and finishing with a return to the less effective technique for A (B to C). Had all resources gone to disease A, we would have followed path OAD, which completely misses the opportunity to reduce mortality due to disease B.

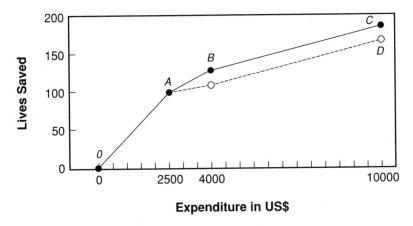

Expenditure in US$

FIGURE 11-1 Examples 1 and 2: visual representation.

Example 3: More Decreasing Returns

There is only one disease, disease A, but there are two possible interventions. For vector control, the cost is $25 per person for the first 100 individuals who benefit and $100 thereafter. This difference in cost may reflect the relative success of focal spraying, which by definition is limited in its applicability, contrasted with control operations that are more widespread and have a lower success rate. The second intervention, passive case detection, can save 200 people for a cost of $10 apiece if they are treated at a clinic. However, if active detection is required, the cost rises to $33.33 per person.

Given the same budget constraint of $10,000, the optimal strategy would be to treat the 200 people who come to the clinic (costing $2,000), conduct focal spraying to save another 100 lives (costing $2,500), and use active case detection methods to exhaust the budget, saving an additional 165 lives. This strategy favors a mixture of techniques as costs increase and returns decrease for single interventions.

Example 4: Average Versus Marginal Costs and Benefits

As in example 3, there are two techniques: vector control and drug therapy. Focal spraying is very effective. It costs $10 per life and can save 200 lives; after that, other vector control techniques are needed which cost $100 to save one life. Drug therapy costs $40 per person. The country's malaria program splits the budget in half, giving $5,000 to vector control and the same amount to malaria clinics for drug procurement. Overall, the policy saves 355 lives (200 from focal spraying, costing $10 per person, 30 from spraying at a cost of $100 per person, and 125 ($5,000/$40) from spending on drug therapy).

An accountant appraises the program and discovers that the average cost of a life saved by vector control is only $21.74 ($5,000/230), while for antimalarial drug therapy, each life saved costs $40. The accountant recommends the vector control operations be expanded at the expense of the clinics.

This is precisely the wrong approach. While the average cost of vector control operations is indeed $21.74, the marginal cost is $100, since the limits of focal spraying (which substantially increased the calculation of average effectiveness) have been reached and the less effective technique of widespread spraying is being used. The correct policy decision would be to reduce vector control spending to $2,000 and use the remaining funds to purchase antimalarial drugs. The number of lives saved would then total 400.

Example 5: Economics and Epidemiologic Paradigms

Depending on the degree of endemicity, control policies have had varying degrees of effectiveness. The most dramatic improvements have occurred in areas of low endemicity, where eradication is at least possible. Even in highly endemic areas, real (though possibly temporary) gains may be possible, and short-run benefits may be worth pursuing. The epidemiologic paradigms in Chapter 10 can be used to determine appropriate malaria control policies. This example illustrates how such polices vary with the particular type of malaria.

Assume that two policies are available: drug therapy and pesticide spraying operations, which can be done in one, two, or three cycles per season. Drug therapy will always save 60 lives per $1,000 spent. On the other hand, the effectiveness of vector operations, in terms of deaths averted per dollar, varies by region. In an urban area where the vectorial capacity is relatively low and spraying can reduce transmission, each round of spraying costs $1,000. A program with one round of spraying saves 100 lives, one with two rounds saves 150 lives, and one with three rounds saves 175 lives. In a forest region, the costs of the program are the same but the numbers of lives saved for the three levels of effort are 10, 15, and 18, respectively. How should these malaria control programs in these areas spend their $3,000 budgets?

In the urban area, the optimal allocation is a single round of spraying, saving 100 lives, with the remainder spent on drug therapy, saving an additional 120 lives, for a total of 220 lives saved. A second round of spraying would have saved only an additional 50 lives for the extra $1,000, compared with 60 lives saved from drugs. The return on the third round of spraying is even worse. In the forest area, even the first round of spraying is not worth the cost. All resources should go to drugs. This will save 180 lives—fewer than in the urban setting, but the best that can be done.

The paradigm approach may also be used to infer the appropriateness of control policies intended to be used in different environments. The inference is not always directly related to overall effectiveness, however, as was true above. In highland fringe areas, which are prone to epidemic malaria, the cost structure may be as follows: a single cycle of spraying saves 75 lives; a second round, 140; and a third round, 170. At every level of spraying effort, vector control in this region yields fewer lives saved than in the periurban areas. However, the appropriate policy in this case is to use two cycles of spraying instead of one. This is because the marginal benefit of the second round of spraying in the epidemic areas is 65 lives per $1,000 (140 - 75), which is still better than the 60 lives saved by drug therapy.

These points are all illustrated in Figure 11-2. For each of the three regions, the number of lives saved by each round of spraying is plotted against costs. For comparison, the number of lives saved by using antimalarial drugs is also plotted as more is spent on therapy (at rate of 60 per $1,000).

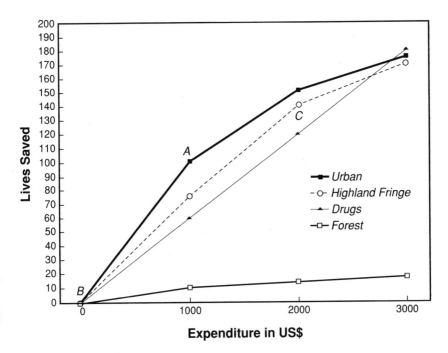

FIGURE 11-2 Example 5: visual representation.

As a rule, vector operations should be expanded as long as the slope of the kinked line is steeper than the line representing drug therapy. The appropriate stopping points are marked A, B, and C, for urban, forest and highland fringe areas, respectively.

RESEARCH AGENDA

The most appropriate malaria control policies will often require a mix of interventions. This mix will vary from one relatively small region to another, and the information needed to assess the effectiveness of each intervention often does not exist.

Decision Making Skills

Malaria is a complicated disease. Malaria control programs need to use a mix of strategies to achieve optimal results, since each instrument is likely to be subject to diminishing returns with expanded use. Further, packages of interventions will be different for each particular type of malaria. Given resource limitations, policymakers need to know the cost and effectiveness of the interventions at their disposal, and they must be aware of the changes in these costs and effects at different scales of implementation and levels of intensity. Unfortunately, the vast majority of policymakers are not aware of these relationships.

> **RESEARCH FOCUS:** Definition of the range of policy choices relevant to malaria control at different levels of decision making, including health care financing, public investments, facility location, education campaigns, and preventive and treatment options.

> **RESEARCH FOCUS:** Assessment of the costs and effectiveness of malaria interventions applied at different levels of intensity in specific areas.

Data Collection

There is a general need for routine collection of economic and financial data related to malaria control. Such information should be epidemiologic in nature, emphasizing the measurement of variables that can be affected by changes in policy, and should be at a level of detail that is useful to decision makers.

> **RESEARCH FOCUS:** Assessment of the fixed and variable costs associated with malaria control programs; de-

termination of how the latter are affected by changes in the level of program effort.

RESEARCH FOCUS: Comparison of the level of effort devoted to malaria control with changes in disease incidence, deaths averted, or cases detected, with the goal of linking specific policy instruments (e.g., houses sprayed and hours worked) to specific epidemiologic types of malaria.

Information, Education, and Communication Programs

IEC programs, or health education generally, may be of great value in improving drug compliance, encouraging women to seek prenatal care, helping people recognize the symptoms of malaria, and encouraging the adoption of personal protection measures. Neither the technology (costs and effectiveness) of providing this information, the effect of this information on behavior, nor the effect of behavior on incidence is well known.

RESEARCH FOCUS: Assessment of the impact of IEC programs on human behavior in different regions.

Resources

The epidemiology of malaria is often shaped by activities in other sectors (e.g., agriculture, industry, and housing). Similarly, malaria often poses an economic cost to activities within these sectors, as discussed in this chapter. Given the limited funds spent on health by many countries, any contribution to malaria control efforts by non-health-related ministries, sectors, and authorities within a malaria endemic country could prove beneficial in the long term. (For example, agricultural extension workers could collect information about water management or insecticide use and its relationship to malaria transmission during their routine activities.)

RESEARCH FOCUS: Determination of how better to take advantage of the resources of both governmental and nongovernmental entities for malaria control within malaria endemic countries.

REFERENCES

Andreano, R., and T. Helminiak. 1988. Economics, health, and tropical disease: a review. Pp. 19-72 in Economics, Health and Tropical Diseases, Herrin, A. N., and P. L. Rosenfield, eds. Manila: University of the Philippines School of Economics.

Audibert, M. 1986. Agricultural non-wage production and health status: a case-study in a tropical environment. Journal of Development Economics 24:275-291.

Barlow, R. 1968. The Economic Effects of Malaria Eradication. Ann Arbor: Bureau of Public Health Economics, University of Michigan.

Barlow, R., and L. M. Grobar. 1986. Costs and benefits of controlling parasitic diseases. PHN Technical Note 85-17. Washington, D.C.: World Bank.

Bhombore, S. R., C. B. Worth, and K. S. Nanjundiah. 1952. A survey of the economic status of villagers in a malarious irrigated tract in Mysore State, India, before and after DDT residual insecticidal spraying. Indian Journal of Malariology 6:355-365.

Brohult, J., L. Jorfeldt, L. Rombo, A. Bjorkman, P.-O. Pehrson, V. Sirleaf, and E. Bengtsson. 1981. The working capacity of Liberian males: a comparison between urban and rural populations in relation to malaria. Annals of Tropical Medicine and Parasitology 75:487-494.

de Castro, B. 1985. Development of Research-Training Project in Socio-Economics of Malaria Eradication in Colombia. Geneva: World Health Organization.

Cohn, E. J. 1973. Assessing the costs and benefits of anti-malaria programs: the Indian experience. American Journal of Public Health 63:1086-1096.

Conly, G. N. 1975. The Impact of Malaria on Economic Development: A Case Study. Washington, D.C.: Pan American Health Organization.

Democratic Republic of Sudan. 1975. National Health Programme 1977/78-1983/84, Khartoum: Government Printing Office.

Doubilet, P., M. C. Weinstein, and B. J. McNeil. 1986. Use and mis-use of the term "cost-effective" in medicine. New England Journal of Medicine 314:253-256.

Ettling, M. B., S. Krachaiklin, K. Thimasarn, and D. Shepard. 1990. Evaluation of Malaria in Maesot, Thailand. Thailand: Malaria Division, Ministry of Public Health.

Foster, S. D. 1990. Improving the Supply and Use of Essential Drugs in Sub-Saharan Africa. PRE Working Paper Series 457. Washington, D.C.: World Bank.

Gandahusada, S., G. A. Fleming, Sukamto, T. Damar, Suwarto, N. Sustriayu, Y. H. Bang, S. Arwati, and H. Arif. 1984. Malaria control with residual fenitrothion in Central Java, Indonesia: an operational-scale trial using both full and selective coverage treatments. Bulletin of the World Health Organization 62:783-794.

Griffith, D. H. S., D. V. Ramana, and H. Mashaal. 1971. Contribution of health to development. International Journal of Health Services 1:253-318.

Hammer, J. In press. To prescribe or not to prescribe: on the regulation of pharmaceuticals in less developed countries. Social Science and Medicine.

Hedman, P., J. Brohult, J. Forslund, V. Sirleaf, and E. Bengtsson. 1979. A pocket of controlled malaria in a holoendemic region of West Africa. Annals of Tropical Medicine and Parasitology 73:317-325.

Jamison, D. T., and W. H. Mosley. 1990. Selecting disease control priorities in developing countries (3rd draft). Pp. 1-66 in Disease Control Priorities in Developing Countries, Jamison, D. T., and W. H. Mosley, eds. Washington, D.C.: Population, Health and Nutrition Division, World Bank.

Kaewsonthi, S. 1989. Costs and performance of malaria surveillance and monitoring in Thailand: a retrospective study based on apportionment of expenditure under budget headings. Social and Economic Research Project Reports No. 5. Geneva: UNDP/World Bank/WHO Special Programme on Research and Training in Tropical Diseases.

Kaewsonthi, S., and A. G. Harding. 1984. Cost and performance of malaria surveillance in Thailand. Social Science and Medicine 19:1081-1097.

Khan, M. J. 1966. Estimate of economic loss due to malaria in West Pakistan. Pakistan Journal of Health 16:187-193.

Lancaster, H. O. 1990. Expectations of Life. New York: Springer-Verlag.

Livadas, G. A., and D. Athanassatos. 1963. The economic benefits of malaria eradication in Greece. Rivista di Malariologia 42:178-187.

Malik, I. H. 1966. Economic advantages of anti-malaria measures amongst the rural population. Publication No. 137. Lahore: The Board of Economic Inquiry.

Mills, A. 1987. Economic study of malaria in Nepal: the cost effectiveness of malaria control strategies. London: Evaluation and Planning Center, London School of Hygiene and Tropical Medicine.

Molineaux, L., and G. Gramiccia. 1980. The Garki Project: Research on the Epidemiology and Control of Malaria in the Sudan Savanna of West Africa. Washington, D.C.: Population, Health and Nutrition Division, World Bank.

Niazi, A. D. 1969. Approximate estimates of the economic loss caused by malaria with some estimates of the benefits of M.E.P. in Iraq. Bulletin of Endemic Diseases 2:28-39.

Ortiz, J. R. 1968. Estimate of the cost of a malaria eradication program. Bulletin of the Pan American Health Organization 64:14-17.

Over, M., R. Ellis, J. Huber, and O. Solon. 1990. The consequences of adult ill-health. Pp. 4.1-4.25 in The Health of Adults in the Developing World, Feachem, R., T. Kjellstrom, C. J. L. Murray, M. Over, and M. Phillips, eds. Washington, D.C.: World Bank.

Quo, W. K. 1959. Malaria Information. Unpublished document. Geneva: World Health Organization.

Rosenfield, P. L., F. Golladay, and R. K. Davidson. 1984. The economics of parasitic diseases: research priorities. Social Science and Medicine 19:1117-1126.

Russell, P. F., and M. K. Menon. 1942. A malario-economic survey in rural South India. Indian Medical Gazette 77:167-180.

San Pedro, C. 1967-1968. Economic costs and benefits of malaria eradication. Philippines Journal of Public Health 12:5-24.

Shepard, D. S., U. Brinkmann, M. Ettling, and R. Sauerborn. 1990. Economic Impact of Malaria in Africa. Arlington: Vector Biology and Control Project, U.S. Agency for International Development.

Sinton, J. A. 1935. What malaria costs India, nationally, socially and economically. Records of the Malaria Survey of India 5:223-264, 413-489.

Sinton, J. A. 1936. What malaria costs India, nationally, socially and economically. Records of the Malaria Survey of India 6:96-169.

Sudre, P., J. G. Breman, D. McFarland, and J. P. Koplan. 1990. Treatment of Chloroquine-Resistant Malaria in African Children: A Cost Effective Analysis. Atlanta: Centers for Disease Control.

Van Dine, D. L. 1916. The relation of malaria to crop production. Scientific Monthly November:431-439.

Walsh, J. A., and K. S. Warren. 1979. Selective primary health care: an interim strategy for disease control in developing countries. New England Journal of Medicine 301:967-974.

Wernsdorfer, G., and W. H. Wernsdorfer. 1988. Social and economic aspects of malaria and its control. Pp. 1421-1471 in Malaria, Principles and Practice of Malariology, Wernsdorfer, W. H., and I. McGregor, eds. New York: Churchill Livingstone.

12

Social and Behavioral Aspects of Malaria

WHERE WE WANT TO BE IN THE YEAR 2010

There is widespread recognition that understanding the human re-sponse to malaria and to control programs is crucial to the success of all malaria control strategies. Because of an improved under-standing of the way people perceive malaria, many social and be-havioral barriers to the acceptance and use of prevention measures will be addressed in the design of malaria control programs. Simi-larly, a better grasp of health-seeking and treatment behavior will lead to more effective health communication strategies for malaria and the promotion of early and effective treatment of clinical cases of malaria, especially among young children. Community represen-tatives will be active participants in the planning and implementa-tion of malaria prevention and control programs. Many communi-ties, particularly those in semiurban areas, will develop innovative ways of reducing larval development sites and at a minimal cost to outside resources, whether governmental or nongovernmental.

WHERE WE ARE TODAY

With the spread of insecticide-resistant vectors and chloroquine-re-sistant *Plasmodium falciparum*, malaria control program planners in many parts of the world are finding that available control measures are either too expensive, not efficacious, or efficacious only under certain conditions. Obtaining high rates of acceptance and use of such interventions, especially those that are marginally efficacious, is crucial to the success of control efforts. Human behavior and social organization—one side of malaria's host-vector-parasite triangle—are clearly vital determinants for the success of control programs. Unfortunately, we do not know enough about how humans respond to malaria to be able to build strong multidisciplinary control programs.

Historically, social scientists have had little or no role in the design and evaluation of malaria control programs. In modern malaria control programs, there is a clear need for applied social science research and the participation of social scientists. The choice of control methods appropriate for a specific community or region requires an understanding of how factors such as deforestation and the movement of populations from one region to another affect the local epidemiology of malaria. Many of these factors have their roots in social and economic change.

It is the behavior of individuals and groups that determines how or whether efforts to prevent or treat malaria will be successful. To attain high rates of acceptance or use of a given control method, attention must be paid to a number of important considerations: (1) local perceptions of malaria and its causes, (2) the manner in which people decide whether a given treatment or preventive measure is efficacious, (3) patterns of treatment-seeking behavior during episodes of malaria, and (4) the role that the community as a whole plays in planning, implementing, and evaluating the control program.

Social science research has often been criticized as anecdotal, unfocused on practical outcomes, and overly academic. These characterizations have little validity today. New research approaches to the social sciences that focus on participatory activities and multidisciplinary problem solving, combined with the adoption of formal and survey research methodologies, have narrowed the gap between the social and natural sciences.

Factors Favoring Malaria Transmission

The constancy of endemic malaria in certain parts of the world, and the resurgence of the disease in areas where eradication efforts were undertaken, are in large measure due to the interplay of broad social, cultural, and economic factors. Three such factors—agricultural development, population movement, and urbanization—are particularly important determinants of patterns of malaria transmission.

Agricultural Development

The link between farming and malaria has a long history. In West Africa some 2,000 years ago, the advent of iron tools and higher-yield crops made the rain forest worth exploiting for agriculture (Livingstone, 1958). The Bantus of the central Benue River valley (what is now Nigeria) were perhaps the first to use iron tools to clear forests for farming. Their "slash-and-burn" and "slash-and-mulch" agricultural techniques may have set the stage for much of the current experience with malaria on the African continent.

Anopheles gambiae mosquitoes account for most of the malaria transmission in Africa south of the Sahara. These insects do not breed in full shade, and it was only after tropical rain forests began to be cleared for crop production that sunlight-exposed pools of standing water, ideal sites for larval development for *An. gambiae*, were created (Coluzzi et al., 1985). Forest clearing also causes soil erosion, which in river valleys can attract mosquitoes to newly formed swamps (Laderman, 1975).

The formation of small towns facilitates malaria transmission as a consequence of farming, which concentrates populations in relatively confined areas. Towns are often located near water supplies or, through change and disruption of the local environment, promote other potential larval development sites. A burrow pit dug at the edge of a village to collect material for construction often fills with water and serves as an ideal haven for mosquito larvae (Bruce-Chwatt and de Zulueta, 1980).

It is no accident that most malaria occurs in rural agricultural communities. Agricultural settlement often brings changes in water use, alters the concentration of domesticated and wild animals, and causes deforestation, all of which can boost the number of larval development sites and increase human-mosquito contact.

Irrigation practices that use canals or pumps to periodically flood fields for crops such as rice have a great impact on mosquito breeding. One type of livestock may attract a particular species of *Anopheles* but not another. The form of ownership of agricultural land and the type of labor utilized, such as sharecropping, also can affect the spread of and exposure to malaria parasites.

Finally, the use of certain chemicals to increase crop production may have an indirect impact on the spread of malaria. High-yield varieties of crops require significant quantities of pesticides and fertilizers. Several studies have cited the use of pesticides in agriculture as a principal contributor to mosquito resistance to DDT in Central America, India, and other regions (Chapin and Wasserstrom, 1981, 1983). Other evidence suggests that DDT resistance can also be caused by antimosquito spraying (Curtis, 1981; Chapin and Wasserstrom, 1983).

Type I and Type II Farming Systems

For the purpose of discussing the interaction between agriculture and malaria, farming systems can be divided into two primary types: type I systems, typically smallholder-subsistence or "minifundia" cash-crop businesses, in which land-use rights are held by the farmers working the land; and larger, type II systems, in which the land is not owned by the people who farm it and frequent use is made of migrant or wage laborers. This distinction is similar to that drawn by Bruce-Chwatt (1987) between "rural areas" and "development projects."

In type II farming, changes in land tenure often occur as land is consolidated into larger parcels. Plantations and capital-intensive agro-industry are two common type II farming arrangements. Poor sanitary conditions among farm workers in type II farming systems favor the transmission of malaria and other diseases that can decimate a work force and make it necessary to import more laborers. For example, the importation of African slaves into Mexico and the establishment of sugarcane plantations there created conditions favorable for *P. falciparum*, to which many Africans already had some natural immunity (Friedlander, 1969). This resulted in an increase in the already high mortality rate among the indigenous Indian workers and a corresponding increased demand for African slaves.

In the early 1900s, the Italian physician Antonio Celli observed that in southern Europe malaria tended to disproportionately affect the poor or landless, especially those who were seasonal laborers on large farms (Celli, 1900; Chapin and Wasserstrom, 1981). Celli reasoned that transmission depended on the flow of nonimmune persons into malarious zones just before the annual peak of the *Anopheles* population.

Packard (1984), in a study of colonial Swaziland, has shown how changes in land ownership and labor utilization can increase malaria transmission. Much of the country's best land was given to European colonial miners, farmers, and land speculators. That, combined with the thinning of cattle herds by an epidemic of rinderpest in 1886 and the decline in traditional Swazi raiding activities, turned the native population from essentially self-sufficient food producers into agricultural wage laborers.

Under this arrangement, it was more difficult to cope with drought, and years of drought became years of famine. The occurrence of major epidemics of malaria in Swaziland in 1923, 1932, 1939, 1942, and 1946 appears to be related not only to the rainfall in the year of the epidemic but also to famine conditions in the preceding year. This suggests that sound land reform and agricultural policies, as well as public health measures, can play an important role in malaria control.

Type II farms are also distinguished by their large-scale use of water. Irrigation is common to almost all forms of type II farming systems. Studies of irrigation projects in India have linked increases in mosquito populations to higher subsoil water tables and to the creation of small side channels suitable for larval development when the canal is refilled (Covell, 1946; Hyma and Ramesh, 1980).

Large dams, which often accompany irrigation projects, create additional opportunities for malaria to gain a foothold. Mosquitoes can breed in the reservoir itself, especially if its edges are not kept clean of vegetation. Seepage from the dam and pooling also can occur, providing new larval development sites. Finally, all large dam projects require that considerable numbers of construction workers be brought to the dam site (Covell, 1946; Hyma and Ramesh, 1980). When nonimmune workers are exposed to malaria, or when malaria is introduced by workers from endemic regions, epidemic malaria may result.

Economic development programs that incorporate dam construction, irrigation, or "green revolution" technologies—also typical of type II farming—likely will change malaria epidemiology. Any development project that alters preexisting relationships between humans and their environment should be evaluated within an ecological framework (Hughes and Hunter, 1970). Careful planning before such projects are undertaken can reduce or eliminate the potential for malaria transmission.

Human Population Movements

The importance of human population movements to malaria control cannot be overemphasized. In fact, such shifts may contribute to the spread of chloroquine-resistant *P. falciparum*. In many African countries, for example, people move from permanent settlements to rural farms during the early months of the wet season, when cultivation, planting, and weeding are carried out (Prothero, 1961). A variation on this pattern is the seasonal movement of pastoralists tending their livestock between mountain and lowland pastures. Religious pilgrimage, need for employment, drought, famine, war, resettlement, and tourism all contribute to the ebb and flow of populations and the spread of malaria.

Population movement increases malaria transmission in four principal ways. First, such movement often introduces nonimmune people into endemic areas or infected people into malaria-free regions. For example, the higher incidence of malaria among Afghan refugees living in Pakistan than among the indigenous population reflects the Afghans' lower level of preexisting immunity (Suleman, 1988).

Second, the living conditions of migrants differ markedly from those of settled populations, resulting in greater exposure to infected mosquitoes.

Housing, if available, is crowded, of poor quality, and often located adjacent to *Anopheles* breeding sites.

Third, the type of work performed by migrants and the conditions under which they work often result in greater exposure to malaria-infected mosquitoes. Much of the work, especially if it is illegal (for example, gem mining, gold prospecting, and drug smuggling), is performed at night, when *Anopheles* mosquitoes are most likely to be biting. In addition, since employment for migrants is usually seasonal or temporary, there are periods when no funds are available for malaria treatment.

Finally, migrant populations rarely are served by government malaria control programs. Even if they are served, most control methods, such as residual application of insecticides to walls of houses, chloroquine prophylaxis for pregnant women, and screening of houses, may be difficult or impossible to implement. For example, gold miners who work along the Madeira River in the Brazilian Amazon live in temporary shelters without walls. The absence of walls makes insecticide spraying impractical and allows mosquitoes to enter freely at night (Coimbra, 1988).

The illegal status of some migrants further complicates efforts at malaria control. During the 1960s, for example, Mozambican laborers were hired to work on sugar estates in Swaziland. When the use of Mozambican laborers instead of indigenous Swazi workers became a political issue, the government of Swaziland imposed restrictions on the use of foreign labor, but Mozambicans continued to migrate and work illegally in the country. Swaziland health authorities had difficulty detecting cases of malaria among these migrants because of their illegal status and the sugar industry's lack of cooperation (Packard, 1986).

Most studies of the dynamics of malaria transmission treat human populations as though they are static. Even research that examines the effects of population movement, such as the Garki project (Molineaux and Gramiccia, 1980), fails to assess such shifts or to adequately distinguish between them.

Urbanization

Diseases transmitted by insect vectors continue to be thought of primarily as illnesses of rural areas. While the insect vectors for some diseases, such as onchocerciasis (river blindness) and African trypanosomiasis (sleeping sickness), are exclusively rural, some of the mosquito vectors that carry malaria, Bancroftian filariasis (elephantiasis), Japanese encephalitis, and dengue hemorrhagic fever have become well adapted to city life (Bang and Shah, 1988; Dunn, 1988). In general, urban areas have higher population densities, which allow for increased rates of disease transmission, large numbers of larval development sites due to water storage practices, and limited methods for disposal of wastewater and refuse.

Anopheles stephensi is the most important vector of urban malaria on the Indian subcontinent. Nowhere else in the world is there a malaria vector so well adapted to urban life. It breeds in wells, cisterns, fountains, ornamental tanks, barrels, and buckets (Bang and Shah, 1988).

During the initial planning of the Indian National Malaria Eradication Program (NMEP), cities and towns with a population of more than 40,000 were considered to have little malaria transmission or to be malaria free (Sharma and Mehrotra, 1986), and malaria control in these communities was turned over to the local government. The result was a precipitous drop in malaria transmission in rural areas with no corresponding drop in urban areas. The proportion of malaria cases occurring in urban areas increased in many parts of India. In the state of Tamil Nadu, for example, 50 percent of malaria cases reported in 1961 were from urban areas; by 1963, this proportion had increased to 95 percent (Sharma and Mehrotra, 1986). The presence of pockets of urban malaria in India was an important contributor to the dramatic resurgence of the disease in the late 1960s. An in-depth evaluation of the NMEP concluded that the absence of control strategies for urban malaria was the program's most important failure (Sharma and Mehrotra, 1986).

At least one other *Anopheles* species, *An. arabiensis*, found in Nigeria, seems to be adapting to living in town or city centers (World Health Organization, 1988). In most of Africa, Latin America, and Asia, however, malaria vectors are primarily confined to rural areas. In these regions, malaria is an important urban disease only in peripherally located communities that are similar in some respects to rural sites. In a study of malaria transmission and urbanization in Brazzaville, Congo, human settlement was initially found to favor the spread of *An. gambiae*, but subsequent increases in population density tended to eliminate larval development sites as open spaces were gradually built up and standing water became too contaminated for *Anopheles* larvae to survive in (Trape and Zoulani, 1987). Since *Anopheles* species breed in fairly clean collections of standing water, such as rice paddies, swamps, and lakes, an increase in fecal or other contamination ruins their suitability for larval development. Malaria, therefore, is more of a problem in semiurban than in truly urban areas.

The proportion of people living in urban and semiurban areas is expanding rapidly. In 1950, almost 30 percent of the world's 2.5 billion inhabitants lived in urban areas. By the year 2000, half of the world's projected 6.2 billion people will live in urban settings, many of them in slums and squatter settlements (World Health Organization, 1988). Although most anopheline mosquitoes do not thrive in urban areas, the fact than an increasing share of the world's population will reside in urban or semiurban locales provides impetus for increased malaria control in those areas.

Finally, it should be pointed out that the social and economic factors that contribute to the appearance of urban malaria are similar to those involved in producing malaria in rural populations and in migrants. The recently settled, low-income neighborhoods on the periphery of urban areas where malaria commonly occurs are usually populated by migrants from rural sites or refugees from war, famine, or changing patterns of land tenure. Many work part of the year in the city as wage laborers and then return to the country.

Implications for Malaria Control Programs

An understanding of the social and behavioral factors that favor malaria transmission may not appear to have any practical implications for malaria control programs. It is difficult to see how these programs can have any impact on processes such as urbanization, deforestation, and migration. Nevertheless, awareness of which of these factors are important in a given area can help in the choice of appropriate control measures and in decisions about how these measures will be implemented.

In choosing control measures, it is important to consider factors such as human population movements, which can make measures such as residual spraying with insecticides to kill mosquitoes both ineffective and difficult to implement because people may not have a permanent home. On the other hand, slight improvements in socioeconomic conditions may make marginally efficacious technologies far more efficacious. In a study in Muheza, Tanzania, it was found that slight improvements in housing conditions significantly improved the efficacy of insecticide-impregnated bednets (Lyimo et al., in press).

Understanding social and behavioral factors which influence transmission can also be helpful to policymakers charged with choosing among malaria control options. For example, the distinction between type I and type II farming systems, even though it is not always clear-cut, can indicate which groups should be involved in control activities. Migrant laborers working in rice production—a type II farming arrangement—may have no control at all over the presence of larval development sites in the field or around housing facilities. In this case, only the landowner or the company can take the appropriate control steps.

Acceptance and Usage of Control Methods

Most malaria control programs are still planned and implemented on the assumption that the major barrier to the adoption of control interventions is lack of knowledge. Posters, pamphlets, radio advertisements, and health education campaigns are all intended to provide information that will change behavior.

Although there is an awareness that other cultural, behavioral, and operational factors may also be acting as barriers to adoption of interventions, they tend to receive less attention for several reasons. First, program planners seldom have the training in qualitative research techniques necessary to investigate these factors. Second, the tremendous diversity in culture and community structure observed in many malarious regions, even between adjacent villages, has led program planners to believe that a serious consideration of these variables would entail the development of a unique control program for each village. This is clearly not a task that can be undertaken with the limited resources of most ministries of health.

Coping with this diversity becomes much less of a challenge when it is realized that certain features of the ways in which people adapt to malaria, including the models used to explain malaria, its causes, and treatments, are found in a broad range of different cultures. As a result, it is possible to describe a set of barriers to the success of control efforts which have been documented in many different parts of the world.

Perceptions of Cerebral Malaria

A major objective of many malaria control programs is to decrease mortality from cerebral malaria. Unfortunately, because of its sudden onset and the presence of neurological symptoms such as convulsions, cerebral malaria is often perceived as a nonmalarious condition. Ramakrishna and Brieger (1987) quote a mother in western Nigeria as saying, "Yesterday I thought my child was having malaria, but today when the convulsion started, I knew it was another disease." This "other disease," which corresponded clinically to cerebral malaria, was identified by the mother to be *ile tutu* or "cold earth," a nonmalarious condition.

The acute mental changes associated with cerebral malaria lead many to believe that it is due to supernatural rather than natural causes. Both Helitzer-Allen (1989) in Malawi and Fivawo (1986) in Tanzania describe a type of fever accompanied by convulsions that is attributed to spirits or witchcraft. The results of such perceptions are twofold. First, cerebral malaria, while seen as dangerous, is not thought to be controllable through vector control or chemotherapy. At the same time, non-cerebral malaria is not seen as an important health threat.

Causes of Malaria

Even among those who view mosquitoes as central to malaria, the presence of mosquitoes may be considered neither sufficient nor necessary for disease transmission. In one survey in the Philippines, 93 percent of respondents agreed that mosquitoes transmit malaria, yet almost half also said the disease could be caused by "germs" in contaminated water, and nearly 30 percent blamed the disease on "microorganisms" (Lariosa, 1986). About 70 percent of respondents believed that malaria was communicable by close contact with a patient.

Some of the reasons that education about the cause-and-effect relationship between mosquitoes and malaria is usually not successful have been listed by Gramiccia (1981). Perhaps the most important is the fact that many mosquito bites may not result in malaria, yet one can get malaria after a few bites or even without being bitten recently, depending on the mosquito species that is biting, the percentage of mosquitoes infected, and the possibility of malaria relapse or recrudescence. Furthermore, someone who installs screens on the house, uses mosquito nets, and eliminates larval development sites around the house may get malaria, while someone who takes none of these precautions may not.

There are many similarities between the explanatory models for the causes of malaria found in different cultures because they are based on observations of similar phenomena. These phenomena include the association of malaria with rain (which increases the number of vector breeding sites), with humidity and heat (which affect mosquito longevity), and with agricultural work (which increases exposure to mosquitoes and often is more intensive during or after the rainy season).

Helitzer-Allen (1989) describes a folk belief for malaria and malaria-like conditions in Malawi. The term *malungo*, which literally means fever and is used to denote malaria, was found to have seven separate subcategories of the disease, each with its own etiology, symptoms, and treatment. They included, by etiology, *malungo* due to mosquitoes; getting wet in the rain or getting cold; hard work; spirits or witchcraft; other airborne methods; dirty water or food; and *kulipuka*, a form of *malungo* in children associated with blisters in the parents.

In the Gambia, MacCormack and Snow (1986) had remarkably similar findings. In the village of Katchang, malaria was thought to be caused not only by mosquitoes but also by getting wet in the rain or getting cold; hard work; eating maize, *kucha*, or fruit of *ningkong* at the end of the rains; not having enough to eat; and lack of sleep due to nuisance mosquitoes.

The significance of perceptions that there are many causes of malaria is that people may feel that there is no way to control malaria. Mosquitoes can be avoided, but it is difficult to avoid hard work, getting wet or cold, or eating "contaminated" food. As a result, people are unwilling to participate in time-consuming malaria control activities. Participants in a study in Liberia, for example, felt that exposure to malaria's causative agents was inevitable, that contracting malaria was determined largely by fate, and that the chance of contracting the illness was unpredictable (Jackson, 1985).

An additional consequence of the perception that mosquitoes are not the only cause of malaria is that people may feel that methods of treatment such as chloroquine do not work for all forms of malaria. In Malawi, Helitzer-Allen (1989) found that only *malungo* attributed to mosquitoes or to airborne dissemination was thought to be treatable with chloroquine. This had the effect of decreasing chemoprophylaxis compliance by pregnant women who underestimated the range of illness episodes that it would be able to prevent.

Water and Mosquitoes

Just as mosquitoes are not believed by many cultures to be the only source of malaria parasites, neither is standing water, such as swamps and drainage ditches, thought to be the exclusive locus of larval development. Indigenous populations commonly believe that mosquitoes originate from almost anywhere in the environment, that the number of potential larval development areas is unlimited, and that mosquitoes are therefore uncontrollable. This view can limit interest in time-consuming mosquito control measures.

Subjects interviewed in Mexico and Honduras expressed the belief that mosquitoes are generated not only by humidity, wind, and rain, but also by plants, mud, earth or waste, and "dirtiness." In Mexico, study participants claimed to have witnessed mosquitoes emerging from leaves (Center for International Community-Based Health Research, 1988; Winch et al., undated); in Honduras, where significant unfamiliarity with mosquito larval stages was found, participants claimed to have witnessed young mosquitoes immediately stretching their wings and flying after hatching (Leontsini, undated).

Distinguishing Malaria from Other Diseases

In regions of the world where malaria is endemic, there is almost always a term that corresponds to clinical malaria. However, there is not always agreement among the patients' perceptions of malaria symptoms, the definition of malaria used in a local health clinic, and the definition used by parasitologists (Jackson, 1985). The result frequently is nosological fusion, a phenomenon in which there is a failure to distinguish between what are biomedically two or more discrete diseases (Young, 1979).

Nosological fusion can affect, in three ways, whether a person feels that a control measure is efficacious. First, if an illness is incorrectly diagnosed as malaria, the patient may conclude that preventive measures taken, such as the use of impregnated bednets, do not prevent malaria. Alternatively, the patient may conclude that an antimalarial medication is ineffective when in fact the drug is inappropriate for whatever disease is present.

Finally, nosological fusion can make local treatments seem effective when they are not. For example, if a viral infection is diagnosed incorrectly as malaria and the patient takes a local remedy and becomes well, the patient may conclude that the treatment is efficacious against malaria when it is not; the viral infection has merely been resolved by the patient's own immune system.

Drug Side Effects and Beliefs About Drug Action

Drug side effects and beliefs about drug action are important determinants of the acceptance of malaria prophylaxis and treatment. When studied, acceptance has usually been found to be low. In one study of compliance with chloroquine prophylaxis among pregnant women in Africa south of the Sahara, rates of compliance ranged from a low of 2 percent in Zaire to a high of 18 percent in the Central African Republic (Breman and Campbell, 1988).

The most common side effect of chloroquine is pruritus (itching). In Saradidi, Kenya, itching due to chloroquine use was reported in about 20 percent of adults (Spencer et al., 1987), and 10 percent of women interviewed stated that they had not taken the chloroquine because of fear of itching (Kaseje et al., 1987). Interestingly, a study of compliance with chloroquine prophylaxis among pregnant women in Malawi found that those who complained about side effects felt that these side effects indicated that the drug was working; side effects were considered more beneficial than harmful (Helitzer-Allen, 1989).

Chloroquine's bitter taste may or may not be a barrier to compliance. In the Saradidi studies and a study conducted in North Mara, Tanzania (MacCormack and Lwihula, 1983), bitterness was not reported as a major barrier to compliance. These findings appeared to be confirmed by the Malawi study, in which women infrequently reported side effects and 99 percent said that chloroquine was not bad for pregnant women. In key informant interviews, however, virtually all participants expressed the view that chloroquine was bad for pregnant women and, because of its bitter taste, was considered to be an abortifacient. A nonbitter formulation, together with improved health education that addressed these perceptions, significantly raised compliance rates (Helitzer-Allen, 1989).

Logistical and Organizational Problems

Many times the failure to achieve a high rate of usage of a malaria control technology is due neither to side effects nor to beliefs but simply to the fact that the technology is unavailable or if it is available, people are unaware that it exists.

MacCormack and Lwihula (1983) show how a program aimed at controlling malaria in children through the use of prophylactic chloroquine failed because of a lack of sensitivity to a series of quite practical problems, including the exclusion of socially marginal families from the program and irregular drug supplies at the local level. While no single problem was insurmountable, together these difficulties threatened the success of an otherwise sound program.

In Saradidi, Kenya, chloroquine prophylaxis was offered free of charge to pregnant women through village health helpers, yet only 29 percent of 357 pregnant women seen in antenatal clinics were taking the drug (Kaseje et al., 1987). Of those women not taking chloroquine, over half said they were unaware that the service was available.

In a study of compliance with malaria chemosuppression regimes in Tanga Region, Tanzania, despite fears of drug side effects and abortifacient properties, the predominant problem was irregular drug supply. Ironically, even when chloroquine became available, it was often not taken because of fears that it might not be available for future needs; mothers were tempted to hoard the drug for use in future malaria episodes instead of using it prophylactically (Matola and Malle, 1985).

Evaluation of the effects of operational and economic barriers to the use of malaria control technologies must take into account explanatory models about malaria and malaria-like illnesses and their causes. If a technology appears to address the problem as it is understood by the community, people may be willing to pay more or endure more inconvenience to obtain it. If, however, it does not appear to address the real problem as elaborated by these models, acceptance may remain low even if the technology is made more available and is less expensive.

Lack of Community Participation

Active community participation in the design and implementation of health and development projects can greatly increase the chances of success. Communities are rarely involved in real decision making and therefore feel that they have little stake in program outcome. Nichter (1984) points out that assumptions regarding what a community wants, needs, or will support are usually made by program planners rather than the community. Rajagopalan and Panicker (1984) state, "Many times such plans are forced upon the villagers and the latter acquiesce passively to their implementation, without participating in them. Their acquiescence is often mistaken for cooperation/participation."

A malaria control program in which community participation was encouraged in the planning and implementation phases was carried out by the Vector Control Research Centre (VCRC) of Pondicherry, India (Rajagopalan and Panicker, 1984). One of the program's initial findings was that the community's objectives did not coincide with those of disease control. To pursue both sets of objectives, a flexible integrated approach was undertaken.

Rather than concentrate strictly on vector control, the VCRC first collaborated with community organizations on issues of concern to the community, including problems related to drinking water and electricity. Once these problems were resolved, attention was given to vector control. VCRC then proceeded to link vector control activities to economic rewards. In the study village, it was found that the presence of algae reduced the number of larval development sites. Since the algae could be used to make cardboard, there was a financial incentive for the villagers to grow, harvest, and sell the algae. A similar economics-based approach was used when it was discovered that the small pools in which mosquitoes thrived could be used to breed prawns.

Even when attempts are made to involve communities actively in program activities, factionalism within communities may limit participation (Schwartz, 1981; Paul and Demarest, 1984; Twumasi and Freund, 1985). Allen and co-workers (1990) describe a malaria chemoprophylaxis program among children in the Gambia in which the drug was administered by village health workers (VHWs). Problems of drug supply and drug side effects had little effect on compliance; however, mothers were unwilling to have their children receive treatment from VHWs or to be cared for by traditional birth attendants if they came from a social or ethnic group different from that of the mother.

Village health workers are often key to the successful operation of malaria control programs. In Latin America, for example, passive case detection networks made up of unpaid community volunteers were established in most countries in the late 1950s. The networks have become the principal tool for malaria surveillance and antimalarial drug treatment in many national malaria programs (Ruebush et al., 1990).

Use of VHWs is not without problems, however. The integration of malaria control into larger national primary health care programs has meant that VHWs have much broader responsibility for health in general, leaving less time for them to address problems specific to malaria (Justice, 1986; Heggenhougen et al., 1987).

Careful selection and training are key to ensuring an effective VHW work force. In a review of VHW activity in Honduras, worker selection was the single most important determinant of the sustainability of local malaria control efforts (Kendall, in press). Unfortunately, selection is often the responsibility of the lowest-level professional health worker, and selection criteria are often ill defined. A manual for the rapid assessment of social and cultural aspects of malaria is now being developed by a working group of the United Nations Development Programme/World Bank/World Health Organization/Special Programme for Research and Training in Tropical Diseases/Social and Economic Research.

RESEARCH AGENDA

The application of social and behavioral science research on malaria (excluding questions of economics and management, which are dealt with in other chapters) should have two main objectives: to help researchers understand and reduce social and behavioral barriers that hinder the acceptance and use of preventive measures; and to promote early and effective treatment of clinical cases of malaria, especially among young children.

Understanding Community Beliefs

Communities often have conflicting beliefs about what causes malaria, where mosquitoes come from, and how best to prevent or treat the disease. For example, because chloroquine tablets are an effective treatment for certain types of malaria but have no demonstrable effect in young children with cerebral malaria, some may conclude that cerebral malaria is not, in fact, a type of malarial illness. Communities and malaria program planners may have widely different views about the nature of the malaria problem and the availability and efficacy of control options.

RESEARCH FOCUS: In-depth studies of community beliefs, observations, and perceptions.

Health-Seeking Behavior

There have been few systematic studies of how episodes of malaria are recognized and treated at the household level. It is essential to know how people, especially mothers and caretakers of young children, make decisions about whether to administer home remedies, consult traditional healers or VHWs, or go to a clinic or hospital. Without information on health-seeking behavior, it will be difficult to develop an integrated strategy for reducing malaria mortality.

RESEARCH FOCUS: Studies of health-seeking behaviors in malaria.

One method that may be especially useful for analyzing health-seeking behavior is the ethnographic protocol. The protocol technique involves interviewing key informants, mothers of children under age three, and health care providers. Relevant data are obtained through free listing of illnesses, narratives of past malaria episodes, hypothetical case scenarios, paired comparisons, severity ratings, and sorting tasks.

> **RESEARCH FOCUS:** Development of an ethnographic protocol on treatment-seeking behavior for episodes of malaria.

Research Methods

Most social science research on malaria is conducted with use of standardized survey instruments, often in the form of knowledge, attitude, and practice questionnaires. Although surveys can be useful when the variables being measured are well defined, such as socioeconomic and demographic data, they are of limited use for examining factors that influence the acceptance and use of malaria control methods. For example, in responding to a questionnaire, individuals may state that mosquitoes are the cause of malaria, but the fact that they believe mosquitoes are considered neither sufficient nor necessary for malaria transmission may be concealed. Multimethod qualitative techniques, which have been used by applied social scientists in research on nutrition and primary care health, need to be adapted to research on malaria.

> **RESEARCH FOCUS:** Development of a malaria rapid assessment procedures guide containing instructions for the use of social science methods, including key-informant interviewing, focus groups, and consensus modeling, as well as other social science data collection methods.

Health Communications

The need for research does not end once barriers to the acceptance and use of interventions have been documented. Research is also needed to determine the best strategy to provide convincing and persuasive means to involve communities in control activities. The traditional approach to malaria education has been to stress biological and medical facts. Mosquitoes are presented as the only route through which malaria parasites can be transferred to humans, and the life cycle of the mosquito is explained repeatedly. The importance of "nonscientific" and traditional theories of illness causation to malaria control should not be underestimated, however, since they summarize the communities' perception of the local epidemiology of malaria and their perception of risk.

RESEARCH FOCUS: Adoption and evaluation of contemporary health communication techniques that use qualitative and quantitative research intensively to define the audiences, behaviors, strategies, channels, and messages for malaria control programs.

RESEARCH FOCUS: Exploration and evaluation of the applicability of contemporary learning models to bring about behavior change in populations at risk.

RESEARCH FOCUS: Evaluation of the role of new channels, such as mass media, and traditional channels, such as theater, as vehicles for health communications on malaria.

Community Participation

Much of the research on community involvement in malaria control has focused on stable rural communities where residents had a significant degree of control over their immediate environment. In urban areas, in areas where agriculture dominates, or within communities whose populations migrate, community participation necessarily will take on a different look. It is often assumed that communities do not exist in urban and migrant settings, and approaches to malaria control in these areas accordingly have often been based on legislation (Bang and Shah, 1988). This strategy has had limited effectiveness, and new approaches will have to be developed for urban and migrant communities that are growing in both number and importance.

RESEARCH FOCUS: Development and evaluation of participatory strategies in malaria control for urban and migrant communities.

Community Involvement in Planning and Evaluation

During the eradication era, intervention strategies were largely predetermined, and there was little room for local input into the decision-making process. Now that choices about what control technologies to use have become less clear-cut, community involvement has become critical. Consultations with the community can reveal whether a certain intervention will be accepted and, if so, to what extent. There may be no point in implementing interventions aimed at decreasing malaria transmission unless a high level of acceptance is expected. Unfortunately, little is known about methods of involving communities in decision making and program evaluation as these activities relate to malaria control.

RESEARCH FOCUS: Development and evaluation of novel ways of involving communities in the planning, implementation, and evaluation of malaria control programs.

REFERENCES

Allen, S. J., R. W. Snow, A. Menon, and B. M. Greenwood. 1990. Compliance with malaria chemoprophylaxis over a five-year period among children in a rural area of The Gambia. Journal of Tropical Medicine and Hygiene 93:313-322.

Bang, Y. H., and N. K. Shah. 1988. Human ecology related to urban mosquito-borne disease in countries of South East Asia region. Journal of Communicable Diseases 20:1-17.

Breman, J. G., and C. C. Campbell. 1988. Combating severe malaria in African children. Bulletin of the World Health Organization 66:611-620.

Bruce-Chwatt, L. J. 1987. Malaria and its control: present situation and future prospects. Pp. 75-110 in Annual Review of Public Health, Breslow, L., J. E. Fielding, and L. B. Lave, eds. Palo Alto: Annual Reviews, Inc.

Bruce-Chwatt, L. J., and J. de Zulueta. 1980. The Rise and Fall of Malaria in Europe. London: Oxford University Press.

Celli, A. 1900. La Malaria Secondo Le Nuove Ricerche [Malaria: According to the New Researches], 2nd ed. London: Longman, Green and Company.

Center for International Community-Based Health Research. 1988. Dengue Control: The Challenge to the Social Sciences. Report of a Workshop, October 20-22, 1988. Baltimore: Center for International Community-Based Health Research, Johns Hopkins University School of Hygiene and Public Health.

Chapin, G., and R. Wasserstrom. 1981. Agricultural production and malaria resurgence in Central America and India. Nature 293:181-185.

Chapin, G., and R. Wasserstrom. 1983. Pesticide use and malaria resurgence in Central America and India. Social Science and Medicine 17:273-290.

Coimbra, C. E. A. 1988. Human factors in the epidemiology of malaria in the Brazilian Amazon. Human Organization 47:254-260.

Coluzzi, M., V. Petrarca, and M. A. Di Deco. 1985. Chromosomal inversion intergradation and incipient speciation in *Anopheles gambiae*. Bolletino di Zoologia 52:45-63.

Covell, G. 1946. Malaria and irrigation in India. Journal of the Malaria Institute of India 6:403.

Curtis, C. F. 1981. Malaria debated. Nature 294:388.

Dubisch, J. 1985. Low country fevers: cultural adaptations to malaria in antebellum South Carolina. Social Science and Medicine 21:641-649.

Dunn, F. L. 1988. Human factors in arbovirus ecology and control. Pp. 281-290 in The Arboviruses: Epidemiology and Ecology, Volume I, Monath, T. P., ed. Boca Raton: CRC Press.

Fivawo, M. 1986. Community response to malaria: Muheza District, Tanzania: 1983-1984; a study in cultural adaptation. Doctoral dissertation. University of Illinois, Urbana.

Friedlander, J. 1969. Malaria and demography in the lowlands of Mexico: an ethno-historical approach. Pp. 217-233 in Proceedings of the American Ethnological Society. Seattle: University of Washington Press.

Gramiccia, G. 1981. Health education in malaria control—why has it failed? World Health Forum 2:385-393.

Heggenhougen, K., P. Vaughan, E. P. Y. Muhondwa, and J. Rutabanzibwa-Ngaiza. 1987. Community Health Workers: The Tanzanian Experience. Oxford: Oxford University Press.

Helitzer-Allen, D. 1989. Examination of the factors influencing the utilization of the antenatal malaria chemoprophylaxis program, Malawi, Central Africa. Doctoral dissertation. Johns Hopkins University School of Hygiene and Public Health, Baltimore, Maryland.

Hughes, C. C., and J. M. Hunter. 1970. Disease and "development" in Africa. Social Science and Medicine 3:443-493.

Hyma, B., and A. Ramesh. 1980. The reappearance of malaria in Sathanaur Reservoir and environs: Tamil Nadu, India. Social Science and Medicine 14D:337-344.

Jackson, L. C. 1985. Malaria in Liberian children and mothers: biocultural perceptions of illness vs clinical evidence of disease. Social Science and Medicine 20:1281-1287.

Justice, J. 1986. Policies, Plans and People. Foreign Aid and Health Development. Berkeley: University of California Press.

Kaseje, D. C. O., E. K. N. Sempebwa, and H. C. Spencer. 1987. Malaria chemoprophylaxis to pregnant women provided by community health workers in Saradidi, Kenya. I. Reasons for non-acceptance. Annals of Tropical Medicine and Parasitology 81(Suppl. 1):77-82.

Kendall, C. In press. The village context of Honduras' village health worker program: 1980-1984. In Community Health Worker Programs—Present Failure But Future Imperative, Frankel, S., ed. Oxford University Press:Oxford.

Laderman, C. 1975. Malaria and progress: some historical and ecological considerations. Social Science and Medicine 9:587-594.

Lariosa, T. R. 1986. Culture, environment and people's perceptions: considerations in malaria control in the Philippines. Southeast Asian Journal of Tropical Medicine and Public Health 17:360-370.

Leontsini, E. Undated. Beliefs about mosquitoes in Honduras: implications for public health campaigns. Unpublished document. Baltimore: Center for International Community-Based Health Research, Johns Hopkins University School of Hygiene and Public Health.

Livingstone, F. B. 1958. Anthropological implications of sickle cell gene distribution in West Africa. American Anthropologist 60:533-562.

Lyimo, E., F. H. M. Msuya, R. T. Rwegoshors, E. A. Nicholson, J. D. Lines, and C. F. Curtis. In press. Trial of pyrethroid-impregnated bednets in an area of Tanzania holoendemic for malaria. Part 3. Impact on the prevalence of malaria parasitaemia and fever. Acta Tropica.

MacCormack, C. P., and G. Lwihula. 1983. Failure to participate in a malaria chemosuppression programme: North Mara, Tanzania. Journal of Tropical Medicine and Hygiene 86:99-107.

MacCormack, C. P., and R. W. Snow. 1986. Gambian cultural preferences in the use of insecticide-impregnated bed nets. Journal of Tropical Medicine and Hygiene 89:295-302.

Matola, Y. G., and L. N. Malle. 1985. Factors affecting the compliance of malaria chemosuppression with chloroquine at some maternal and child health clinics in Tanga Region, Tanzania. East African Medical Journal 62:720-724.

Molineaux, L., and G. Gramiccia. 1980. The Garki Project: Research On the Epidemiology and Control of Malaria in the Sudan Savanna of West Africa. Geneva: World Health Organization.

Nichter, M. 1984. Project community diagnosis: participatory research as a first step toward community involvement in primary health care. Social Science and Medicine 19:237-252.

Packard, R. M. 1984. Maize, cattle and mosquitoes: the political economy of malaria epidemics in colonial Swaziland. Journal of African History 25:189-212.

Packard, R. M. 1986. Agricultural development, migrant labor and the resurgence of malaria in Swaziland. Social Science and Medicine 22:861-867.

Paul, B. D., and W. J. Demarest. 1984. Citizen participation overplanned: the case of a health project in the Guatemalan community of San Pedro La Laguna. Social Science and Medicine 19:185-192.

Prothero, R. M. 1961. Population movements and problems of malaria eradication in Africa. Bulletin of the World Health Organization 24:405-425.

Rajagopalan, P. K., and K. N. Panicker. 1984. Feasibility of community participation for vector control in villages. Indian Journal of Medical Research 80:117-124.

Ramakrishna, J., and W. R. Brieger. 1987. The value of qualitative research: health education in Nigeria. Health Policy and Planning 2:171-175.

Ruebush, T. K. I. I., R. Zeissig, H. A. Godoy, and R. E. Klein. 1990. Use of illiterate volunteer workers for malaria case detection and treatment. Annals of Tropical Medicine and Parasitology 84:119-125.

Schwartz, N. B. 1981. Anthropological views of community and community development. Human Organization 40:313-322.

Sharma, V. P., and K. N. Mehrotra. 1986. Malaria resurgence in India: a critical study. Social Science and Medicine 22:835-845.

Spencer, H. C., D. C. O. Kaseje, A. D. Brandling-Bennett, A. J. Oloo, and W. M. Watkins. 1987. Epidemiology of chloroquine-associated pruritis in Saradidi, Kenya. Annals of Tropical Medicine and Parasitology 81(Suppl. 1):124-127.

Suleman, M. 1988. Malaria in Afghan refugees in Pakistan. Transactions of the Royal Society of Tropical Medicine and Hygiene 82:44-47.

Trape, J. F., and A. Zoulani. 1987. Malaria and urbanization in Central Africa: the example of Brazzaville. Part III. Relationships between urbanization and the intensity of malaria transmission. Transactions of the Royal Society of Tropical Medicine and Hygiene 81(Suppl.):19-25.

Twumasi, P. A., and P. J. Freund. 1985. Local politicization of primary health care as an instrument for development: a case study of community health workers in Zambia. Social Science and Medicine 20:1073-1080.

Winch, P., L. Lloyd, E. Puigserver-Castro, G. Barrientos-Sanchez, and C. Kendall. Undated. Beliefs about biting insects and disease transmission in Merida,

Mexico. Unpublished document. Baltimore: Center for International Community-Based Health Research, Johns Hopkins University School of Hygiene and Public Health.

World Health Organization. 1988. Urban vector and pest control. Eleventh report of the WHO Expert Committee on Vector Biology and Control. WHO Technical Report Series No. 767. Geneva: World Health Organization.

Young, A. 1979. The dimension of medical rationality: a problematic for the psychosocial study of medicine. Pp. 67-85 in Towards a New Definition of Health, Ahmed, P. I., and G. V. Coelho, eds. New York: Plenum Press.

Appendix A

TYPES OF MALARIA

1. African wet savannah
2. Forest
3. Irrigated agriculture
4. Highland fringe
5. Desert fringe and oasis
6. Urban malaria
7. Plains—traditional agriculture
8. Coastal

DETERMINANTS

1. Level of endemicity

   * Highly endemic: perennial transmission
   * Moderately endemic: perennial transmission
   * Modestly endemic: seasonal transmission
   * Highly endemic: seasonal transmission
   * Low endemicity: seasonal transmission
   * Epidemic transmission

2. Parasite species

* *Plasmodium falciparum*
* *P. vivax*
* *P. malariae*
* *P. ovale*

3. Population characteristics

* Immune status (high, low, none)
* Movement (settled, resettled, transient); if transient: organized, nomads, random
* Population density and settlement patterns

4. Social, behavioral, and economic characteristics

* Housing
* Occupation
* Water utilization
* Health-seeking behavior
* Sleeping habits
* Customs and taboos
* Income and wealth
* Local understanding of malaria
* Access to health care

5. Health infrastructure

* National health budget
* Status of governmental health care delivery system
* National malaria control program (type, budget, and efficiency)
* Importance of non-governmental services (i.e. missions, private voluntary organizations)
* Availability of private health care
* Importance of health care delivery by family, market, etc.

6. Use of drugs

* Cost
* Availability
* Drug-use patterns
* Effectiveness (degree of resistance)

7. Vector considerations

* Behavior (breeding, feeding, resting)

* Susceptibility to insecticides
* Cost, safety, and acceptability of effective insecticides
* Availability and cost of bed nets
* Feasibility of bed net impregnation with insecticides
* Availability and cost of repellents and fumigant coils

8. Development projects

* Government development projects (dam construction, road building)
* Unofficial or illegal activities (mining, gemming)
  -organized
  -random

TOOLS

1. Vector control

* Personal protection
  -nets or curtains with or without insecticide
  -screens
  -house siting (where the house is physically located)
  -repellents
  -smoke coils
* Environmental management
  -source reduction
  -flushing, sluicing
  -clearing vegetation
  -water management
  -reforestation
* Larvicides
  -chemical
  -mechanical
  -biological
* Adulticiding (killing the adult forms of the mosquito)
  -residual spraying
  -fogging
  -large-scale ULV (ultra low volume spraying)
* Zooprophylaxis

2. Medical resources

* Diagnosis
  -clinical
  -microscopic

* Treatment facilities
  -inpatient
  -outpatient
  -market
* Prophylaxis
* Mass chloroquine-primaquine administration for epidemics

3. Information, education, and communication

* Public
  -individuals, households, and communities
  -school curricula
  -radio
  -newspapers
  -television
  -local media (songs, theater, etc.)
* Health care providers

4. Surveillance

* Diagnosis and treatment
  -morbidity
  -incidence of severe malaria
  -mortality
  -prevalence of parasitemia
* Epidemic early warning
* Vector information
  -insecticide resistance
  -behavioral changes
* Antimalarial drug resistance

Appendix B

DISSENTING OPINION

The following is my dissenting opinion on the report on malaria research, prevention, and control:

As you know, the Institute of Medicine (IOM) was asked to undertake this study because of the recent deterioration in the global malaria situation. The terms of reference for the multidisciplinary committee, of which I am a member, was to assess the current status of malaria research, prevention, and control, and to make recommendations on strategies to control the malaria problem. The committee, in defining the malaria problem in Chapter One, under "Conclusions and Recommendations," made the following important statements and observations:

1. ". . . More importantly, however, many malarious countries do not have the resources, either human or financial, to carry out even the most meager efforts to control malaria. . . ."

2. ". . . In most malarious regions of the world, there is inadequate access to malaria treatment. Appropriate health facilities may not exist, or if they exist, may be inaccessible to affected populations, may not be supplied with effective drugs, or may be staffed inappropriately or by untrained personnel."

These statements truly reflect the current situation. It is, therefore, more logical to correct these discrepancies by strengthening the health services of these countries in general and their malaria control programs in particular, as a higher priority than searching only for new tools, products, and methods of vector control, since the currently available tools are not effectively used for the very reasons mentioned above. However, this does not mean that the development of new tools is not necessary. Due to widespread problems of drug resistance, research efforts on drug discovery and development do require increased funding and commitment.

I participated in the three meetings of the IOM committee and expressed my concern during two of these meetings that too much emphasis was being placed on malaria research and too little on its prevention and control. The committee's final report reflects that imbalance. There are recommendations on all aspects of research, including risk factors for severe malaria, social and cultural aspects, pathogenesis of severe and complicated malaria, vaccine development, drug discovery, and development and vector studies to interrupt transmission. There are also recommendations for malaria control, such as improvement of treatment guidelines and improving communication, but these do not address the fundamental issues of building the capabilities of endemic countries for malaria control.

Apart from theoretical discussion and limited exchange of ideas among the committee members, there was no in-depth discussion or review of country malaria control programs in Africa and South America. From Asia, an officer of the malaria control program in Thailand gave a presentation on the status of malaria control in his country. According to the data he presented, the malaria control program in Thailand is having an impact using currently available tools (the mortality rate decreased from 200/10,000 in 1949 to 1.5/10,000 by 1987). In spite of problems of drug resistance in Thailand, it seems that the developed infrastructure, national commitment, and the size of external assistance to the Thai program have made a difference. It seems to me that the solution to malaria control should be primarily concentrated on correcting the present lack of resources and the nonresponsive, underdeveloped health care delivery systems that prevail in most malaria-endemic countries, and not only on searching for new strategies and tools. Investment in additional research to generate new tools and products for the future, while useful, will not by any means help to correct the precarious malaria situation that exists today.

It is also unrealistic to expect that the malaria situation will be improved through the establishment of an advisory panel in the United States, with a core of experts to advise donor agencies concerning allocation of funds for surveillance, impact assessment, operational research, support of senior malaria control managers, etc., unless fundamental action is taken to improve health infrastructure and to support control programs in a meaningful way.

I do not agree with the concept that there are four priority areas for malaria control, as if each area could stand by itself and from which donors could choose to support or not. For various reasons, one strategy or approach, by itself, cannot bring about the desired impact; instead, it will be important to think of an integrated approach. I am also concerned with the order of these priorities. For example, it will be important to encourage individual and community-based preventive measures such as the removal of mosquito breeding places by environmental modification and/or manipulation, use of biological control agents for larval control whenever feasible, and use of bednets and mosquito-proofing of houses. These preventive measures should be applied in an integrated and coordinated manner and should not be presented as independent and separate measures.

In addition to the above, there are situations such as epidemics or large-scale irrigation projects, etc., where residual spraying can be effective. The collective use of the above preventive antimalarial activities will significantly reduce the incidence of malaria cases. At the same time, it will be imperative for countries to develop their health services systems to ensure prompt diagnosis and treatment. This approach will also facilitate the development of community involvement in malaria preventive measures.

As a result of rapid ecologic, socioeconomic, demographic, and environmental changes, due to various reasons, many countries are increasingly affected by large-scale malaria epidemics. It is important that countries get sufficient support to establish surveillance mechanisms for prevention or early detection of incipient epidemics and for undertaking control measures in the event of epidemics.

I do not agree with the recommendation that donor agencies be required to involve an advisory body from the United States and a core of experts to plan malaria control activities for endemic countries. I would recommend instead that these resources be utilized to train people from endemic countries to assume that responsibility.

I participated in a two-day meeting in Montreux, Switzerland at which nine professionals from the World Health Organization, one from the World Bank, and an IOM staff member were present to discuss the paradigm approach. Indeed, the classification of the malaria problem into a certain number of major types or paradigms is a process of stratification. What is different is that this classification is based on previous experience and accumulated knowledge. Such an approach has been previously discussed by J. A. Najera (1989).

In view of the constraints associated with the classical stratification approach, it was found necessary to simplify the method by using as few variables as possible. Kouznetsov et al. (1989) went to the other extreme and classified the malaria situation in Africa into nine strata using characteristics of transmission and indicated possible control measures for each of the nine stratum. Najera (1989), on the other hand, presented the view that the analysis of a situation need not always start from general principles by involving a series of variables "if reference can be made to a well-defined problem prototypes and associated control paradigms." The author described malaria problems associated with forest fringe, agricultural activities, and open gem mining in forest areas, large scale irrigation projects, etc., and recommended further devlopment of the process.

The Ethiopian Malaria Control Programme, having stratified the malaria situation into various categories on the basis of the above concept, has developed control strategies for each particular situation. While this approach is useful, it will only be relevant if there will be sufficient resources to implement the strategies developed on the basis of an epidemiological approach.

It is also important to note, as I tried to stress in the Montreux meeting, that this epidemiologic/paradigm approach is not a strategy but a process that will be useful for a better understanding of the malaria situation and, therefore, will lead to improved planning. Thus, the meeting was more one of promoting a simplified version of stratification. I do not agree with the recommendation that the paradigm approach will require field validation. Instead, I would recommend that countries be supported in classifying their malaria problems into epidemiologic types, developing an appropriate control strategy for each paradigm, and undertaking control activities accordingly.

Most of the descriptions and examples given for each paradigm are recent additions and the information is not complete and could be misleading. For example, "forest malaria" is not a uniform, single paradigm and the recommended control measures are not applicable to all forest situations. For these reasons, I recommend that only the list of the paradigms be retained in the report, not the descriptions.

The deteriorating malaria situation must not be seen as a justification for undertaking more research as a solution to the prevailing malaria problem, but as a warning that the situation may worsen further unless the international community and donor agencies participate in the control of malaria in a meaningful way to bring about fundamental changes.

In summary, my concerns are that there is too much emphasis in this report on malaria research while little attention is given to malaria prevention and control. The strategy for control is not well developed and the concept of four priority areas for intervention is misleading. The concept of stratification of malaria problems into major types or paradigms has been oriented into a research focus, instead of a tool to be used in actual control.

In view of the above, I would like to recommend that an in-depth review of malaria prevention and control be undertaken, in order to come up with fundamental and realistic solutions.

A. Teklehaimanot

REFERENCES

Najera, J. A. 1989. Global Malaria Situation. Geneva: World Health Organization. WPR/MAL (1)/89.14. Unpublished.

Kouznetsov, R. L., L. Molineaux, and P. F. Beales. 1989. Stratification and selection of anti malaria measures in tropical Africa in malaria and planning for its control in tropical Africa., P. F. Beales and V. S. Orlov, editors. Geneva: World Health Organization. Unpublished.

Glossary

actin a protein that is a major constituent of cell microfilaments.

adjuvant a compound, injected as a mixture with an antigen, that serves to intensify the immune response.

AIDS acquired immunodeficiency syndrome.

allele one of two or more alternative forms taken by a gene that occupies corresponding sites on structurally similar (homologous) chromosomes. The allelic forms differ in DNA sequence.

allotypes antigenic markers on immunoglobulin chains or other serum proteins that are not common to normal members of a species; the markers are controlled by allelic genes.

amino acid protein subunits; there are 20 found universally in proteins.

anopheline used when referring to *Anopheles* mosquitoes.

anthropophilic attracted to humans as a source of food.

antibody a protein produced by the immune system in response to the introduction into the body of a substance (an antigen) recognized as foreign by the body's immune system. The purpose of the antibody is to interact with other components of the immune system and render the antigen harmless, although for various reasons this may not always occur.

antigen a molecule capable of eliciting an immune response.

antigenic diversity the ability of an organism to change its antigenic makeup in response to environmental factors.

antigenic variation see **antigenic diversity.**

apical complex a group of organelles, thought to be involved in the red blood cell invasion process, at the apical (tip) end of the malaria parasite.

asexual reproduction a stage in the life cycle of the malaria parasite in humans.

biotinylated a process in which DNA probes are labeled with biotin.

B lymphocyte same as B cell. One of two types of lymphocytes (white blood cells) involved in the humoral immune response in humans. When instructed to do so by T lymphocytes, B lymphocytes produce antibodies against specific antigens.

buffy coat a layer, composed of white blood cells, that occurs upon centrifugation of whole blood under specific conditions.

carrier protein an immunogenic molecule to which an incomplete antigen (one that cannot induce an immune response by itself) is attached, rendering the antigen capable of inducing an immune response.

cDNA complementary or copy DNA, produced from an RNA template transcribed from the DNA that is being copied.

cell-mediated immunity a type of immune response in which subpopulations of T cells (helper T cells and killer T cells) cooperate to destroy cells in the body that bear foreign antigens, such as parasite-infected red blood cells.

chemoprophylaxis the use of drugs to prevent infection or progression of infection to illness.

chromosome DNA-containing genetic material in the nucleus of a cell. Each organism has a specific number of chromosomes, each responsible for transmitting distinctive characteristics to the organism's progeny.

circumsporozoite protein a protein located on the surface of the sporozoite that is thought to be important in host cell recognition and invasion.

clone genetically engineered replicas of DNA sequences.

congenic a situation in which two members of the same genus have an identical genetic makeup.

conserved sequence an amino acid or nucleotide sequence that has not changed (or has changed only slightly) over a period of time.

cytoadherence the ability of red blood cells, infected with *Plasmodium falciparum*, to adhere to the endothelial cell lining of brain capillaries.

cytokine specific compounds that, when present, induce the proliferation of immune cells.

cytotoxic T lymphocyte same as cytotoxic T cell. A lymphocyte that binds and kills foreign cells.

DDT 1,1,1-trichloro-2,2-bis(*p*-chlorophenyl)ethane or chlorophenothane, a pesticide.

DNA deoxyribonucleic acid, a carrier of genetic information (i.e., hereditary characteristics) found chiefly in the nucleus of cells.

Duffy antigen blood group antigens on the surface of erythrocytes that serve as receptors for *Plasmodium vivax*, rendering individuals who are Duffy negative refractory to vivax malaria. Most peoples of African descent are Duffy negative.

efflux the process in which an antimalarial drug is transported out of the parasite.

EIR see **entomological inoculation rate**.

electrophoresis the process by which substances, such as serum, are separated into their components by the application of an electrical field to a suspension containing the substance. An example is gel electrophoresis, in which the substance is suspended in a gel.

ELISA enzyme-linked immunosorbent assay. An immunological technique used for the quantitation of antigen or antibody. In the assay, enzyme-labeled antigen or antibody is bound to a solid surface (such as beads, tubes, or microplate wells). After addition of the patient specimen and substrate, the presence of the desired antigen, antibody, or antigen-antibody complex is indicated by a color change based on an enzyme-substrate reaction.

endemic the condition in which a disease is present in a community at all times. There are four subcategories of endemicity: holo-, hyper-, meso- and hypoendemic.

endophilic associated with humans and their domestic environment.

entomological inoculation rate (EIR) a measure of the number of infective bites each person receives per night. A direct measure of the risk of human exposure to the bites of infective mosquitoes.

epidemic the condition in which a disease spreads rapidly through a community in which the disease is normally not present or is present at a low level.

epidemiology study of the distribution and determinants of a disease within a given population.

epitope a small segment (structural component) of an antigen responsible for specific interaction with antibody molecules elicited by the same or a related antigen.

erythrocyte red blood cell; oxygen-carrying cell. Invaded by malaria merozoites during malaria infection.

exchange transfusion the process by which the blood of a person is replaced with blood taken from others; used in cases of severe malaria where the parasite has caused such damage to the red blood cells that they are unable to carry sufficient oxygen to the individual's cells.

exflagellation   the formation of microgametes by extrusion of nuclear material into peripheral processes of gametocyte cytoplasm. These processes resemble flagella.

exoerythrocytic   applies to stages of development of the malaria parasite that occur in cells other than red blood cells.

Fab fragment   either of two segments of an antibody molecule (IgG). Each Fab fragment remains capable of combining with the antigen that elicited its production.

falciparum malaria   malaria caused by the parasite *Plasmodium falciparum*.

gamete   mature germ cell. In malaria, there are two types, micro- and macrogametes. These develop from male and female gametocytes and fuse within the mosquito midgut to form a zygote.

gametocyte   the sexual-stage precursors of the malaria parasite. The micro- and macrogametocytes (male and female) develop within the human host and are picked up by the mosquito while in the act of biting. In the mosquito, the gametocytes develop further into micro- and macrogametes.

gene   the biological unit of heredity, located on chromosomes.

gene-cloned vaccine   see **recombinant vaccine**.

genetic diversity   differences in genetic makeup within a species.

genomic library   a random collection of fragments of the DNA of a given species inserted into a corresponding collection of vectors and cloned in a suitable host. Such a collection includes all the unique nucleotide sequences of the genome.

genotype   the genetic makeup of an organism, as distinguished from its physical appearance or phenotype.

hepatocyte   a liver cell invaded by the malaria sporozoite.

heterologous   a disparity in antigenic makeup between two or more antigens.

HIV   human immunodeficiency virus, the agent that causes AIDS.

holoendemic   the condition in which malaria is present in a community at all times and with a very high transmission rate, resulting in a population (particularly adults) that has considerable immunity to the disease.

homologous   corresponding in structure, such as homologous antigens.

humoral immunity   immunity based on the interaction of antibody with antigen. Involves both T and B cells and may be present in the company of cell-mediated immunity.

hyperendemic   the condition in which malaria is present in a community at all times and with a high incidence.

hypnozoite   latent sporozoite that undergoes a period of dormancy in the host's liver, eventually giving rise to a relapse of the disease.

hypoendemic   the condition in which malaria is present in a community at low levels, resulting in a population that generally has little or no immunity.

hypoglycemia an abnormally low level of sugar in the blood, which may result in shaking, cold sweats, hypothermia, headache, and potentially convulsions and coma.

IgA immunoglobulin A; a class of immunoglobulin found in external body secretions such as saliva, tears, and sweat, and on the surface of cell membranes.

IgG immunoglobulin G; the predominant immunoglobulin involved in the secondary immune response.

IgM immunoglobulin M; the predominant immunoglobulin found in the primary immune response.

immune system a natural defense mechanism of the body, in which specialized cells and proteins in the blood and other body fluids interact to eliminate or neutralize infectious microorganisms and other foreign substances.

immunodominant the central or dominant epitope on an antigen.

immunogen a substance, or antigen, capable of eliciting an immune response.

immunoglobulin antibody secreted by plasma cells (mature lymphoid cells). There are five classes of immunoglobulin: IgG, IgM, IgA, IgE, and IgD.

incidence as used in epidemiology, the number of new cases of a disease that occur within a specified time period.

in vitro biological processes that occur in isolation from the whole organism, such as in a test tube or in cell culture; in the laboratory.

in vivo biological processes that occur within in the body of a living organism.

kilodalton a unit of mass equal to one thousand daltons or approximately 1.65×10^{-21} grams.

ligand a molecule (such as oxygen) that binds to a complementary site on a given structure (such as hemoglobin).

loading dose the dose used at the initiation of therapy to rapidly establish the desired blood and tissue levels of the drug; also known as a priming dose.

macrogametocyte see **gametocyte**.

macrophage a large, phagocytic, mononuclear lymphocyte found in tissues but derived from blood monocytes. Depending on the tissue they are locating in, macrophages are called histiocytes (connective tissue macrophages), Kupffer's cells (liver macrophages), or alveolar macrophages (lungs). Involved in the immune response to antigens, the macrophages process antigens and present them to the lymphocytes.

marginal benefit the extra benefit attributed to an extra unit of output.

marginal cost   the extra cost incurred for an extra unit of output.

merozoite   the stage of the parasite, in the human host, that infects the red blood cells.

mesoendemic   the condition in which malaria is present in a community at low levels, with occasional epidemics resulting from the generally low level of immunity in the population.

microgametocyte   see **gametocyte**.

monoclonal   derived from a single clone of cells.

monoclonal antibody   immunoglobulins derived from a single clone of plasma cells. Monoclonal antibodies constitute a pure population, as they are produced by a single clone in vitro and are chemically and structurally identical.

monocyte   the largest lymphocyte found in the blood; they are phagocytic.

nucleotide   one of the compounds into which a nucleic acid is split by the action of a nuclease; nucleotides are composed of a base, a sugar, and a phosphate group.

oligonucleotide   a polymer composed of more than three nucleotides.

oocyst   the encysted or encapsulated ookinete in the wall of an infected mosquito's stomach.

ookinete   the fertilized form of the malaria parasite in the mosquito's body.

parasitemia   the level of parasites in the blood.

parenteral   a method in which a drug or vaccine is introduced into the body, other than by oral ingestion.

passive protection   disease-specific immunity produced by the injection of antibody-containing serum from a donor with active immunity to the disease.

PCR   polymerase chain reaction. A method of amplifying low levels of specific DNA sequences in a sample, thus allowing one to detect very low levels of antigen or antibody in the sample.

phenotype   the entire physical, biochemical, and physiological makeup of an organism as determined by both genetics and the environment.

point mutation   a mutation caused by the substitution of one nucleotide for another.

polyclonal   antibodies generated by more than one clone of B lymphocytes in response to an antigen; i.e., arising from more than one clone.

prevalence   as used in epidemiology, the total number of cases of a disease in existence at a specific time and within a well-defined area.

reading frame alteration   a change in a nucleotide sequence that results in the insertion or deletion of a nucleotide in newly formed DNA strands during replication.

receptor   a specific chemical grouping, on the surface of an immunologically competent cell, with the capability of combining with a specific antigen. Also may refer to a receptor for antibodies.

recombinant vaccine a vaccine prepared by recombinant DNA technology in which a a host organism (expression vector) is directed to synthesize specific molecules as the result of insertion of DNA segments from another organism (such as the malaria parasite). In this manner, vaccines that are directed against specific antigens within the parasites can be made.

recombination the formation of new combinations of genes as a result of crossing over (sharing of genes) between structurally similar chromosomes, resulting in progeny with different gene combinations than in the parents.

recrudescence recurrence of a disease after a brief intermission.

relapse recurrence of disease symptoms after a period of improvement.

returns to scale the proportionate increase in output resulting from proportionate increases in all inputs.

RIA radioimmunoassay. A highly sensitive assay for antigen in which the concentration of an unknown, unlabeled antigen is determined by comparing its inhibitory effect on the binding of radioactively labeled antigen to specific antibody with the inhibitory effect of known standards.

schizogony the process in which sporozoites develop into merozoites within the liver hepatocytes.

schizont a multinucleate parasite that reproduces by schizogony.

sensitivity the ability of a test to detect small differences in the level of antigen or antibody in a sample.

sequestration the situation in which the malaria parasite resides in and obstructs the capillaries of the brain, apparently causing cerebral malaria.

seronegative negative result in a serological test; i.e., the inability to detect the antibodies being tested for.

seropositive positive result in a serological test.

serum the clear liquid remaining after blood has clotted.

sexual reproduction refers to the stage of the parasite's life cycle that begins in the vertebrate host and is completed in the mosquito.

specificity refers to the relative ability to differentiate among different organisms or strains of an organism.

sporogony that portion of the sexual reproduction of the parasite that takes place in the mosquito.

sporozoite a stage of the malaria parasite that is transmitted to humans by the mosquito. Sporozoites are released from oocysts on the mosquito's stomach, travel to the salivary glands, and are transmitted when the mosquito bites.

subunit vaccine a vaccine prepared from parts of a whole organism. The concept is to use those portions of the organism that are immunogenic, leaving out those that produce pathologic manifestations.

synthetic vaccine a vaccine manufactured by biochemical means, to simulate the immunogenic portions of the organism against which the vaccine is being prepared.

tandem repeats duplications of tandem combinations.

T lymphocyte same as T cell. An immunologically competent white blood cell that direct the production of antibody by B lymphocytes; are responsible for cell-mediated immunity and immunological memory.

trophozoite the stage, between the ring stage and the schizont, that occurs in the red blood cell.

tubulin a principal protein component of microtubules (which play key roles in cell division and morphogenesis). Alpha- and beta-tubulins have been described.

vector the mosquito that transmits the malaria parasite from one host to another.

vector competence refers to the relative ability of a vector (relative to another vector) to transmit a specific infective agent from one host to another, implying that a competent vector is one that takes in sufficient numbers of an agent to ensure infection, supports the development or multiplication of the agent, and is able to deliver a large enough inoculum to an appropriate site in a new host to ensure infection.

vivax malaria malaria caused by the malaria parasite *Plasmodium vivax.*

zoophilic prefer to feed on animals.

zygote an organism produced by the union of two gametes.

Index